RY

9

Rehabilitation of the Foot and Ankle

Rehabilitation of the Foot and Ankle

G. James Sammarco, M.D., F.A.C.S.
Volunteer Professor
University of Cincinnati Medical Center
Cincinnati Orthopaedic Clinic
Cincinnati, Ohio

with 255 illustrations

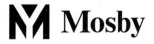 **Mosby**

St. Louis Baltimore Berlin Boston Carlsbad Chicago London I
Naples New York Philadelphia Sydney Tokyo Toronto

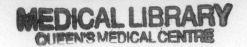 Mosby

Dedicated to Publishing Excellence

Editor: Robert Hurley
Developmental Editor: Christine Pluta
Project Manager: Linda Clarke
Project Editor: Vicki Hoenigke
Designer: Sheilah Barrett
Manufacturing Supervisor: Theresa Fuchs
Cover art: Nancy McDonald

Printed in the United States of America
Composition by The Clarinda Company
Printing/binding by Maple Vail Press

Mosby-Year Book, Inc.
11830 Westline Industrial Drive
St. Louis, Missouri 63146

Library of Congress Cataloging-in-Publication Data

Rehabilitation of the foot and ankle / [edited by] G. James Sammarco.
    p.   cm.
    Includes bibliographical references and index.
    ISBN 0-8016-7771-8 (alk. paper)   100063530I
    1. Foot—Wounds and injuries.   2. Ankle—Wounds and injuries.
 I. Sammarco, G. James.
    [DNLM: 1. Foot. 2. Ankle. 3. Fractures—rehabilitation.
 4. Sprains and strains—rehabilitaion. 5. Athletic Injuries—
rehabilitation. 6. Foot Diseases—rehabilitation. 7. Foot
Deformities—rehabilitation. 8. Sports.   WE 880 R345 1995]
 RD563.R44 1995
 617.5'8503—dc20
 DNLM/DLC
 for Library of Congress   94-37892
                     CIP

95 96 97 98 99 / 9 8 7 6 5 4 3 2 1

Contributors

Richard V. Abdo, M.D.
Orthopaedic Specialties
Clearwater, Florida

Donald E. Baxter, M.D.
Clinical Professor of Orthopaedics
Baylor College of Medicine
Methodist Hospital
Houston, Texas

John H. Bowker, M.D.
Professor and Associate Chairman
Department of Orthopaedics and
  Rehabilitation
University of Miami
Director, Foot and Ankle Amputee Services
Jackson Memorial Hospital
Miami, Florida

Stephen F. Conti, M.D.
Assistant Professor
University of Pittsburgh Medical Center
Medical Director
Foot and Ankle Center
Pittsburgh, Pennsylvania

Jean Bloecher Cooper, P.T.
Physical Therapist
University of Connecticut Health Center
Farmington, Connecticut

Paul Cooper, M.D.
Assistant Professor
Department of Orthopaedics
University of Connecticut Health Center
Farmington, Connecticut

Pamela F. Davis, M.D.
Trinity Medical Center
Moline, Illinois

Timothy R. Derrick, M.S.
University of Massachusetts
Amherst, Massachusetts

Betsy K. Donahoe, M.S., P.T., P.C.S.
Physical Therapist II
Children's Hospital Medical Center
Cincinnati, Ohio

Rafael F. Escamilla, Ph.D., C.S.C.S.
Biomechanist
Auburn University
American Sports Medicine Institute
Birmingham, Alabama

Keith S. Feder, M.D.
Clinical Instructor
University of California, Los Angeles, School
  of Medicine
Chief of Arthroscopic Surgery and Sports Medicine
Harbor-UCLA Medical Center
West Coast Center for Orthopaedic Surgery
  and Sports Medicine
Chief of Orthopaedic Surgery
Daniel Freeman Memorial Hospital
Manhattan Beach, California

Carol C. Frey, M.D.
Associate Clinical Professor of Orthopaedic Surgery
University of Southern California
Director, Orthopaedic Foot and Ankle
  Center
Orthopaedic Hospital
Los Angeles, California

Marilyn T. Geier, B.S., P.T.
Children's Hospital Medical Center
Cincinnati, Ohio

Joseph Hamill, Ph.D.
Professor
Director of Biomechanics Laboratory
  University of Massachusetts
  Amherst, Massachusetts

Thomas J. Herrmann, Ed.D., A.T., C.
Head Athletic Trainer
  Department of Orthopaedic Surgery
  University of Cincinnati
  Cincinnati, Ohio

Kenneth G. Holt, Ph.D., P.T.
Assistant Professor
  Department of Physical Therapy
  Boston University
  Boston, Massachusetts

Dennis J. Janisse, C.Ped.
President and Chief Executive Officer
  National Pedorthic Services, Inc.
  Milwaukee, Wisconsin

Kimberly A. Kuhnell, M.S., P.T.
Physical Therapy I
  Children's Hospital Medical Center
  Cincinnati, Ohio

Janet C. Limke, M.D.
Assistant Professor of Physical Medicine and
Rehabilitation
  University of Cincinnati
Attending Physician
  University of Cincinnati Medical Center
  Cincinnati, Ohio

Marika Molnar, M.S., P.T.
Director, Westside Dance Physical Therapy
Director, Physical Therapy Services
  New York City Ballet and School of
    American Ballet
  New York, New York

Arleen Norkitis, P.T.
Clinical Coordinator
  Diabetic Foot Clinic
  Pleasant Gap, Pennsylvania

Anna Buechele Pati, M.S., L.P.T.
Instructor
  Department of Physical Medicine and
    Rehabilitation
  Baylor College of Medicine
Research Coordinator
  Physical and Occupational Therapy
    Department
  Methodist Hospital
  Houston, Texas

J. Christopher Reynolds, M.D.
Director, Foot Clinic
  Brackenridge Hospital
  Austin, Texas

Lew Charles Schon, M.D.
Associate Director of Foot and Ankle Fellowship
Director, Dance Medicine Program
  Department of Orthopaedics
  Union Memorial Hospital
  Baltimore, Maryland

Thomas C. Skalley, M.D.
Orthopaedic Surgeon
  The Everett Clinic
  Everett, Washington

David A. Stone, M.D.
Assistant Professor of Orthopaedic Surgery
  Sports Medicine Division
Staff
  Presbyterian University Hosptial
  Montefiore University Hospital
  Pittsburgh, Pennsylvania

Mariann L. Strenk, P.T.
Physical Therapist
  Children's Hospital Medical Center
  Cincinnati, Ohio

To my family, my teachers, and my students

Preface

Injury to the foot accounts for 20% of all orthopaedic admissions to the hospital. However, the majority of foot care is provided by family practitioners and constitutes more than 50% of all foot care. Orthopaedic surgeons and podiatrists also provide a large percentage of foot care. The help and assistance of athletic trainers, physical therapists, and other allied health professionals including nurse practitioners and physician assistants is necessary in order to achieve successful outcomes in the treatment of foot disease. An important part of treatment of acute and chronic injuries and diseases includes rehabilitation. This book is presented as a guide for the physician, surgeon, therapist, coach, and trainer to achieve a successful outcome in foot care, return patients to their pre-disease or injury level as quickly as possible, and to give treatment with the least pain and discomfort in the shortest time. It is hoped that it will serve as an easy to use reference. The book is divided into sections which include basic science, therapy modalities, trauma, sports, pediatrics, orthotics, and prosthetics. It is clear, concise, and direct so that the information can be put directly to use and not require additional references. An evaluation of patients in each section is provided so that the practitioner will understand the progress of his or her patient. Einstein once said that today's complex problems cannot be solved with the solutions which were available when those problems first were encountered. So it is with rehabilitation of the foot. The problems and patient needs are different today than they were a generation ago. This book is our response to that need.

G. James Sammarco

Acknowledgments

There are many people who have helped in the preparation of this manuscript. My heartfelt thanks goes to the many authors who have donated their time, energy and expertise to create chapters which are useful and relevant to today's patient needs. I wish also to thank my office staff including Kay Dickerson, transcriptionist, who helped collate the chapters, Dr. Hiram Carrasquillo who proofread some of the chapters, and Mosby, whose support and encouragement helped to bring this book to fruition. Thanks go to my wife, Ruthann, and my children, Alissa, Jim, Alex, Anne and Natalie, who had the patience and who allowed me the flexibility in our family commitments to complete this book. Their support was an inspiration to me. A special thanks goes to Drs. Paul Cooper, Steve Conti, Carol Frey, Pam Davis, Keith Feder, Lew Schon, Rick Abdo, Tom Skalley and Dave Stone, rising young orthopaedists, who bring new ideas to medicine. Dr. Janet Limke contributed an excellent chapter on the rehabilitation of the soccer player. The therapists Jean Cooper, Arleen Norkitis, Betsy Donahoe, Kim Kuhnell, Mariann Strenk, Marilyn Geier, Kenneth Holt, and Annie Pati were also of great help giving special information on therapy.

Dennis Janisse has given special advice with respect to pedorthic management of foot deformity. Thanks to Drs. Chris Reynolds, Don Baxter and John Bowker for sharing their mature outlook and experience. They were of great help as was Marika Molnar who gave insight in dance rehabilitation. The trainers, biomechanists, and exercise physiologists, Timothy Derrick, Rafael Escamilla, Joseph Hamill, and Tom Herrmann brought science and medicine into perspective with respect to bone, ligament, and muscle function and the athlete's recovery. Finally, I wish to thank my mother and father who instilled in me the desire to learn and to teach and to never give less than my best effort.

Contents

Rehabilitation of the Athlete's Foot and Ankle

Taping, Shoe Modifications, Orthoses, Arthrodeses

1 Anatomy and Physiology

1

Anatomy of the Foot and Ankle

G. James Sammarco

The basis on which an understanding of the leg, foot, and ankle is founded is anatomy. With a background in understanding physical structure and function, the reader is then prepared to gain knowledge of the principles determining lower extremity disease and its treatment. The study of rehabilitation begins with a foundation in basic anatomy, physiology, and the study of foot and ankle function. What is presented in this chapter will be used throughout the book as both background knowledge and as a reference resource in order to understand the disease process and to rationalize treatment modalities to bring about a successful outcome for care.

The Ankle

The tibia, fibula, and talus are the bones of the ankle. The *tibia* has a triangular shaft. A bony crest runs down the anterior border. The shaft expands into a metaphysis distally with a medial malleolus extending downward to become the medial bony support of the ankle joint. The lateral surface expands forming a slight depression

This chapter is adapted from a chapter originally published in Sammarco GJ: *Foot and ankle manual,* Philadelphia, 1991, Lea & Febiger.

for the fibula. The undersurface, the tibial plafond, articulates with the talar dome. It is more narrow medially where it is continuous with the articular surface of the medial malleolus. The posterior surface of the tibia is broad and grooved to accommodate the posterior tibialis, flexor digitorum longus, and flexor hallucis longus tendons.

The *fibula* lies lateral to the tibia. Proximally the head has a facet medially, which articulates at the knee with the tibia. The shaft is triangular, and its medial surface attaches to the interosseus membrane. At the ankle, the medial border flattens in the tibiofibular syndesmosis. Below the syndesmosis is the triangular articular surface of the lateral malleolus. The lateral malleolus is tapered distally and grooved posteriorly. The peroneal tendons pass behind the ankle here.

There are 26 major bones in the foot: seven tarsals, five metatarsals, and 14 phalanges (Fig. 1-1). The hindfoot consists of the talus and calcaneus.

The *talus* consists of three parts, the body, neck, and head. It transmits forces from the foot through the ankle joint to the leg. It consists of mostly articular surfaces and has no muscular or tendinous attachments.

The body of the talus is at a 25-degree angle medially to the sagittal plane. Its saddle-shaped

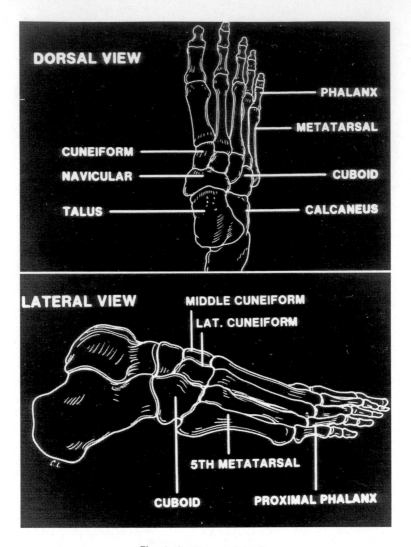

Fig. 1-1 Bones of the foot.

dome is narrower posteriorly and articulates with the tibia and fibula. The radius of curvature on the medial aspect is less than that of the lateral side. The medial and lateral articular surfaces are slightly concave. At the posterior border, a small groove is present for the flexor hallucis longus tendon. The os trigonum accessory bone, present in 6% to 8% of the population, articulates with the tip of the posterior process. The posterior facet on its inferior surface lies at a 45-degree angle to the frontal plane of the leg.

The talar neck is directed medially and downward. Beneath the neck is the sinus tarsi canal,

between the talus and calcaneus. The blood supply to the talus enters through the artery of the sinus tarsi from below and from small arteries behind the posterior facet.

The head of the talus is anteromedial to the ankle joint and is convex. The posterior plantar medial surface articulates with the sustentaculum tali of the calcaneus. The anterior portion of the talus forms part of the anterior facet of the subtalar joint, and the medial portion lies on the plantar calcaneal ligament. The distal ovoid articular surface articulates with the tarsal navicular. The talus functions passively, being held in a sling of tendons connected to adjacent bones by a series of ligament complexes.

The *calcaneus* is the largest bone in the foot, occupying the most posterior position. It provides a lever arm for the Achilles tendon. Dorsally, there are three surfaces. The dorsal roof lies posteriorly with a fat pad above it. On the anterior portion of the dorsal surface lie attachments of the posterior capsule of the ankle. The midportion of the calcaneus contains the convex posterior facet of the subtalar joint and the floor of the sinus tarsi. It also contains the articular surface of the sustentaculum tali medially. Anteriorly it forms the anterior articular facet of the subtalar joint. The anterior surface of the calcaneus contains a concavoconvex surface, which articulates with a cuboid. The medial surface of the calcaneus is concave, containing the sustentaculum tali, which is grooved beneath for the tendon of the flexor hallucis longus. Laterally, a slightly concave surface is present with a ridge, processus trochlearis above and below which the peroneal tendons pass. The inferior tuberosity of the calcaneus accepts the posterior attachment of the plantar aponeurosis.

The *tarsal navicular* (scaphoid) lies anterior to the talus and medial to the cuboid. It is the keystone atop the longitudinal arch of the foot. The proximal surface is concave, articulating with the talar head. The distal surface has a facet for each of the three cuneiforms. A small facet articulates with the cuboid. The tibialis posterior tendon inserts on the tuberosity medially.

The *cuboid* articulates with the calcaneus proximally and the fourth and fifth metatarsals distally. Medially there is a small facet, which opposes the tarsal navicular. Its infralateral surface is grooved for the peroneus longus tendon.

The medial, middle, and lateral *cuneiforms* are wedge-shaped, with the apex of each bone pointing inferiorly. They articulate with the first three metatarsals distally. The medial and lateral cuneiforms project farther distally than the intermediate cuneiform. A notch is created into which the base of the second metatarsal fits, creating a stable keylike mortise.

There are five *metatarsals,* all tapered distally and all articulating with proximal phalanges. The first metatarsal is the shortest and widest. Its base

articulates with the medial cuneiform and is cone-shaped. The head of the first metatarsal also articulates with two sesamoids on its plantar articular surface. The second metatarsal extends beyond the first proximally. It articulates with the intermediate cuneiform as well as with the medial and lateral cuneiforms in a keylike configuration that promotes stability, making the second ray the stiffest portion of the foot. The third, fourth, and fifth metatarsals are broad based, narrow in the shaft, and have dome-shaped heads. The fifth has a prominent styloid, proximally at its base, on which the peroneus brevis tendon inserts.

There are two *phalanges* for the hallux and three for each lesser toe. All phalanges are concave on their plantar surface. The heads of the proximal and middle phalanges are saddle-shaped. The middle phalanges are shorter and broader than the proximal phalanges. The distal phalanges are smaller yet, with a tuft of bone distally. These distal expansions at the tip anchor the toe pads.

Two constant *sesamoids* are present beneath the first metatarsal head. There are multiple variations in their ossification. The tibial and fibular sesamoids lie within the tendons of the flexor hallucis brevis muscle. They articulate with the inferior surface of the first metatarsal head. Occasionally, lateral metatarsals have sesamoids present at the metatarsophalangeal joint. The tibialis posterior and the tibialis anterior as well as the peroneus longus tendons also occasionally have a sesamoid bone within them.

Joints and Ligaments

The *ankle joint* consists of the distal tibia and tibial plafond, including its posterolateral border (posterior malleolus), the medial malleolus and the distal fibula (lateral malleolus), and the talus (Fig. 1-2). The joint is saddle-shaped. The larger circumference of the talar dome is lateral, and the smaller lies medial. The dome itself is wider anteriorly than posteriorly. As the ankle extends (dorsiflexes), the fibula rotates externally through the tibiofibular syndesmosis to accommodate the

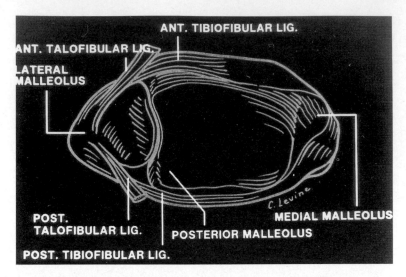

Fig. 1-2 Ankle joint. Tibial plafond as viewed from below.

widened front of the talar dome. The foot also rotates externally during dorsiflexion.

The ankle achieves its stability both in flexion and extension by means of its saddle shape. Additional stability is maintained through the ligaments and capsule. The capsule itself is thin anteriorly and posteriorly but is thicker for medial and lateral support.

The *deltoid ligament* (medial collateral ankle ligament) is fan-shaped and is divided into a deep and a superficial portion (Fig. 1-3). The superficial portion has three parts: the anterior tibionavicular portion, which helps stabilize the anterior portion of the joint; the tibiocalcaneal portion, which contributes to stability of both the ankle and subtalar joints; and the tibiotalar, or posterior, portion. The deep portion of the deltoid ligament has two short portions and attaches from beneath the tip of the medial malleolus to the medial talus.

The *lateral ankle ligament complex* has three major parts (Fig. 1-4). The anterior talofibular ligament extends from the anterior portion of the lateral malleolus to the lateral neck of the talus. The fibulocalcaneal ligament passes from the inferior tip of the lateral malleolus across the subtalar joint to insert on the lateral calcaneus. The posterior talofibular ligament lies almost horizontal to the ankle joint.

The distal *tibiofibular syndesmosis* is supported by the anterior tibiofibular ligament and the posterior tibiofibular ligament. These may be disrupted with injury to the ankle.

The inferior portion of the talus has two articular surfaces, a large posterior concave surface, a separate joint, and a smaller talocalcaneonavicular joint (Fig. 1-5).

There are three major ligaments of the *subtalar joint* in addition to medial and lateral talocalcaneal ligaments: the anterior ligament of the posterior facet in the sinus tarsi, the interosseous talocalcaneal ligament, and the cervical ligament, which covers the lateral aspect of the sinus tarsi. The interosseous talocalcaneal ligament within the sinus tarsi prevents excessive eversion of the foot.

The anterior facet is multiaxial. The convex head of the talus articulates with this facet as well as with the navicular. There is a thin talonavicular ligament dorsally. Plantarward lies the strong plantar calcaneonavicular ligament (spring ligament). This connects the sustentaculum tali to the inferior navicular. Laterally, the bifurcate ligament connects the calcaneus to the navicular. The *sustentaculum tali* lies medial and articulates with the rearmost part of the anterior facet. It supports the talus beneath the medial talar process.

Anatomy and Physiology

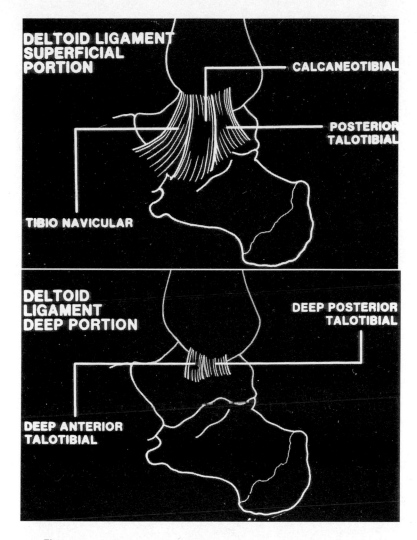

Fig. 1-3 Deltoid ligament. **A,** Superficial portion. **B,** Deep portion.

The *calcaneocuboid joint* is saddle-shaped and is associated with the *talonavicular joint*. This combined joint is called Chopart's joint (Fig. 1-6). The talocalcaneocuboid joint moves with the subtalar joint.

Ligaments surrounding the joint include the long plantar ligament, which runs from under the calcaneus to the cuboid and also terminates on the metatarsals, and the short plantar ligament, which connects the calcaneus to the cuboid. These ligaments help maintain the longitudinal arch. Dorsolaterally the bifurcate ligament is a major supporter of the joint. Motion in this important complex includes flexion, extension, and rotation of the midfoot and forefoot.

The distal navicular has a facet for each of the cuneiforms. This *cuneonavicular joint* is a synovial joint and is contiguous with the intercuneiform joints, the cuneocuboid, the second and third cuneometatarsal, and the intermetatarsal joints. Motion here is minimal. Some flexion and extension is permitted, but this is restricted by interosseous dorsal and plantar ligaments. The limited motion of these joints maintains a longitudinal arch while permitting some motion to maintain the overall flexibility of the foot.

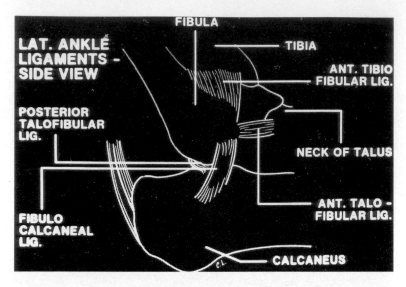

Fig. 1-4 Lateral ankle ligaments, side view.

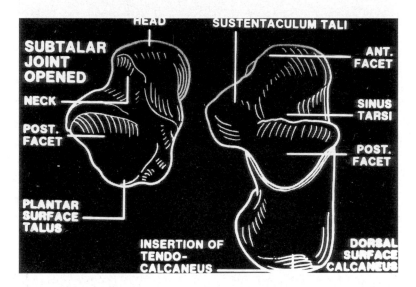

Fig. 1-5 Subtalar joint (opened). calcaneus is viewed from above. Talus is viewed from below.

The *first cuneometatarsal joint* is a separate synovial joint and may be round or ovoid. The four lateral *tarsometatarsal joints,* however, are continuous and surrounded by a single synovial membrane that connects to the intercuneiform and cuneonavicular joints. These joints are commonly referred to as *Lisfranc's joint* (Fig. 1-7).

The base of the second metatarsal lies proxi-

mal to the first and third metatarsals, articulating with the intermediate cuneiform. In doing so the joint between the tarsal and metatarsal bones is stabilized. There are strong plantar and dorsal ligaments as well as interosseous cuneometatarsal ligaments. They aid in maintaining the longitudinal arch. The joints have a small excursion during walking. There are also *intermetatarsal joints* proximally. The first and fifth metatarsals

Anatomy and Physiology

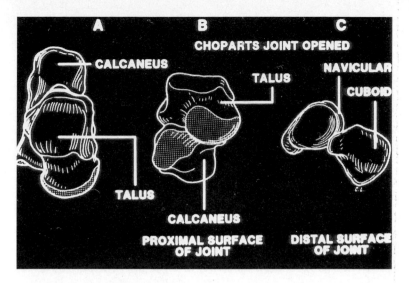

Fig. 1-6 Chopart's joint (opened). **A,** Viewed from above. Joint lies at bottom of diagram. Joint surfaces **(B)** viewed from front. **C,** Viewed from behind.

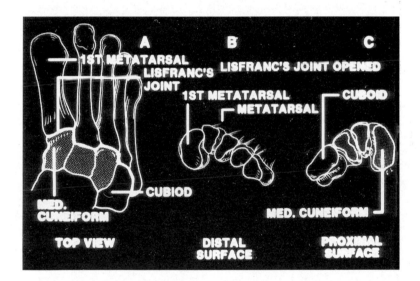

Fig. 1-7 Lisfranc's joint. **A,** Viewed from above, cuneiforms are marked. **B,** Metatarsals viewed from behind. **C,** Tarsals viewed from front, cuneiforms are marked.

are not firmly connected to their adjacent metatarsals, giving flexibility to the forefoot.

The general shape of the metatarsal heads is round. The *first metatarsophalangeal joint* of the hallux has a wide dorsal excursion and a range of motion greater than 90 degrees. This accommodates the toe-off part of stance during walking. Plantarflexion of the joint is about 40 degrees. There are strong medial and lateral ligaments supported by muscles to maintain power and control. The plantar surface of the metatarsal head articulates with two sesamoids, each imbedded in a tendon of the flexor hallucis brevis (Fig. 1-8).

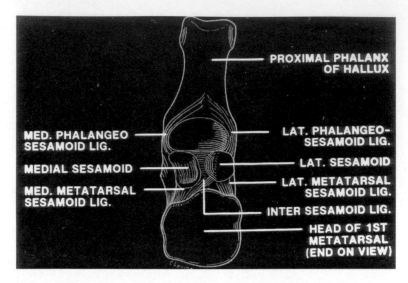

Fig. 1–8 First metatarso phalangeal joint (opened from above). Tibial medial and fibular lateral sesamoids within flexor hallucis brevis are exposed.

The intersesamoidal ligament bridges the two sesamoids. Ligaments that align the sesamoids to the metatarsals include the medial metatarsal sesamoid ligament and the lateral metatarsal sesamoid ligament. Medially the abductor hallucis and laterally the adductor hallucis stabilize the position of the sesamoids. As the hallux extends during the last portion of the stance phase of gait, the sesamoids are pulled distally so that weight-bearing is maintained through them and the metatarsal head.

The *metatarsophalangeal joints* of the second to fifth toes also have stabilizing collateral ligaments. The plantar plate of each toe is strong and limits joint extension, aiding in the transfer of forces between the plantar pad, flexor tendons, and metatarsal heads. The small toes extend to 90 degrees. The metatarsal heads are ovoid, and the opposing proximal phalanx is concave. The plantar aspect of the metatarsal heads is more prominent than the dorsal part. The dorsal capsule is thin. The extensor digitorum longus and the extensor digitorum brevis join at the metatarsophalangeal joint to protect and reinforce it dorsally. Intermetatarsal ligaments maintain the alignment of all the metatarsal rays.

Aponeuroses and Retinacula

The retinacula serve as retainers so that appropriate vital structures, including neurovascular bundles and tendons, can be protected and guided to their areas of function.

The *superior extensor retinaculum* has attachments on the anterior lateral malleolus and anterior tibia. It is attached to the deep fascia of the leg proximally and holds within it the tendons of the tibialis anterior, extensor hallucis longus, extensor digitorum longus, and peroneus tertius. The neurovascular bundle, consisting of the anterior tibial artery and deep branches of the peroneal nerve, runs beneath it. There may be a separate tunnel for the tibialis anterior tendon.

The *inferior extensor retinaculum* is shaped like a Y. It has two lateral attachments on the calcaneus and two medial attachments, one to the medial malleolus and one to the plantar aponeurosis. Laterally, the *superior peroneal retinaculum* contains both peroneal tendons. It is attached to the lateral malleolus, the lower portion of the tendocalcaneus (Achilles tendon), and lateral calcaneus. The *inferior peroneal retinaculum* is a con-

Anatomy and Physiology

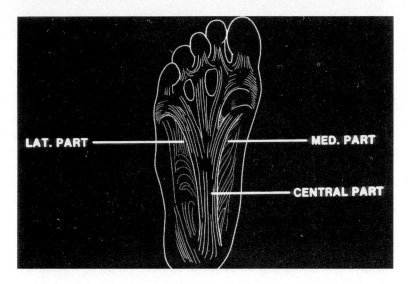

Fig. 1-9 Plantar aponeurosis has three parts. The thickest is the central part.

tinuation of the inferior extensor retinaculum. It has a superficial and a deep portion and attaches to the lateral calcaneus forming portions of tunnels through which the peroneal tendons pass. Its inferior attachment is on the lateral calcaneus.

Located at the posteromedial ankle, the *upper tibiotalar tunnel* has a deep and a superficial portion, which are continuations of the aponeurosis of the leg. It retains the tibialis posterior, flexor digitorum longus, and flexor hallucis longus muscle and tendons as well as the posterior tibialis artery veins and nerve.

The *flexor retinaculum* (laciniate ligament) is attached at the medial malleolus. Its base covers the abductor hallucis muscle medially. Anteriorly, its fibers attach to the extensor retinaculum and the anterior tibia. Its base is attached to the calcaneus.

The *tarsal tunnel* houses the posterior tibial tendon. It passes medial to the talus, behind the deltoid ligament, above the calcaneonavicular and inferior calcaneonavicular ligaments, beneath the flexor retinaculum.

The flexor digitorum longus tunnel is deep to the posterior tibial artery behind the ankle. It joins the tunnel of the flexor hallucis longus distally in the foot. The neurovascular bundle containing the posterior tibial artery, nerve, and ve-

nae comitantes lies between the flexor digitorum longus and flexor hallucis longus at the posterior ankle, then passes posterior to the flexor digitorum longus against the medial calcaneus.

The *plantar aponeurosis* has three parts (Fig. 1-9). The central portion is important in maintaining the longitudinal arch of the foot. It is triangular and attached proximally at the posterior calcaneal tuberosity. It passes distally as a single structure, dividing and spreading into five slips beneath the metatarsal heads. Distally, long sagittal septae are attached into the sole of the foot, creating tunnels for the long flexor tendons. Distally the plantar aponeurosis inserts through the longitudinal septa into the proximal phalanges as well as into the skin and natatory ligaments. Through these connections the aponeurosis tightens as the toes are extended. The medial and lateral portions are thinner. The special attachments between the calcaneus, proximally, and the ligaments and skin, distally, allow the plantar aponeurosis to perform an important function through a "windlass" mechanism. When the toes are dorsiflexed, as in the last portion of stance prior to toe-off, the aponeurosis is pulled distally. When this occurs, it tightens, and the bones of the foot are held tightly so that the foot functions as a single unit.

Longitudinal septa pass between the medial

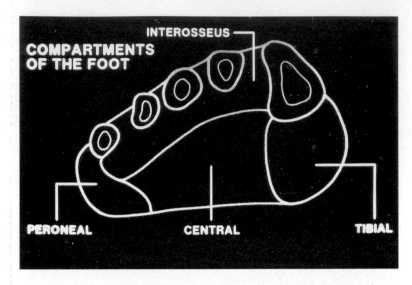

Fig. 1-10   Compartments of the foot.

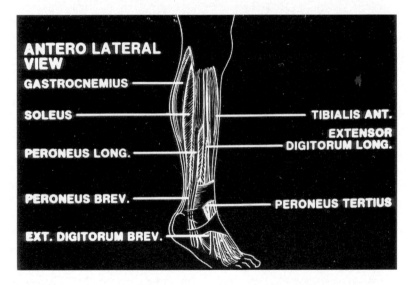

Fig. 1-11   Muscles of the lower leg and foot viewed from anterolaterally.

and central portions, and the central and lateral portions of the plantar aponeurosis to the interosseous ligaments along the lateral side of the first metatarsal and medial portion of the fifth metatarsal. These create compartments within the foot: a central compartment, an interosseous compartment, a peroneal compartment, and a tibial compartment (Fig. 1-10).

Muscles

The muscles of the foot are divided into those of extrinsic origin, and those that arise within the foot, of intrinsic origin. Many muscles in the foot span more than a single joint and in some cases span several joints (Fig. 1-11).

There are four compartments for muscles in the leg. The *superficial posterior compartment* for the flexors of the ankle lies posterior to the deep compartment. Two of the three muscles in this compartment begin on the femur and one on the proximal tibia. The femoral component includes the origins of the two heads of the *gastrocnemius,* one from each condyle, and the *plantaris* muscle, from the lateral femoral condyle. The *soleus* arises below the knee from the posterior aspect of the tibia and fibula, proximally. These muscles are innervated by branches of the tibial nerve and flex the ankle and foot. The gastrocnemius muscle also aids in knee flexion.

The *plantaris* is a small muscle immediately forming a tendon, which courses between the soleus and gastrocnemius medially to insert distally on the medial portion of the Achilles tendon. The largest tendon in the body is the *tendo calcaneus* (Achilles). It is formed from the soleus muscle deep in the calf and from the gastrocnemius muscle through a long musculotendinous junction. Tendon fibers from the soleus are situated anteriorly in the proximal portion of the tendon, while the tendon fibers from the gastrocnemius are posterior.

The *deep posterior compartment* contains the *tibialis posterior,* which originates on the posterior tibia interosseous membrane. At the ankle it passes through a groove posterior to the medial malleolus in a fibrous tunnel. It courses over the medial aspect of the talus beneath the inferior calcaneonavicular ligament (spring ligament) lying superficial to the deltoid ligament. Its major insertion is on the navicular tuberosity, the navicular-cuneiform joint and the medial cuneiform, with a middle insertion under the middle and lateral cuneiforms, cuboid, and lesser metatarsals, and a posterior portion at the anterior sustentaculum tali. The tibialis posterior inverts and adducts the foot and flexes the ankle. It supports the longitudinal arch of the foot.

The *flexor digitorum longus* arises from the middle three fifths of the tibial interosseous membrane, passes with its common tendon into its own canal at the ankle, and lies lateral to the tibialis posterior at the talus. It passes medial to the sustentaculum tali in its own canal and crosses plantar to the flexor hallucis longus, beneath the talus, dividing into four slips. The flexor hallucis longus sends a tendinous slip to the flexor digitorum longus. Each tendon slip also receives a part of the insertion of the quadratus plantae muscle. A lumbricalis arises from the medial side of each of four tendinous slips. Each tendon slip courses through the arch of the plantar aponeurosis. Each tendon then passes through the bifurcation in the flexor digitorum brevis tendon to insert on the distal phalanx. The function of the flexor digitorum longus is to flex the ankle, elevate the arch, and flex the toes.

The *flexor hallucis longus* takes origin on the interosseous membrane and the posterior tibia, tibialis posterior, and peroneal muscles. It is the most lateral muscle in the posterior deep compartment. The muscle fibers have the lowest origin in the leg. The tendon lies in the medial ankle at the posterior talus. It passes in its own tunnel beneath the sustentaculum tali deep to the flexor digitorum longus tendon into the medial compartment of the foot. It passes through the arch of the plantar aponeurosis and the fibrous flexor tunnel between the sesamoids to insert on the distal phalanx. It flexes the ankle, elevates the arch, and flexes the great toe.

The *lateral compartment* contains the *peroneus longus muscle,* which lies superficial to the peroneus brevis muscle and arises from the upper two thirds of the lateral fibula, anterior and posterior intermuscular septa, and fascia. The tendon lies posterior to the peroneus brevis tendon at the tip of the lateral malleolus passes into its own tunnel beneath the processus trochlearis on the lateral calcaneus. At the lateral border of the cuboid it courses medially to insert on the first metatarsal and the medial cuneiform. It functions to plantarflex the first metatarsal and to flex the ankle as well as abduct the foot. A sesamoid os peroneum is present within the tendon at the lateral cuboid 20% of the time.

The peroneus brevis muscle arises from the lower two thirds of the fibula and anterior and posterior intermuscular septae. It courses posteriorly against the lateral malleolus and lies in the common tunnel with the peroneus longus tendon. It passes into its own canal above the processus trochlearis on the lateral calcaneus. It lies superficial to the calcaneofibular ligament and inserts on the styloid process of the fifth metatarsal. It functions to flex the ankle and evert the foot.

The *anterior compartment* contains the *tibialis anterior muscle,* which takes origin from the lateral condyle and upper anterior tibia, interosseous membrane, and interosseous septum. It courses beneath the extensor retinacula, often within its own tunnel, to insert at the medial border of the foot on the first metatarsal and medial cuneiform. This muscle functions to extend (dorsiflex) the ankle, invert the foot, and actively support the arch.

The *extensor hallucis longus muscle* arises from the middle two thirds of the anterior fibula and interosseous membrane, passing beneath the extensor retinaculum. The anterior tibial artery and deep peroneal nerve lie between it and the tibialis anterior muscle. It lies medial to the neurovascular bundle at the ankle. The tendon passes along the dorsal aspect of the first metatarsal to insert at the base of the distal phalanx of the hallux. It functions to extend the ankle and great toe and to invert the foot.

The *extensor digitorum longus* muscle takes origin from the lateral tibial condyle, interosseous membrane, and intermuscular septa. Its tendon splits into several slips just above the inferior extensor retinaculum, lateral to the dorsalis pedis artery. It passes over the dorsal aspect of the foot to form an extensor hood at the metatarsophalangeal joint. It joins the tendons of the extensor digitorum brevis at the second, third, and fourth toes. Each tendon divides at its insertion into a central and two lateral slips. The central slip inserts on the base of the middle phalanx. Each lateral slip on the tibial side receives the insertion of a lumbrical muscle. The extensor hood formed from these tendons then passes over the middle phalanx to insert on the dorsal aspect of the distal phalanx. The extensor digitorum longus extends the metatarsophalangeal joints through direct attachment on the joint capsule and its extensor sling. It also extends the proximal interphalangeal and distal interphalangeal joints by means of the extensor hood and along with the intrinsic muscles, which also attach to the hood.

The peroneus tertius muscle is often considered part of the extensor digitorum longus muscle. It is the most lateral muscle in the anterior compartment and takes origin from the distal fibula and interosseous membrane. Its tendon lies lateral to the extensor digitorum longus and inserts on the base of the fifth metatarsal. It extends the ankle and everts the foot.

The single muscle on the dorsal aspect of the foot is the *extensor digitorum brevis*. It takes its origin partly from the superolateral calcaneus anteriorly and the sinus tarsi. It lies in the dorsolateral aspect of the midfoot. The lateral three tendons pass medially and insert on the lateral side of the second, third, and fourth tendons of the extensor digitorum longus muscle. The first tendon (extensor hallucis brevis) passes over the neurovascular bundle and inserts on the dorsolateral aspect of the base of the hallux proximal phalanx. It is innervated by a lateral branch of the deep peroneal nerve.

There are four layers of muscles on the plantar aspect of the foot. These layers differ from the compartments of the foot, which are separated from one another by interosseous and intermuscular membranes. The muscle layers are related to their position with respect to the sole.

All muscles in the first layer arise from the calcaneus and insert on the proximal phalanges. They have active control over the height of the longitudinal arch. They lie just beneath the plantar aponeurosis and are innervated by medial or lateral branches of the plantar nerve (Fig. 1-12).

The *abductor hallucis* muscle rises from the medial border of the calcaneus, forming a portion of the calcaneal canal. The flexor digitorum longus and flexor hallucis longus tendons pass deep to its belly. It inserts on the medial base of the proximal phalanx with the lateral head of the flexor hallucis brevis. At the hallux metatarsophalangeal joint, it blends with the medial capsule.

The *flexor digitorum brevis* muscle arises from the calcaneus, deep aspect of the plantar aponeurosis, and intermuscular septum. It forms four tendons, which pass through arches of the vertical septa of the plantar aponeurosis. They penetrate the fibroosseous tunnel beneath the metatarsals, where each tendon then divides to allow the flexor digitorum longus to pass through it.

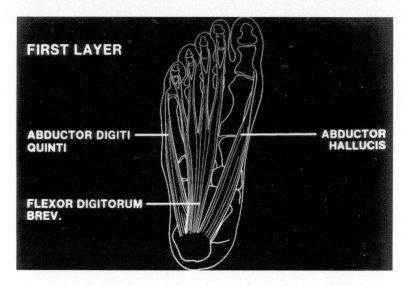

Fig. 1-12 First muscle layer of the foot viewed from below.

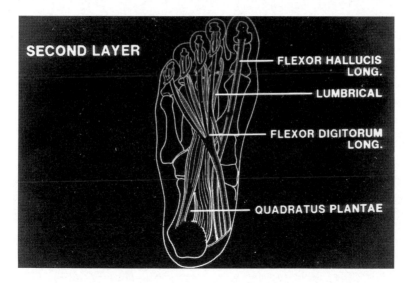

Fig. 1-13 Second muscle layer of the foot viewed below; first muscle layer is removed.

The tendons insert on the plantar aspect of the middle phalanx. The function of the flexor digitorum brevis is to flex the toes through flexion of the proximal interphalangeal joints and to maintain the longitudinal arch of the foot.

The *abductor digiti minimi* (quinti) arises from the lateral aspect of the calcaneus plantar aponeurosis and lateral intermuscular septum. It passes through the plantar aponeurosis to insert on the lateral proximal aspect and the plantar plate on the fifth toe. It abducts and flexes the small toe and helps maintain the longitudinal arch of the foot.

The second layer consists of muscles for controlling toe motion (Fig. 1-13).

The *quadratus plantae* origin has two heads. The lateral tendinous head arises from the calcaneal tuberosity, long plantar, and calcaneocuboid

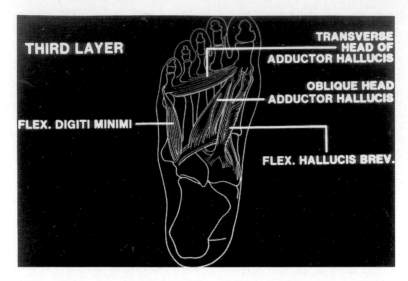

Fig. 1-14 Third muscle layer of the foot viewed from below; first and second muscle layer is removed.

ligaments. The medial head arises from the medial calcaneus and long plantar ligament. The two heads unite and then the muscle inserts on each of the tendons of the flexor digitorum longus. The quadratus plantae aids flexion of the toes through the flexor digitorum longus tendons.

There are four *lumbricals*. These are small fusiform muscles that arise from the segmented tendons of the flexor digitorum longus shortly after their division from the common tendon. They pass along the medial aspect of each metatarsal head and beneath the deep transverse metatarsal ligament to insert on the medial aspect of the extensor hood along with the interosseous muscles. They extend the proximal interphalangeal joints.

The third layer is related to the first and fifth toes (Fig. 1-14).

The *flexor hallucis brevis* muscle takes its Y-shaped origin medially from the tibialis posterior tendon and its lateral head from the cuboid and lateral cuneiform and medial intermuscular septum. It divides into two parts. The smaller lateral head lies in a groove of the first metatarsal.

It courses distally to attach to the fibular sesamoid along with the adductor hallucis muscle beneath the metatarsal head. It then inserts on the base of the proximal phalanx along with the adductor hallucis. The other head passes forward to attach to the medial plantar plate and the tibial sesamoid. It is joined by the tendon of the abductor hallucis muscle and inserts on the medial plantar part of the proximal phalanx. It flexes and stabilizes the metatarsophalangeal joint of the hallux.

The *adductor hallucis* has an oblique head and a transverse head. The oblique head has a long origin from the base of the cuboid, the second, third, and fourth metatarsal bases, and the sheath of the peroneus longus muscle. The transverse head takes origin from the plantar plates and the transverse metatarsal ligaments of the third, fourth, and fifth toes. The belly of the oblique portion of the muscle is near the flexor hallucis brevis muscle. The muscle passes dorsal to the transverse metatarsal ligament. It inserts through a conjoined tendon on the lateral aspect of the lateral sesamoid as well as on the plantar lateral aspect of the base of the proximal phalanx and part of the extensor aponeurosis. The muscle functions to flex and adduct the hallux.

The *flexor digiti minimi* muscle arises from the medial base of the fifth metatarsal, the sheath of the peroneus longus tendon, and the cuboid. It inserts on the plantar plate and the base of the proximal phalanx near the insertion of the abductor digiti minimi. It aids in the control of the fifth toe.

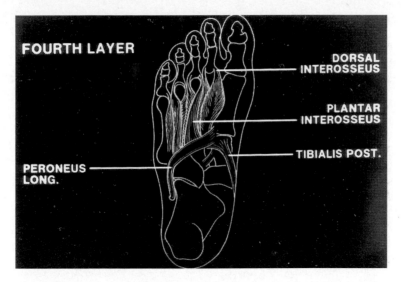

Fig. 1-15 Fourth muscle layer of the foot viewed from below. The three plantar muscle layers have been removed.

The fourth layer consists of the *interossei muscles*. They are divided into two groups, four dorsal interossei and three plantar interossei. They are named according to their function with respect to the second metatarsal (Fig. 1-15). Those that move the toes toward the longitudinal axis of the second metatarsal are adductors, and those that move the toes away from the axis are abductors. The tendons of two additional muscles are included in the fourth layer, the tibialis posterior tendon entering from the medial side and the peroneus longus tendon from the lateral side.

The interossei arise from both metatarsals in the intermetatarsal space from which they take origin. Each muscle passes distally, dorsal to the transverse metatarsal ligament at the level of the metatarsal heads.

The dorsal interossei arise from all metatarsals. They insert on the abductor sides of the second, third, and fourth proximal phalanges and into the extensor hood of each toe. The first dorsal interosseous muscle forms an arch at its origin. The dorsalis pedis artery passes through this arch from the dorsum of the foot between the first and second metatarsals to the deep plantar arterial arch.

The three plantar interossei take origin from beneath the dorsal muscles and are smaller in size.

They take origin from the third, fourth, and fifth metatarsals and insert on the adductor sides of the third, fourth, and fifth phalanges and the extensor hoods also.

The interossei flex the metatarsophalangeal joints and, through their attachments to the extensor hood, extend the proximal interphalangeal and distal interphalangeal joints.

Nerves

The *saphenous nerve* is a terminal branch of the femoral nerve that has its origin in the second to fourth lumbar segments of the spinal cord. At the knee, it lies deep to the sartorius muscle, pierces the fascia lata between the sartorius and gracilis muscles, and then passes medial to the tibia in the leg, just posterior to the greater saphenous vein. There are two branches distally. The smaller one terminates at the ankle; the larger one gives sensation anterior to the medial malleolus and along the medial border of the foot (Fig. 1-16).

The cutaneous and muscular innervation to the leg, ankle, and foot is derived from the *sciatic nerve*. Its origin includes a peroneal portion

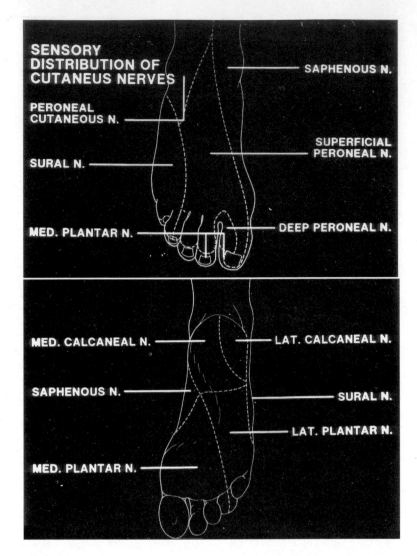

Fig. 1-16 Sensory distribution of cutaneous nerves. **A,** Dorsal. **B,** Plantar.

from the posterior divisions of the ventral rami of the lumbosacral plexus, originating from the fourth lumbar to the second sacral segments of the spinal cord (Fig. 1-17). The tibial portion derives from the fourth lumbar to the third sacral nerve roots and forms from the anterior divisions of the ventral rami of the lumbosacral plexus.

The main sensory nerve of the leg is the *sural nerve,* a branch of the tibial nerve arising in the posterior superior popliteal fossa. It passes down the posterior aspect of the calf, piercing the posterior fascia in the middle of the calf. It communicates with the cutaneous branch of the lat-

eral popliteal nerve at the posterolateral border of the lateral malleolus, 1 cm from the tip. Its distribution is to the lower and posterior portion of the lateral malleolus and the lateral foot.

The *common peroneal nerve* is the smaller of the two branches of the sciatic nerve that separate at the popliteal fossa. It courses laterally over the biceps femoris tendon and lateral head of the gastrocnemius, beneath the posterior and lateral aspect of the knee joint. It then passes beneath the head of the fibula into the anterior portion of the leg, where it divides into a superficial and a deep branch.

Anatomy and Physiology

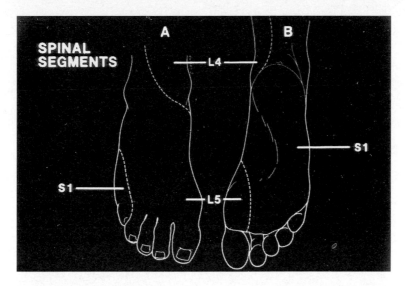

Fig. 1-17 Lumbosacral innervation to the foot.

The *superficial peroneal nerve* branches off the common peroneal nerve between the peroneus longus muscle and the neck of the fibula. It descends the anterior aspect of the leg, innervating the peroneus longus and peroneus brevis muscles, and then pierces the fascia 10 to 15 cm above the lateral malleolus. It continues subcutaneously and 6 cm above the lateral malleolus splits into a medial dorsal cutaneous branch and an intermediate dorsal cutaneous branch. These branches give sensory innervation dorsally to the first to fifth toes.

The *deep peroneal nerve* (anterior tibial nerve) passes into the anterior compartment following the branching of the superficial peroneal nerve. Motor branches pass to the extensor hallucis longus, tibialis anterior, extensor digitorum longus, and peroneus tertius muscles. The sensory nerve descends along the lateral side of the anterior tibial artery, deep to the extensor retinaculum behind the extensor hallucis longus, and passes with the dorsalis pedis artery onto the dorsum of the foot. It lies between the extensor hallucis longus and extensor digitorum longus tendons 2 cm above the ankle joint. It lies beneath the extensor hallucis longus at the ankle and divides into a medial and a lateral branch 1 cm above the ankle joint. These branches innervate the ankle joint anteriorly.

The medial branch then lies lateral to the dorsalis pedis artery and passes to the second toe to give sensory innervation to the first web space.

The lateral branch gives off a motor branch to the extensor digitorum brevis and sensory branches to joints of the forefoot. The cutaneous distribution of the deep branch of the peroneal nerve is variable, but most variations include sensation to the first web space. When decreased sensation is present in the first web space, a differential diagnosis must include deep peroneal nerve–impaired function, as with anterior compartment syndrome or peroneal nerve palsy.

The tibial nerve is the larger portion of the sciatic nerve (Fig. 1-18**A**). It begins in the popliteal fossa following the branching of the common peroneal nerve and passes superficial to the popliteal artery and vein at the popliteus muscle. It enters the deep posterior compartment of the calf and then passes beneath the soleus muscle with the posterior tibial artery and vein. In the lower leg it gives off a branch to the flexor hallucis longus muscle, which lies lateral to it. It courses along the medial border of the Achilles tendon.

The *medial calcaneal nerve* branches from the tibial nerve in the leg. It courses inferiorly and anterior to the Achilles tendon toward the medial and posterior heel. There is an anterior branch and a plantar branch, which innervate the sole and the medial aspect of the foot. The tibial

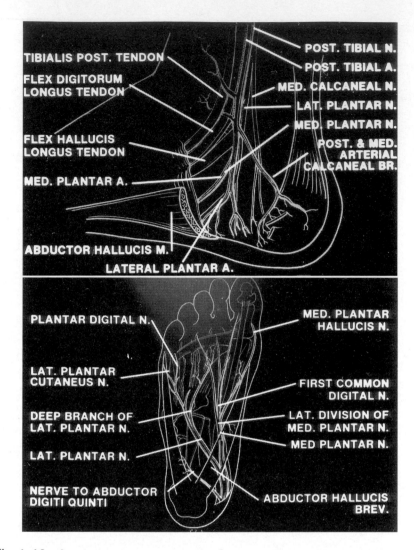

Fig. 1-18   **A,** Tibial nerve and its branches. **B,** Nerves of the plantar aspect of the foot.

nerve branches into the medial and lateral plantar nerves 1 cm above the medial malleolus.

The *medial plantar nerve* is larger and more anterior than the lateral. It passes with the tibial artery and vein into the upper calcaneal canal and contains motor branches to the abductor hallucis brevis, flexor digitorum brevis, and first lumbrical muscles (Fig. 1-18**B**).

The *proper digital nerve* is a branch of the medial plantar nerve. It sends a motor branch to the flexor digitorum brevis and also gives sensation to the medial aspect of the hallux, the sole, and the ball of the foot. The motor branches enter the lateral sides of the abductor hallucis and

flexor digitorum brevis along the wall of the medial compartment at the base of the first metatarsal.

The *first common digital nerve* lies between the flexor hallucis longus tendon and the flexor digitorum longus tendon. It gives sensation to the lateral side of the hallux and the medial side of the second toe. A motor branch passes to the first lumbrical. The second and third common digital nerves anastomose with the fourth common digital nerve. Each of the nerves bifurcates in the fatty soft tissue at the level of the metatarsal heads. Each digital nerve passes along the plantar medial or plantar lateral side of the respective toe. These are sensory nerves to the plantar aspects and tufts of the toes.

The *lateral plantar nerve* passes into the lower calcaneal canal posterior to the tibial artery. The first branch passes laterally to the abductor digiti quinti, arising at the medial border of the flexor digitorum brevis between that muscle and the quadratus plantae. It also gives its motor branch to the quadratus plantae muscle. It has two branches. The superficial branch contains a sensory branch to the outer sole area and also gives a motor branch to the short flexor of the fifth toe. Occasionally a branch goes to the interossei of the fourth metatarsal space. The fourth and fifth common digital nerves are formed from this nerve. It ultimately becomes the lateral plantar cutaneous nerve. Occasionally, it provides anastomotic branches to the third common digital nerve.

The deep branch follows the lateral plantar artery into the lower calcaneal canal and passes between the adductor hallucis and the interossei muscles. It gives small motor branches to the lateral three lumbricals and to the interossei muscles of the second, third, and fourth spaces and the transverse head of the adductor hallucis.

Arteries and Veins

The arteries of the leg arise from the popliteal artery at the knee, which divides into three parts. The *anterior tibial artery* branches from the popliteal artery at the lower border of the popliteus muscle and passes over the interosseous membrane and the tibialis posterior muscle. Along with venae comitantes, it lies on the anterior surface of the interosseous membrane, between the tibialis anterior and extensor digitorum longus muscles and then between the tibialis anterior and extensor hallucis longus muscles. It passes beneath the extensor retinacula, where it becomes the dorsalis pedis artery. It gives off anterior branches to the ankle and anastomoses with tarsal arterial branches to form a collateral circulation about the ankle.

The *dorsalis pedis artery* begins at the ankle joint (Fig. 1-19**A**). It lies medial to the deep branch of the peroneal nerve. It sends a branch laterally to the sinus tarsi and the first dorsal metatarsal artery. It also gives off the arcuate artery, after which it passes to the plantar aspect of the foot at the proximal first intermetatarsal space. In the foot, it becomes the first plantar metatarsal artery and connects with the deep arterial arch.

The popliteal artery becomes the *posterior tibial artery* at the inferior border of the popliteus muscle (Fig. 1-19**B**). It passes deep to the soleus muscle and along the medial border of the Achilles tendon along with the tibial nerve and veins. It then passes beneath the flexor retinaculum between the flexor digitorum longus medially and the flexor hallucis longus laterally. Here the artery lies medial to the nerve and divides into the medial and lateral plantar arteries, divided by the transverse septum at the calcaneal canal.

The *medial plantar artery* passes deep to the abductor hallucis and flexor digitorum brevis muscles parallel to the flexor hallucis longus tendon. It gives off a superficial branch, which lies on the plantar side of the flexor hallucis brevis muscle and on the tibial side of the flexor hallucis longus tendon. This anastomoses with the first plantar metatarsal artery and supplies the first three intermetatarsal spaces and the medial four toes. The small deep branch terminates on the deep plantar arch.

The *lateral plantar artery* passes into the lower calcaneal canal and into the middle compartment of the foot. It passes under the quadratus plantae muscle and forms the plantar vascular arch, anastomosing with the dorsalis pedis artery from the dorsal aspect of the foot in the proximal first intermetatarsal space.

A superficial plantar arterial arch is formed when the common digital arteries anastomose with one another. The digital plantar arteries arise from this more distal anterior arch. The *peroneal artery* branches from the posterior tibial artery 3 cm beyond the branching of the anterior tibial artery in the deep posterior compartment of the leg. It runs along the posterior border of the fibula beneath the flexor hallucis longus muscle. At the lateral malleolus it anastomoses with the lateral malleolar branches of the anterior tibial artery. There is great variability in the size and position of this artery.

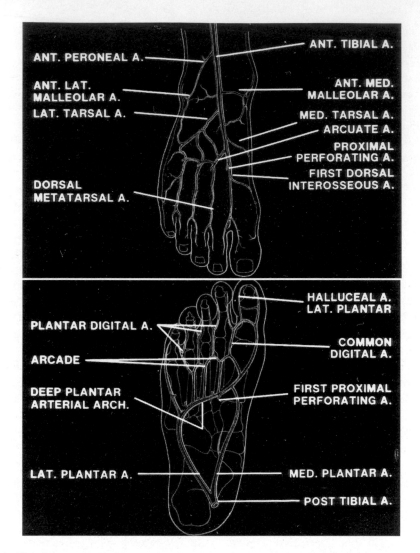

Fig. 1-19 **A,** Anterior of the dorsum of the foot, **B,** Anterior of the plantar aspect of the foot.

The venous system of the ankle and foot is quite variable. On the dorsum of the foot, two groups exist, a superficial and a deep system. The superficial venous system lies above the superficial fascia and includes the saphenous veins. These veins drain the dorsal aspect of the toes and form the dorsal venous arcade on the dorsum of the foot. The veins converge at the anterior ankle and also lead into the deep venous system.

The *greater saphenous vein* is the largest vein draining blood from the dorsum of the foot. It lies just anterior to the medial malleolus at the ankle. Its valves prevent reflux of blood into the foot. It courses along the medial aspect of the calf in the subcutaneous tissue, receiving communicating branches from the deep calf to end in the femoral vein. The *lesser saphenous vein* lies posterior and lateral to the lateral malleolus. Smaller than the greater saphenous vein, it drains blood from the lateral aspect of the foot and the lateral arch. These veins are easily visualized and fairly constant in their position.

The deep venous system of the dorsal foot consists of the *venae comitantes* of the dorsalis pedis artery and its tributaries. Such major arteries

Anatomy and Physiology

often have two veins accompanying them. They communicate with the greater and lesser saphenous veins through the malleolar and metatarsal veins by means of perforating veins.

The plantar aspect of the foot also has two systems of veins. The superficial system is intradermal and subdermal and consists of a thin mesh of vessels on the sole, which drain the medial and lateral margins of the foot. This system is valveless and communicates with the deep plantar venous system. The deep plantar veins accompany the medial and lateral plantar arteries and form a deep plantar venous arch. This drains the metatarsal veins.

The lymphatic system of the foot and ankle consists of a superficial and deep system. The superficial system drains the skin of the toes, the sole, and the heel. There is a large plexus of minute vessels on the dorsum of the foot. These vessels follow the course of the greater and lesser saphenous veins to terminate at the inguinal lymph nodes and less frequently at the popliteal node.

Skin

The skin on the dorsum of the foot is thin and supple. Loose attachments to the underlying subcutaneous tissue permit it to be moved easily over tendons. There are cleavage lines, which are oriented obliquely along the lateral border of the foot but longitudinally along the medial border.

The skin of the sole of the foot is thick and closely adherent to the subcutaneous tissue. Thickness of the epidermis approaches 5 mm over the areas of increased weight-bearing on the heel and ball of the foot. Skin here lacks sebaceous glands and epocrine glands. Eccrine glands, however, are profuse on the sole. These are sensitive to both adrenergic and cholinergic stimuli. The sensitivity of the sole is greater than that of the dorsum of the foot.

The skin of the sole is closely bound to the plantar aponeurosis through septa. These septa run from the dermis to the aponeurosis in the ball and toes. Between these septa are fat globules, which act as a cushion during walking. In the heel, septa connecting the calcaneus to the skin are arranged in a layered, counterspiralling fashion to act as shock absorbers during heel strike.

Nails

The *toenails* consist of three layers and function to protect the distal toes. The medial and lateral borders of the nail lie in a nail groove. The germinal portion of the nail lies 4 mm proximal to the cuticle border. Trauma, infection, or surgery in this area can affect the germinal tissue, permanently altering the shape of the nail. The nail of the great toe grows the most slowly of all the nails, requiring from 9 months to 1 year to regenerate following removal.

Bibliography

1. Edwards EA: Anatomy of the small arteries of the foot and toes, *Acta Anat (Basel)* 40:81, 1960.
2. Grant JCB: *An atlas of anatomy,* ed 4, Baltimore, 1956, Williams & Wilkins.
3. Greenfield GB: *Radiology of bone disease,* Philadelphia, 1969, JB Lippincott.
4. Huber JF: The arterial network supplying the dorsum of the foot, *Anat Rec* 80:373, 1944.
5. Kelikian H: *Functional anatomy of the forefoot in hallux valgus, allied deformities of the forefoot and metatarsalgia,* Philadelphia, 1965, WB Saunders, pp. 27-42.
6. Kosinski C: The course, mutual relations and distribution of the cutaneous nerve of the metazonal region of the leg and foot, *J Anat* 60:274, 1926.
7. Laidlaw PL: The varieties of the os calcis, *J Anat Physiol* 38:138, 1904.
8. Mann RA: Rupture of the tibialis posterior tendon. In Murray JA, editor: *Instructional course lectures,* vol 33, 1984, American Academy of Orthopedic Surgeons, Rosemont, IL.
9. Manter JT: Distribution of compression forces in the joints of the human foot, *Anat Rec* 96:313, 1946.
10. Nathan H, Gloobe H: Flexor digitorum brevis: anatomical variations, *Anat Anz* 135:295, 1974.
11. Sammarco GJ: Biomechanics of the foot. In Nordin M, Frankel VH, editors: *Basic biomechanics of the musculoskeletal system,* Philadelphia, 1989, Lea & Febiger.
12. Sarrafian SK: *Anatomy of the foot and ankle, descriptive, topographic, functional,* Philadelphia, 1983, JB Lippincott.
13. Woodburne RT: *Essentials of human anatomy,* New York, 1961, Oxford University Press.

2

Biomechanics of the Foot and Ankle

Joseph Hamill

Kenneth G. Holt

Timothy R. Derrick

The foot and the ankle make up a complex structure consisting of 26 irregularly shaped bones and 57 joints coupled with over 100 ligaments and 32 muscles. All of these structures must interact harmoniously to provide a smoothly functioning unit. The foot and ankle contribute significantly to the function of the lower extremity, the foot providing for the dynamic interaction of the body with the ground. The foot-ankle structure is specialized for support and bipedal locomotion but performs multiple functions that often conflict with one another. It has the general functions of balance, support, and propulsion. This anatomic structure is remarkable in that it must adapt to many types of terrain, including changes in surface consistency and shape, while sustaining great weight-bearing stresses. The foot-ankle complex must aid in accepting the body weight in collisions with the ground and also act to provide effective push-off during locomotion. It must continually provide a successful interaction between the body and its environment.

In sporting activities, the foot must adapt to many types of playing surfaces and must accomplish many tasks that result in many different types of footfall patterns. For example, in straight-ahead locomotion, such as running, there are three identifiable footfall patterns exhibited by runners. However, in other sports such as tennis, racquetball, and basketball, lateral movements are employed, which require the foot to move in a completely different footfall pattern from that of straight-ahead running. In many sports the participant must jump and land safely on the playing surface. The result is a unique landing footfall pattern.

In this chapter, we discuss the functional anatomy and biomechanics of the foot in each of these footfall patterns—running, lateral movements, and landing from a jump—as they relate to sports.

Regions of the Foot

The foot-ankle complex is generally divided into three structural/functional units: the hindfoot, the midfoot, and the forefoot. These divisions, while somewhat artificial, have biomechanical significance and are generally useful in describing normal and pathological foot function (Fig. 2-1). The hindfoot is composed of the talus and the calcaneus and is generally the first point of contact of the foot with the ground in many locomotor activities. The calcaneus is the site of insertion of the calf muscles and the origin of the plantar fascia. In terms of research on the foot, the hindfoot area has received by far the most attention. The midfoot is composed of the navicular, cuboid, and cuneiform bones. This system of bones forms the bridge between the hindfoot and the forefoot. It is difficult to assess the movements of each bone within this unit, but the function of this system of bones is critically important. The forefoot is composed of the metatarsals, which are referred to as *rays*. These rays fan out from a constricted beginning in the midfoot, with the relative movement between them increasing as they fan out.

Joints of the Foot–Ankle Complex

There are several joints in the foot–ankle complex that determine the myriad actions of the foot during sports activities. These joints are the ankle (talocrural) joint, the subtalar joint, the talocalcaneonavicular joint, the transverse tarsal joint, the tarsometatarsal joints, and the metatarsophalangeal joints.

Ankle Joint

The traditionally named ankle joint is more correctly named the talocrural joint. This hinge joint is the articulation between the talus and the distal tibia and the talus and the fibula (Fig. 2-2). From a biomechanical point of view, the ankle joint is designed for stability rather than mobility, being most stable when forces are absorbed through the limb. The ankle joint may be considered to have a single axis of movement, or 1 degree of freedom, although it has been suggested that rotation of the talus in the transvere plane occurs.[19A] When the ankle joint is in a neutral position, the axis of the joint passes through the medial malleolus and the talus and just below the lateral malleolus. Since the lateral malleolus lies more distally than the medial malleolus, the axis of the ankle joint is rotated laterally 20 to 30 degrees in the frontal plane. The resulting motions of the ankle joint are plantarflexion and dorsiflexion; however, the rotation of the axis results in motion across two planes. The dorsiflexor action brings the foot up and slightly abducted, while the plantarflexor action brings the foot down and slightly adducted. The normal range of motion of the ankle joint is generally accepted as 20 degrees of dorsiflexion from the neutral position and from 30 to 50 degrees of plantarflexion.[12]

Subtalar Joint

The subtalar or talocalcaneal joint is located between the talus and the calcaneus and has three separate articulations, of which the posterior ar-

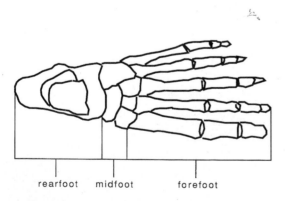

Fig. 2-1 Functional segments of the foot.

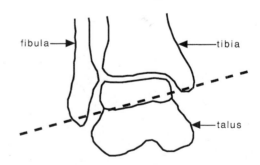

Fig. 2-2 Frontal view of the ankle joint showing orientation of the axis of the ankle joint.

ticulation is the largest (Fig. 2-3). The subtalar joint has the functions of absorbing the rotation of the lower extremity during support, via the actions of pronation and supination, and attenuating the impact of shock during support, via pronation. The axis of rotation of the subtalar joint runs from the posterior, lateral plantar to the anterior, dorsal, medial surface of the talus and is directed approximately 23 degrees medially from the sagittal plane and tilted 42 degrees upward from the transverse plane.[12] Greater variability appears to be associated with the degree of tilt of the axis from the transverse plane. The actions associated with the subtalar joint are pronation and supination. The subtalar joint is considered to have *triplanar motion;* that is, component motions about the cardinal axes of eversion/inversion, abduction/adduction, and plantarflexion/dorsiflexion. However, Edington and colleagues[6] have suggested that the motion of the subtalar joint is triplanar only if the planes being considered are the cardinal planes of the body. They state that this characterization implies that the axis of the subtalar joint is not aligned with any of the cardinal axes. Thus, when pronation at the subtalar joint occurs, if viewed from the

cardinal planes, it will appear to have the components of internal rotation, dorsiflexion, and calcaneal eversion, and supination will have the components of external rotation, plantarflexion, and calcaneal inversion. The range of motion for pronation and supination is 20 to 62 degrees, with the supination movement about double the range of pronation.

Talocalcaneonavicular Joint

This joint is a compound joint that combines the functionally related talonavicular and the subtalar joints. They are related since the talus moves simultaneously on both the calcaneus via the subtalar joint and the navicular via the talonavicular joint. The talus is a unique bone in that it has no muscular attachments and thus acts like a ball-bearing between the tibia/fibula superiorly, the calcaneus inferiorly, and the navicular anteriorly. The axis for this compound joint is very similar to that of the subtalar joint, with an inclination of 40 degrees upward anteriorly and 30 degrees medially which is slightly more medial than the subtalar joint (Fig. 2-4). The talocalcaneonavicular joint thus also enables the actions of pronation and supination.

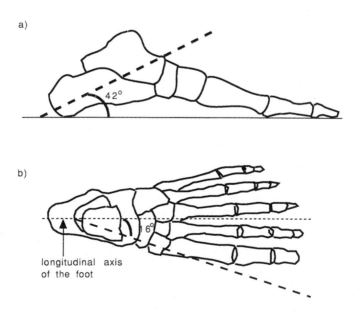

a)

42°

b)

16°

longitudinal axis of the foot

Fig. 2-3 Axis of the subtalar joint. **A,** From a medial sagittal view. **B,** From an anterior view.

Biomechanics of the Foot and Ankle

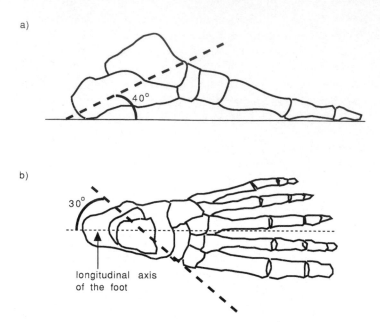

a)

40°

b)

30°

longitudinal axis
of the foot

Fig. 2-4 Axis of the talocalcaneonavicular joint. **A,** From a medial sagittal view. **B,** From an anterior view.

Transverse Tarsal Joint

The transverse tarsal or midtarsal joint is a compound joint formed by the talonavicular and calcaneocuboid joints. The talonavicular joint is therefore a part of both the talocalcaneonavicular joint and the midtarsal joint. These two joints form an S-shaped structure that divides the hindfoot from the midfoot and provides the transition from the hindfoot to the forefoot. Since the cuboid is fixed during weight-bearing, the motion of the midtarsal joint is that of the talus and the calcaneus on the navicular and the cuboid bones. The midtarsal joint is considered to move about two independent axes, a longitudinal anteroposterior axis and an oblique axis (Fig. 2-5). The longitudinal axis is slightly inclined upward and medially. Motion about this axis is pronation/supination. The oblique axis of this joint is almost parallel to that of the talocalcaneonavicular joint, also providing pronation/supination actions. The motion about these two axes together provides about one third of the range available at the talocalcaneonavicular joint so that the joint may be considered an adjunct to the previously discussed joints. Movement at the midtarsal joint is dependent on the subtalar position.

Tarsometatarsal Joints

The tarsometatarsal joints are gliding planar joints formed by the intersection of the distal tarsal row and the bases of the metatarsals. These joints are numbered one through five, with the first metatarsal intersecting the medial cuneiform, the second the middle cuneiform, the third the lateral cuneiform, and the fourth and fifth the cuboid. Each of these joints and their associated structures is referred to as a *ray,* although the ray is formed only by the metatarsal itself in the fourth and fifth rays. The axes of the first and fifth rays are oblique (Fig. 2-6). The axis of the first ray allows dorsiflexion accompanied by inversion and adduction, and conversely, plantarflexion is accompanied by eversion and abduction. The movements of the fifth ray do not undergo the same range and have the opposite arrangement. That is, dorsiflexion is accompanied by eversion and abduction, and plantarflexion is accompanied by inversion and adduction. The axes of the second and fourth rays are also oblique but not as oblique as the first and fifth ray axes. The axes of these rays are thought to be intermediate to the adjacent rays. The axis for the third ray allows the predominant motion of plantarflexion/dorsiflexion.

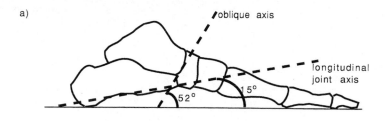

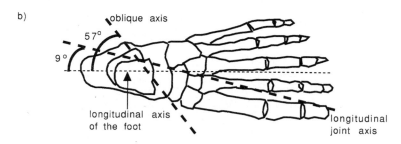

Fig. 2-5 Longitudinal and oblique axes of the transverse tarsal joints. **A,** From a medial sagittal view. **B,** From an anterior view.

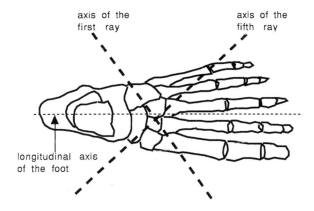

Fig. 2-6 Axes of the first and fifth rays of the tarsometatarsal joints from an anterior view.

Metatarsophalangeal Joints

There are five metatarsophalangeal joints. Each is a biaxial joint, thus allowing 2 degrees of freedom, which results in both dorsiflexion/plantarflexion and abduction/adduction movements, with plantarflexion/dorsiflexion being the predominant movement. The range of motion of these joints varies greatly depending on whether the motions occur in weight- or nonweight-bearing activities. These joints allow the foot to "bend" or "hinge" in order that the heel may be lifted off the ground.

Coordinated Actions of the Foot Joints

While it may appear that each of the joints of the foot has individual actions, these individual actions are in fact highly coordinated, allowing the foot to function dynamically as a unit. The actions of the joints are highly integrated, and action at one joint usually results in a functional compensatory movement in another joint. The pronation/supination actions of the foot illustrate these compensatory movements. Pronation of the subtalar and talocalcaneonavicular joints results in a position of mobility and movement at the midtarsal joint that is dependent on the pronatory position. When the hindfoot is pronating, the two axes of the midtarsal joint are parallel, which unlocks the joint, creating hypermobility in the foot, allowing the foot to be very mobile in absorbing the shock of impact with the ground and also in adapting to uneven surfaces. These actions also allow the forefoot to flex freely. In the support phase of locomotion, for example, the motion at the midtarsal joint is unrestricted from heel contact to foot flat as the foot moves toward the surface. In addition, if the foot is to remain on the ground, the tarsometatarsal joints must undergo a counteracting supination.

During supination of the hindfoot, the two axes running through the midtarsal joint converge and are no longer parallel. This locks the joint, creating a rigidity in the foot that is necessary for efficient force application. In locomotion, the midtarsal joint becomes rigid and more stable from foot flat to toe-off. It is usually stabilized creating a rigid lever at 70% of the stance phase. At this time there is also a greater load on the midtarsal joint, making the articulation between the talus and the navicular more stable.

Arches of the Foot

The bones of the foot are arranged to form one transverse arch and one longitudinal arch, although the longitudinal arch may be considered two separate arches. The longitudinal arches are designated according to their position relative to the longitudinal axis of the foot. The medial longitudinal arch consists of the calcaneus, talus, navicular, three cuneiforms, and the three medial metatarsals (Fig. 2-7A). This is a relatively high arch and keeps the medial portion of the foot from touching the ground. It is much more flexible than the lateral longitudinal arch and plays a significant role in shock attenuation upon con-

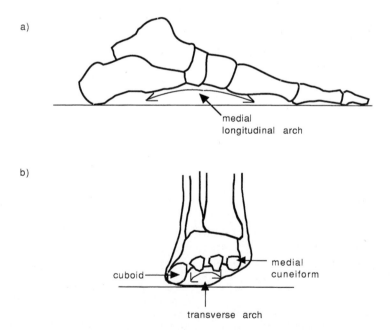

a)

medial longitudinal arch

b)

cuboid — medial cuneiform

transverse arch

Fig. 2-7 Arches of the foot. **A,** Medial longitudinal arch. **B,** Transverse arch.

tact with the ground. The lateral longitudinal arch is not as high as the medial longitudinal arch, and the lateral portion of the foot actually touches the ground. It consists of the calcaneus, the cuboid, and the two lateral metatarsals. The transverse arch is perpendicular to the longitudinal arches. It is most evident at the bases of the metatarsals, but it can also be seen at the level of the anterior tarsals (Fig. 2-7B). These arches are supported by ligaments, muscle tendons, the plantar fascia, and by many small intrinsic muscles.

The plantar fascia is a strong, fibrous aponeurosis that is extremely complex in structure and function. It is attached to the calcaneus and extends forward spanning the tarsal and metatarsophalangeal joints to the proximal phalanges. The resulting structure is like a mechanical truss whose tether is the plantar fascia.[19B] The plantar fascia acts like a cable or truss between the heel and toes, whose elongation is a shock-absorbing mechanism. The plantar fascia also prevents collapse of the longitudinal arch during standing support by preventing passive flexion of the toes. Passive flexion of the toes would cause the fascia to relax and the longitudinal arch to flatten.

The plantar arches are adapted to serve the weight-bearing functions of the foot. The foot could perform some biomechanical functions if it had no arches or a fixed arch structure, but it could not perform the functions of attenuating the shock of weight-bearing and adapting to changes in the terrain. The arches, therefore, function as shock absorbers and give resilience to the foot. During weight-bearing the arches flatten, and they rebound to their original shape during a nonweight-bearing state.

Muscles of the Foot

There are 32 muscles, 13 extrinsic and 19 intrinsic, that control the actions of the foot. All of the extrinsic muscles, except for the gastrocnemius, soleus, and plantaris, act across both the subtalar and midtarsal joints. The muscles of the foot play an important role in sustaining impacts of high magnitude. The passive structures—ligaments, tendons, and muscle fascia—store some energy to return it later in the movement.

Extrinsic Muscles

The extrinsic muscles of the calf include the gastrocnemius, the soleus, the plantaris, the flexor hallucis longus, the flexor digitorum longus, and the tibialis posterior. The gastrocnemius and the soleus are muscles that combine to form the strongest of the plantarflexors. Their function is mediated through the subtalar joint, which transmits the force to the talus and the foot. The plantaris also acts as a weak plantarflexor of the foot. The deep posterior muscles—flexor hallucis longus, flexor digitorum longus, and tibialis posterior—act like pulleys by passing around bony projections on the tibia and the calcaneus and insert on the plantar surface of the foot. The tibialis posterior is active in standing and is important in controlling the stability of the foot while also actively supporting the longitudinal arch. The flexor hallucis longus and flexor digitorum longus control flexion of the toes during locomotion.

The lateral extrinsic muscles of the leg include the peronei muscles: the peroneus longus, brevis, and tertius. Their tendons pass pulleylike under the lateral malleolus of the fibula. The tendon of the brevis inserts into the base of the fifth metatarsal, while the tendon of the longus inserts into the base of the first metatarsal and the cuneiform. The peronei muscles are evertors of the foot, while the longus is also a plantarflexor of the transverse tarsal joint.

The extrinsic anterior muscles of the leg are referred to as the dorsiflexors of the foot and extensors of the toes. These muscles are the tibialis anterior, the extensor digitorum longus, and the extensor hallucis longus. The tibialis anterior is the major dorsiflexor of the foot with the added function of inverting the foot. The extensor digitorum longus is a weak dorsiflexor of the foot and a strong extensor of the second through fifth toes. The extensor hallucis longus originates on the fibula and inserts into the base of the hallux. Its primary function is extension of the big toe, but it also acts as a dorsiflexor and evertor of the foot.

Intrinsic Muscles

The major intrinsic muscles of the foot are the flexor hallucis brevis, the extensor digitorum brevis, and the abductor digiti minimi. These muscles do not have general functions like many of the extrinsic muscles but have very specific functions. The flexor hallucis brevis flexes the proximal phalanx of the first toe; the extensor digitorum brevis extends the proximal phalanges of the medial four toes; and the abductor digiti minimi abducts and flexes the fifth toe. Beneath the tendons of the flexor hallucis brevis are the two sesamoid bones of the hallux. These are located beneath the head of the first metatarsal and act to transfer loads from the ground to the metatarsal heads. There are several other intrinsic muscles of the foot, but they have little importance in the overall biomechanical function of the foot.

Kinematics of the Foot

Running
Footfall Patterns

Although it is the predominant view that the heel-toe footfall pattern is characteristic of "slow" running and the forefoot strike pattern is characteristic of "fast" running, there is little evidence to support this contention. Cavanagh and Lafortune[3] suggested that there is a continuum of initial contact points that cover the entire posterior 60% of the shoe length. Mason,[14] however, identified three general footfall patterns used by runners, which he classified according to the point on the foot that first contacts the ground, and referred to these as heel-toe (HT), toe-heel-toe (THT), and forefoot (FF) patterns. In this study, he pointed out that these patterns constituted a continuum, with the HT and FF patterns the extremes. The majority of runners fell into the HT footfall type. Runners generally did not change their footfall pattern even when they increased their running speed. If they did change, it was only to the pattern adjacent to the preferred pattern. For example, an HT runner would not change to an FF pattern. Slavin and Hamill[20] conducted a study in which HT runners were forced to run in an FF pattern and FF runners in an HT pattern. They reported that the energy cost of running in an HT pattern was less than in the FF pattern regardless of the preferred footfall pattern. Generally the majority of recreational athletes run with an HT pattern.

In the THT footfall pattern, the initial contact is made in the midfoot with the heel immediately coming down to contact the ground during the impacting phase. During the propulsive phase, the pressure center moves in the anterior direction toward the toes. Mason[14] reported that the stride length of runners using this footfall pattern was significantly longer than that of runners using an HT pattern. In addition, the time until the total body center of mass passed over the base of support was significantly shorter than in the HT footfall pattern.

In the FF footfall pattern, the initial contact is made on the lateral portion of the forefoot. Although the heel drops toward the ground, it never makes contact with the ground. The heel drop is necessary to produce a stretch in the leg extensor muscles resulting in a more propulsive contraction during takeoff. FF footfall pattern runners are characterized by long stride lengths.[14]

Kinematics

The support portion of the running stride is generally broken down into three distinct phases: the impact phase, the midstance phase, and the pushoff phase. Figure 2-8 is a graphic representation of the hindfoot motion during the support period of a running stride. In a running gait classified as an HT footfall pattern, the impact phase begins with initial heel contact with the ground. This initial contact is made by the lateral aspect of the heel with the foot in a slightly supinated position. This would appear to be the result of the swing of the leg toward the line of progression. The touchdown velocity of the foot is mostly vertical, about 0.8 to 1.5 m/sec, but also slightly forward, about 0.5 to 1.0 m/sec. Immediately after this initial contact, the foot starts to pronate rapidly with a maximum angular velocity as high as 800 degrees/sec. The impact phase functions to attenuate the impact shock and to distribute the load as evenly as possible

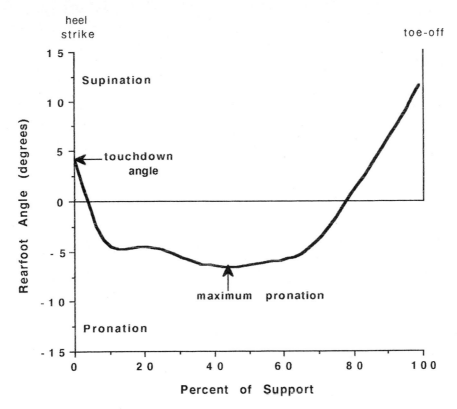

Fig. 2-8 Graphic representation of a frontal view hindfoot angle during the support phase of a running footfall.

on different structures of the locomotor system.[13]

Midstance is defined as the time during which the entire foot is on the ground. At about 20% of the support phase, the subtalar joint passes from a supinated to a pronated position. However, the occurrence of this event shows considerable variation depending on the anatomic structure of the foot. Pronation then continues to about 85% of the support phase, with maximum pronation occurring between 35% and 45% of the support phase. Values of maximum pronation range from 4.5 degrees to 25.5 degrees.[5] However, these values are greatly influenced by external factors such as shoe type and shoe inserts. At maximum pronation, the foot changes from a force-attenuating structure to one that propels the body forward to the next airborne phase.

The pushoff phase begins when the heel rises

from the ground and ends when the toes leave the ground. In this propelling phase, the foot begins to supinate, forming a more rigid structure that helps to maximize the push off the support leg. Luethi and Stacoff[13] identified three different types of takeoff positions: (1) the heel rises up with no varus or valgus tilt, (2) the foot remains in a pronated position, and (3) the foot supinates and the heel rotates externally. They suggested that in the latter two cases, the force distribution on the Achilles tendon is not homogeneous and may lead to high force concentrations on locally small areas of the tendon.

Since the majority of runners utilize an HT footfall pattern, most of the research on the sagittal view kinematics of running has been done on this pattern. A typical sagittal view ankle profile is presented in Figure 2-9. In this convention, dorsiflexion angles are positive, plantarflexion angles are negative, and the neutral ankle po-

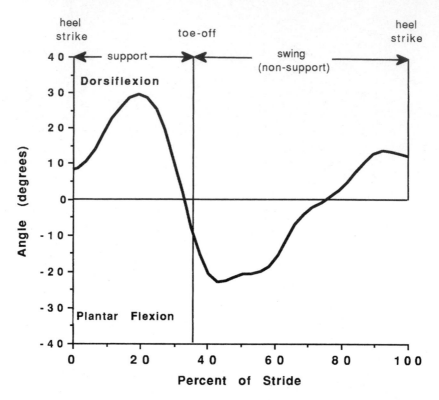

Fig. 2-9 Graphic representation of a sagittal view ankle angle during the support phase of a running footfall.

sition is 0 degrees. At footstrike, the ankle is slightly plantarflexed. The forward swing of the leg results in this slight plantarflexion of the subtalar joint in addition to adduction of the forefoot and inversion of the calcaneus. This position brings the forefoot closer to the running surface, thus increasing the range of motion and allowing for a greater time period over which to absorb the force of impact. Following the initial contact, the foot is placed flat on the surface via an eccentric action of the anterior tibialis. The leg then rotates forward relative to the foot segment, resulting in about 20 degrees of dorsiflexion at the ankle. The ankle continues to dorsiflex until it reaches a maximum at midstance. At this point, the ankle begins to plantarflex to a maximum of −20 degrees shortly after toeoff.

Lateral Movements
Footfall Patterns

In lateral movements, footfall patterns are almost as varied as they are in running. Stuessi et

al[23] suggested ways in which a change in lateral direction (i.e., braking and starting in another direction) can take place when viewed from the perspective of functional anatomy. It was assumed that the greatest strain in this type of movement occurred during the braking and/or rotation motions when the foot is fixed relative to the floor. These types of movements result in extreme supination of the foot. In the first case, the foot lands on either the heel or the forefoot, with the foot placed perpendicular to the direction of motion. This requires motion of the subtalar joint and the ankle joint and exposes the muscles and lateral ligaments to considerable strain. In another case, the foot lands on the lateral edge at the level of the ball of the foot with the tibia internally rotated. These researchers also presented a case, called the forward lunge, in which the foot is positioned in the direction of motion with the axis of the foot and of the knee perpendicular to the direction of motion. The thigh-leg-foot can act to decelerate the total body at the knee or the ankle and thus prevent a lateral strain on the foot. It was noted in this paper that these three braking movements can occur in a variety of combinations.

Lateral Movement Kinematics

In fast lateral movements, the initial point of foot contact is on the medial portion of the forefoot. This is followed by a rapid supination action of the forefoot and a lowering of the heel to the ground. Stacoff et al[21] reported that maximum supination in a lateral movement occurred within the first 50 ± 20 ms after touchdown. They suggested that this time span is of the same magnitude as that reported for pronation in running. In another study on lateral movements, Sussman[25] reported foot contact angles of 12 to 13 degrees of supination with maximum supination angles of 17 to 25 degrees depending upon shoe type. Less supination was assumed to indicate increased lateral stability, while greater supination was thought to represent decreased lateral stability. In this study, however, the time to maximum supination was considerably longer than in the previous study, possibly due to the difference in locomotor speed.

Landings from Jumps
Footfall Patterns

When landing from a jump, the foot-ankle complex is the first point in the kinematic chain where the force incurred from the jump can be attenuated. The actions of plantarflexion/dorsiflexion and, to a lesser extent, pronation accomplish this task. In an investigation on landings from jumps of basketball players, Valiant and Cavanagh[27] identified two distinct types of landings. The majority of the subjects (80%) in this study were in a greatly plantarflexed position at the instant of foot contact and therefore made initial contact with the forefoot. Upon initial contact, the heel of the foot was lowered to contact the surface. The remaining subjects landed in a fairly flatfooted position. These results were verified in a later study conducted by Sussman et al[26] in which only 9 of 160 trials were of the flatfooted type.

Landing Kinematics

In landing from a jump, the lower extremity structures and most importantly the foot must act to decrease the downward velocity of the center of mass, thus attenuating the impact force. Since the foot is the initial point of impact, the foot must be placed in a position to attenuate the shock. The foot, therefore, is generally in a plantarflexed position prior to impact. At impact, shock attenuation is accomplished by dorsiflexing at the ankle and pronating the foot. The angular velocity of dorsiflexion has been reported to increase with increased distance from which the individual falls, with values ranging from 578 degrees/sec to 1025 degrees/sec from heights of 20 cm and 60 cm respectively.[1]

Few studies have reported values for foot orientation in the frontal plane during landings. Sussman[25] reported values ranging from 12.1 to 24.2 degrees of supination at touchdown depending upon the type of prophylactic ankle taping. At maxmimum pronation, the pronation values ranged from 3.2 to 3.5 degrees, with maximum pronation occurring about 200 ms after impact.

Kinetics of the Foot

Kinetics is the measurement and analysis of factors that cause motion. In reference to the human body these factors include internal forces such as muscle forces, friction between internal structures, and elastic energy from ligaments, tendons, and connective tissue. External forces such as gravity, ground reaction forces (GRFs), and external friction must also be included in a complete kinetic analysis.

Running
Ground Reaction Forces

GRFs are exerted by the supporting surface on the body. Newton's third law states that these forces are equal in magnitude but opposite in direction to the forces that the body exerts on the supporting surface. These forces are a reflection of the acceleration of the center of mass of the body. GRFs are generally measured with a force platform that resolves the forces into three orthogonal components: vertical, anteroposterior, and mediolateral. In addition to the forces, the force platform measures moments of force about the three primary axes. From this information it is possible to calculate the point of force application, which is commonly referred to as the center of pressure (COP).

Much research has been directed at establishing norms for GRFs and identifying the influential variables. Vertical GRF patterns have been given the most attention because of their relatively higher magnitudes in running. During running, peak vertical force values range from 1.5 to 3.0 times body weight (BW), while mediolateral forces range from 0.1 to 0.2 BW, and anteroposterior forces range from 0.35 to 0.75 BW. Vertical running GRF curves portray a bimodal pattern when the typical HT or THT footfall style is used (Fig. 2-10). The initial high-frequency "passive" peak is the result of the heel striking the ground. The peak is termed passive because it is the result of the foot colliding with the ground. The lower frequency "active" peak is thought to be under muscular control and indicates pushoff. The less common midfoot strikers who contact the ground with the middle lateral portion of the foot produce a single peak in their vertical GRF curves and typically have greater mediolateral GRFs.[3]

It has been suggested that the magnitude of the impact peak or the rate of loading may be linked to running injuries. Force platform studies have revealed that this impact peak increases with the velocity of the runner, while the active peak is not affected.[8] The time to peak impact does not change with increasing velocity. This results in an increased loading rate, which may create symptoms that do not appear at lower velocities.

COP information calculated from force platform output contains limited information about the forces experienced by the foot structures. The COP is the point of application of the resultant GRF. If half of the force is distributed in the forefoot region and half in the heel region, the COP will be in the midfoot region. In this example there is no pressure where the COP is located. The COP has been used to differentiate between footfall types (Fig. 2-11). In individuals who run with an HT footfall pattern, the COP moves rapidly toward the midline of the shoe for the first 18% to 20% of stance. At approximately 22% to 24% of stance, the COP progresses anteriorly to 50% of the shoe length. The COP then remains within 50% to 80% of the shoe length from the heel until the end of the support phase. For those with a THT footfall pattern, the first contact is made at approximately 50% of the shoe length. The COP then moves anteriorly briefly and then posteriorly and toward the midline of the shoe. The most posterior migration of the COP occurs at about 10% to 14% of stance. The COP then progresses anteriorly for the rest of the stance period.

It is possible, however, to directly measure the pressures (force per unit area) under the foot. Pressure-sensitive sensors that measure the distribution of forces over the entire foot surface have been used to identify the anatomical locations that experience the greatest pressures. When these sensors are inserted into the shoe, they have the advantage over GRFs of directly measuring the forces the body experiences rather than the forces at the shoe/ground interface. Peak pressures during running are generally seen in the heel region, with additional high pressures mainly on the hallux and to a lesser extent on the metatarsals (Fig. 2-12). Approximately 50% of the load under the foot is on the heel region, and 50% is transmitted across the metatarsal heads during the stance phase of gait. In-shoe pressure systems have been used clinically to diagnose abnormal foot function. Any alteration in foot structure that disrupts the distribution of the load under the foot can cause serious injury to the runner. For example, a flexible flat-arched foot tends to distribute the forces into the midfoot area, and a rigid high-arched foot concentrates the forces in the heel and forefoot regions. Pressure sensors provide an ideal means to identify high pressure areas as well as test the success of a treatment.

Moments of Force

Joint moments of force and the joint reaction forces are the net result of all internal and external forces that act to alter the joint position. Calculating joint moments and forces involves a

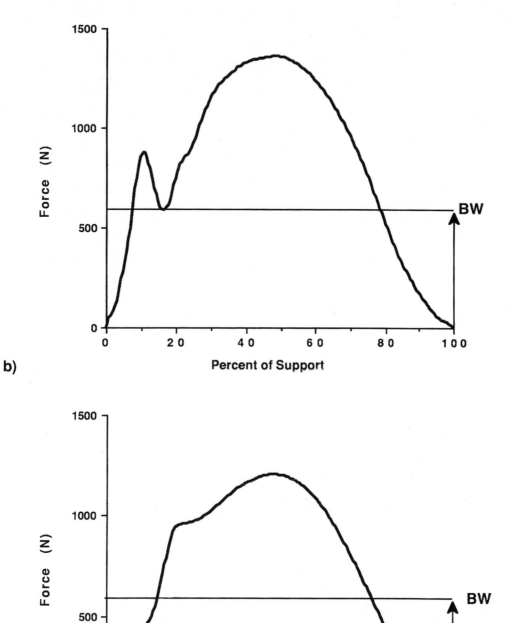

2-10 Graphic representations of the vertical ground reaction force component during a running footfall. Heel-toe footfall pattern. **B,** Midfoot contact footfall pattern.

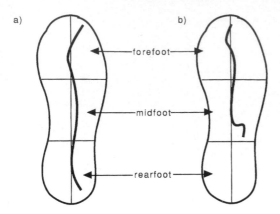

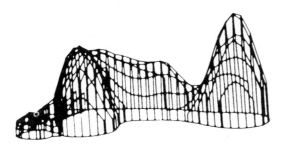

Fig. 2-11 Center of pressure paths during running. **A,** Heel-toe footfall pattern. **B,** Midfoot contact footfall pattern.

Fig. 2-12 Peak plantar pressure patterns in a "normal" foot during running. (From Cavanagh PR: The biomechanics of running and running shoe problems. In Segressor B and Pforringer W, editors: The shoe in sport, Chicago, 1989, Year Book Medical Publishers; with permission.)

process of inverse dynamics in which the moments of force are determined from the combination of kinematic, kinetic, and anthropometric data. The anthropometric data required for these calculations consist of the mass, length, center of mass, and moment of inertia of each relevant body segment. The ankle joint moment during running activities is predominantly plantarflexion, with peak values of approximately 3 Nm/kg occurring at 50% to 75% of stance (Fig. 2-13). This peak value increases with the velocity of running. The moment is initially eccentric as the ankle musculature stops the downward acceleration of the body and then turns concentric during propulsion. Sometimes there is a

small inconsistent dorsiflexion moment at the beginning of stance that may serve to control the foot or to help rotate the shank over the foot. Ankle joint reaction forces have been reported to be 8.97 and 4.15 times BW for the compressive and shear components respectively.[11]

Fewer attempts have been made to determine the joint moments or reaction forces at any foot joints other than the ankle joint. Procter and Paul[18] considered the moments and reaction forces at the ankle and the talocalcaneonavicular joints. They reported peak residual moments of force of 40 nm at the talocalcaneonavicular joint and peak forces of 3.88 and 2.43 BW at the ankle and talocalcaneonavicular joints respectively.

Lateral Movements

Whenever the ground is used to change the direction of motion or velocity of the body, the GRF will increase. Lateral movements, pivoting, starting, stopping, and running along a curved path increase vertical and shear reaction forces and may cause asymmetric loading of the lower extremity. During straight-line running, the vertical GRF is responsible for most of the external load placed on the body, but when anteroposterior or mediolateral velocity changes occur, the shear forces should also be assessed. Hamill et al[9] found that the outside foot of a runner performing a track turn experiences a higher impact peak than the inside foot. Also, the mediolateral force value of the inside foot was found to be greater than that of the outside foot. The authors suggested that these stressors would be greater if the radius of the turn was smaller.

Landing from a Jump

When assessing injury potential by measuring the forces acting on the body, the magnitude of the force is not the only factor to consider. As an example, consider a basketball player who has jumped into the air for a rebound. The amount of force that will be required to stop the downward progression of the body mass is determined by the height of the center of mass. This total amount of force cannot be altered during the airborne phase of the jump, but the effects of the force can be modified in three ways. First, the force can be distributed over a larger area. This

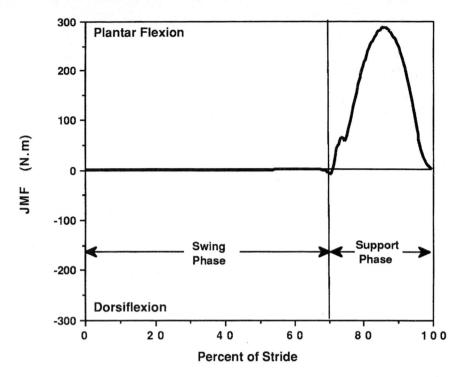

Fig. 2-13 Graphic representation of a sagittal plane ankle moment of force during a running stride. Note that the moment of force is almost zero during the swing or nonsupport phase.

decreases the pressure underneath the foot and decreases the injury potential. The basketball player may accomplish this reduction in pressure by landing on both feet instead of just one. Secondly, the force required to stop the body mass can be applied over a greater period of time. This will decrease the rate of loading as well as the maximum force. Lastly, a basketball player who lands with improper kinematics may be more susceptible to injury even if the forces are not excessive. For instance, too much supination at contact could result in a sprained ankle even though the force of landing may be moderate.

Ground Reaction Force

Foot contacts that occur during a landing from a jump also produce a bimodal vertical GRF pattern. However, the impact portion of the curve results from contact on the forefoot region of the foot rather than the heel, as it would in certain running footfalls (Fig. 2-14). Panzer et al[17] measured the vertical GRF during the landing phase of a double back somersault and found average values of 9.33 BW and 10.55 BW for the first peak and second peak respectively. Although the number of repetitive landings is much reduced compared to the thousands of footfalls experienced during a running session, the magnitude of these forces indicates the potential for injury.

Valiant and Cavanagh[27] reported that some basketball players will land flat-footed rather than in the typical toe-heel pattern. Individuals who used the flat-footed technique landed with peak vertical forces of 6.0 BW compared to 4.1 BW for the toe-heel landers. Peak pressures were also greater in the flat-footed group, with average values of 1.55 MPa as opposed to 0.77 MPa for the toe-heel group. The peak values for both groups occurred in the heel region. Even though the toe-heel strategy appears to have the advantage of lesser peak vertical forces, it has not been shown that a person with a natural flat-footed landing style will reduce peak vertical forces by changing this landing strategy. Caution should

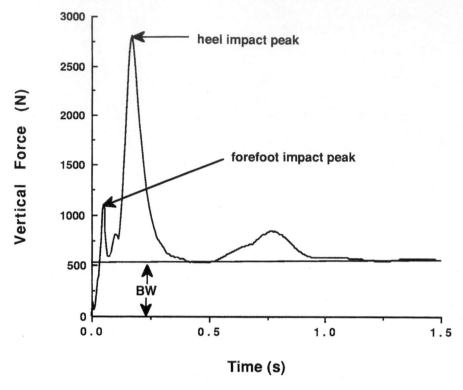

Fig. 2-14   Graphic representation of a vertical ground reaction force component during a landing from a jump. Initial foot contact is on the forefoot.

be emphasized whenever the natural strategy of the individual is modified since it is thought that individuals tend to choose a strategy optimal for themselves.

Another landing technique that has been shown to modify vertical GRFs is the control over joint stiffness. Joint stiffness is controlled by the amount of joint flexion and the amount of muscular contraction that opposes joint flexion during contact. A very stiff joint will show very little flexion at contact and will produce larger vertical GRFs than a less stiff landing.

Moments of Force

Ankle moments during landings tend to plantarflex the ankle joint. Typical peak values when the landing is followed by a counter-jump range from 3.5 to 7.5 Nm/kg and occur at the start of pushoff. In landings on surfaces of different stiffnesses, the ankle joint moments ranged from 209 to 251 Nm on soft and hard surfaces respectively.[7] These values depend on the amount of time given to reverse the downward path of the center of gravity. The longer the period of time, the smaller the value of the peak moment.

Variations in Foot–Ankle Function

In this chapter, normal foot-ankle function has been discussed for movements of this structure during running, lateral movements, and landings from a jump. If we consider the performer and the movement environment as a system, there are four sources of variation that could lead to an alteration in foot function: (1) the foot structure, (2) the performance of the activity, (3) the footwear, and (4) the activity surface.

Anatomy and Physiology

Variation in Foot Structure

While "normal" foot function has been described in this chapter, there are many variations in foot structure that can influence the various functions of the foot-ankle complex. One structural problem, for example, arch height, is thought to be associated with discrepancies in foot function. Subotnick[24] associated the flat arch (pes planus) with a highly flexible and thus a hyperpronated foot. In the "normal" foot the subtalar joint axis is 42 to 45 degrees, whereas in the low-arched foot the axis is closer to horizontal. Thus for any given internal rotation of the tibia, there is greater internal rotation of the foot, resulting in more pronation. The high-arched foot, pes cavus, has been associated with a rigid foot that does not adapt well to the surface, resulting in shock-absorbing types of injuries. In the high-arched foot, the subtalar joint axis is more vertical, being greater than 45 degrees. The resulting effect is that for any given internal rotation of the tibia, there is less internal rotation of the foot, creating less pronation. Many research studies have been conducted to substantiate these effects, but as yet no definitive results have emerged.

Other abnormal foot structures that misalign the hindfoot and forefoot also result in biomechanical problems. These variations in foot structure are discussed further in the next chapter.

Variation in Performance of the Activity

Of the sources of variation that can alter foot function, change in performance is probably the least influential. Williams and Ziff[28] manipulated step length, step width, and shoulder rotation to evaluate the effects on hindfoot motion. Although step width reduced the amount of pronation, the authors suggest that runners attempt to maintain some aspects of running mechanics despite major alterations to other elements of running style. For example, it has been suggested that runners not usually alter their footfall pattern.[14,20] In fact many of the actions of the foot-ankle could be considered passive movements in that they do not come under muscular control. Hamill et al[10] reported that subtalar joint pronation did not change as a function of a 15-minute run at a speed corresponding to 90% of maximum oxygen uptake, indicating that pronation may not be under muscular control.

Variation in Footwear

It has been widely demonstrated in the biomechanics literature that foot function can be influenced by the footwear worn by the performer. In running, changes in foot actions, particularly subtalar joint movement, as a function of shoe structure have been demonstrated by many researchers.[2,10,15,16,22] Many design variables of shoes interact to produce kinetic and kinematic adaptations of the foot during athletics. Although the interactions are complex, several specific effects are attributed to shoe design characteristics. These characteristics include midsole density, heel flare, and stability devices.

The density of the midsole can influence the degree of hindfoot pronation (Fig. 2-15). For example, a soft shoe designed for maximum cushioning may deform on the medial side when loaded, resulting in increased hindfoot motion. A hard midsole deforms less than a softer one upon impact. However, initial ground contact in a hard midsole shoe is more lateral than in a soft midsole shoe, creating a longer moment arm with respect to the subtalar joint axis. The leverage effect increases hindfoot angular displacement.[15,22] Multidensity midsoles, with a softer material on the lateral side and a firmer material on the medial side, have been used to control hindfoot motion.

Heel flare on the lateral and medial sides of a shoe has decidedly significant effects on foot function. Increasing the flare on the lateral side increases the moment arm about the subtalar joint axis. Studies have reported that pronation decreased as lateral heel flare decreased.[16] On the other hand, medial flare can reduce the degree of hindfoot pronation by improving medial support.[5]

Stability devices in shoes have been used to reduce hindfoot pronation. Devices such as a stiff heel counter, rigid arch supports, orthotic inserts, and upper stiffeners have been used to increase hindfoot stability in sports shoes. Reports on the use of these devices are mixed, but some research studies and clinics have verified their effectiveness. Robinson and associates[19] reported signifi-

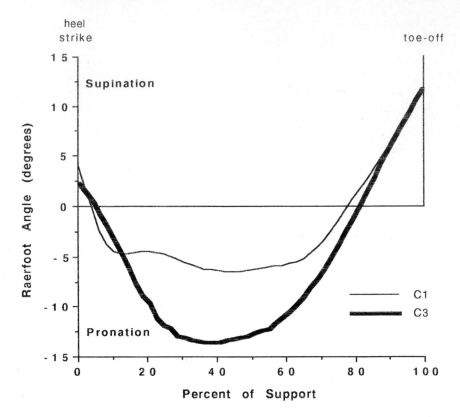

Fig. 2-15 Graphic representation of frontal plane hindfoot angles of the same individual running in shoes with different midsole densities (C1 = hard midsole, C3 = soft midsole).

cant reduction in range of motion of the ankle and subtalar joints and decreased performance in a movement task as the ankle was restricted by stiffeners placed in the upper of a basketball shoe. However, there are so many different devices, all reporting success, that it is difficult to determine exactly why these devices work.

Variation in Activity Surface

A number of characteristics of activity surfaces can influence the function of the foot as it contacts the ground. In describing foot function, we presume that athletes function on level terrain or that the surface is of a constant texture or hardness. This is not necessarily true, especially in activities such as road running. Variations of the activity surface can have a profound effect on foot function. For example, if runners do not take into consideration the camber of a road during a run, their foot function will change as a result of the camber. While running on the right-hand side of the road, the runner will tend to pronate more than usual on the left or uphill foot and less than usual on the right or downhill foot. A similar effect results for runners who continually run in the same direction around a track.

The other critical factor that can alter foot function is the frictional characteristics of the surface. These characteristics are dependent on the material and the properties of the contacting surfaces. Depending on the type and objective of the movement, different friction characteristics are required. For example, any movement that requires a sudden fixation of the foot, such as the takeoff in jumping, should have a relatively high static coefficient of friction. If the frictional characteristics are not sufficient for the activity, foot action during movements may change, and injury may result.

Summary

In this chapter, the biomechanics of the foot and ankle were presented. The foot-ankle structure is a complex biomechanical unit. The foot acts as the interface between the rest of the body and the ground. It has the general functions of balance, support, and propulsion. There are three structural regions of the foot, referred to as the hindfoot, the midfoot, and the forefoot. A number of joints are associated with each of the regions in the foot and give the foot the ability to perform its varied functions. The joints act in concert to make the foot either a flexible adapter to the activity surface or a rigid structure for propulsion. The muscles of the foot determine the actions at these joints. The foot structure results in both longitudinal and transverse arches, which are critical in shock attenuation during impact with the ground.

In athletics, a number of footfall patterns are required depending on the activity. These range from a straight-ahead locomotor footfall, as in running, to lateral movements and landings from jumps, as in basketball. This chapter reviewed the biomechanics of the foot actions in these patterns from both a kinematic and kinetic perspective. Finally, viewing the performer and the environment as a system, there are several variations in the system that may result in alterations in foot function. These include variations in anatomy, performance of the activity, footwear, and playing surface.

References

1. Bobbert MF, Huijing PA, and van Ingen Schenau G: Drop jumping II: the influence of dropping height on the biomechanics of drop jumping, *Med Sci Sports Exerc* 19:339, 1987.
2. Cavanagh PR: The running shoe book, Mountain View, Calif, 1980, Anderson World.
3. Cavanagh PR and Lafortune MA: Ground reaction forces in distance running, *J Biomechanics* 13:397, 1980.
4. Cavanagh PR: The biomechanics of running and running shoe problems. In Segesser B and Pforringer W, editors: The shoe in sport, Chicago, 1989, Year Book Medical Publishers.
5. Clarke TE, Frederick EC, and Hamill C: The study of rearfoot movement in running. In Sports shoes and playing surfaces, Frederick EC, editor: Champaign, Ill, 1984, Human Kinetics.
6. Edington CJ, Frederick EC, and Cavanagh PR: Rearfoot motion in distance running. In Cavanagh PR, editor: Biomechanics of distance running, Champaign, Ill, 1990, Human Kinetics.
7. Fukuda H: Biomechanical analysis of landing on surfaces with different stiffnesses. In DeGroot G et al, editors: Biomechanics VII-B, Amsterdam, 1988, Free University Press.
8. Hamill J et al: Variations in ground reaction force parameters at different running speeds, *Hum Movement Sci* No. 2, 47-56, 1983.
9. Hamill J, Murphy MV, and Sussman DH: The effects of track turns on lower extremity function, *Int J Sport Biomech* 3:276, 1987.
10. Hamill J et al: Effects of shoe type and cardiorespiratory responses and rearfoot motion during treadmill running, *Med Sci Sports Exerc* 20:515, 1988.
11. Harrison RN et al: Bioengineering analysis of muscle and joint forces acting in the human leg during running. In Jonsson B, editor: Biomechanics X-B, Champaign, Ill, 1987, Human Kinetics.
12. Inman VT: The joints of the ankle, Baltimore, 1976, Williams & Wilkins.
13. Luethi SM and Stacoff A: The influence of the shoe on foot mechanics in running. In van Gheluwe B and Atha J, editors: Current research in sports biomechanics, Basel, 1987, Karger.
14. Mason BR: A kinematic and kinetic analysis of selected parameters during the support phase of running, doctoral dissertation, Eugene, 1980, University of Oregon.
15. Nigg BM and Morlock M: The influence of lateral heel flare of running shoes on pronation and impact forces, *Med Sci Sports Exerc* 19:294, 1987.
16. Nigg BM et al: The influence of running velocity and midsole hardness on external impact forces in heel-toe running, *J Biomechanics* 20:951, 1987.
17. Panzer V et al: Lower extremity loads in landings of elite gymnasts. In DeGroot G et al, editors: Biomechanics VII-B, Amsterdam, 1988, Free University Press.
18. Procter P and Paul JP: Ankle joint biomechanics, *J Biomechanics,* 15:627, 1982.
19. Robinson JR, Frederick EC, and Cooper LB: Systematic ankle stabilization and the effect on performance, *Med Sci Sports Exerc* 18:625, 1986.
19a. Sammarco GJ, Burnstein AH, Frankel VH: Biomechanics of the ankle: A kinetic study. *Clin North Am* 1(4): 75-96, 1973.
19b. Sammarco GJ: Biomechanics of the foot. In Basic Biomechanics of the Musculoskeletal System 2 ed. In: Nordin M and Frankel VH, eds. Lea and Febiger, Philadelphia, 1989, p 163-207.
20. Slavin MM and Hamill J: Alteration of foot strike pattern in distance running. In Tant CL, Patterson PE, York SL, editors: Biomechanics in Sports IX, Ames, 1991, Iowa State University Press.
21. Stacoff A, Stussi E, and Sonderegger D: Lateral stability

of sport shoes. In Winter DA et al, editors: Biomechanics IX-B, Champaign, Ill, 1985, Human Kinetics.

22. Stacoff A et al: Running injuries and shoe construction: some possible relationships, *Int J Sports Biomech* 4:342, 1988.

23. Stuessi A, Stacoff A, and Tiegermann V: Rapid sideward movements in tennis. In Segesser B and Pforringer W, editors: The shoe in sport, St. Louis, 1989, Mosby–Year Book.

24. Subotnick SI: The flat foot, *Physician Sports Med* 9:85, 1981.

25. Sussman DH: The effect of high and low cut basketball shoes on subtalar joint pronation and supination, doctoral dissertation, Carbondale, 1987, Southern Illinois University.

26. Sussman DH, Hamill J, and Miller MK: Effect of shoe height and prophylactic taping on ankle joint motion during simulated basketball rebounding. In DeGroot G et al, editors: Biomechanics XI-B, Amsterdam, 1988, Free University Press.

27. Valiant GA and Cavanagh PR: A study of landing from a jump: implications for the design of a basketball shoe. In Winter DA et al, editors: Biomechanics IX-B, Champaign, Ill, 1985, Human Kinetics.

28. Williams KR and Ziff JL: Changes in distance running mechanics due to systematic variations in running style, Int J Sport Biomech 7:76-89,

3

Foot and Ankle Function in Sports

Carol C. Frey

The function of the foot and ankle in sports is a dynamic one that is extremely important to athletic performance. As the speed and intensity of the sport increase, not only is the speed of foot and ankle mechanisms increased but also the magnitude of the force involved. This chapter covers important aspects of foot and ankle function that are necessary for the performance of specific sports.

Running

Running is a repetitive motion that involves the entire body and a sequence of support and airborne phases. The support phase includes heel strike, midstance, and toe-off. The airborne phase includes follow-through, forward-swing, and foot descent. Runners' feet make contact with the ground approximately 5000 times per mile, over 50 to 70 times per minute for each foot, creating a force of two to three times the body weight.[13] The impact is absorbed by the running shoe and transmitted up the body. Minor anatomic or biomechanical abnormalities that are of little significance in walking can lead to injury while running.

The long-distance runner usually lands heel-toe or flat-footed. In the elite runner, the ball of the foot and the heel can touch the ground simultaneously. However, most joggers and sports runners land on the lateral aspects of the heel. For these runners, the heel-toe gait provides more shock absorption than a flat-footed gait (Fig. 3-1).

Pronation and supination are complex motions that involve the subtalar joint as well as other structures in the lower extremity. Pronation unlocks the foot, allowing adaptation to various terrains and shock absorption during running. Supination locks the foot, allowing stabilization of the foot at heel strike and toe-off. Approaching heel strike, the foot is supinated and the tibia is externally rotated. After heel strike, the foot pronates for 55% to 60% of the support phase. The subtalar joint then supinates before toe-off and stays in this position throughout the airborne phase. During pronation, the tibia rotates internally on the talus proportional to the amount of pronation.

The quadriceps angle (Q angle) is the angle formed by the line of the pull through the quadriceps muscle and the line of the patellar tendon where they intersect at the center of the patella. The angle changes with pronation and supination. At heel strike, the tibia is externally rotated and the patellar tendon angulates laterally. When

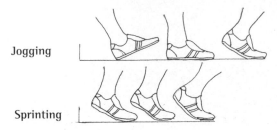

Jogging

Sprinting

Fig. 3-1 A long-distance runner usually lands heel-toe or flat-footed. The ball of the foot and the heel may touch the ground simultaneously in the elite runner. Most joggers, however, land on the lateral aspects of the heel. For most sprinters, landing and propulsion are carried out on the ball and middle part of the foot.

offered from friction between the shoe and the ground. Increased friction may be great enough to prevent most of the abduction, but the running athlete will nonetheless have the tendency to rotate the upper part of the shoe in relation to the sole.[8]

Anatomically, the structure of the foot shows a range from pes cavus to pes planus. Functionally, this can be described as the foot going from rigid to hypermobile. Pressure distribution is also affected by anatomic variation. With pes cavus, high pressure is typically seen at the heel and little at the midfoot. In contrast, the normal foot and pes planus show high values at the midfoot and forefoot. In general, the pes cavus foot is rigid and does not absorb shock well, while the pes planus foot can adapt its structure and absorb shock. Because of these differences, these two types of feet have different shoe requirements.[3]

the foot pronates, the Q angle indicates the amount of internal tibial rotation.

If pronation is prolonged or exaggerated, the ankle sags medially, with an increase in internal tibial rotation that places increased strain on the knee and the foot. Excessive pronation also makes it more difficult for the foot to return to the more stable supinated position for toe-off. Hyperpronation may be a compensatory mechanism for tibia vara, tight Achilles tendon, tight gastrocnemius and soleus muscles, or hindfoot and forefoot varus.

Some runners toe in or toe out, which can affect the amount of pronation and internal tibial rotation. The amount of foot rotation at midstance is determined primarily by the amount of external or internal rotation at the hips, the amount of torsion in the hips, and femoral neck anteversion.

The typical motion sequence in running begins with contact between the ground and the lateral edge of the shoe followed by pronation at the subtalar joint, bringing the plantar surface of the shoe in further contact with the ground.

A small amount of abduction of the foot can be seen just before the foot is lifted off the ground, depending on the amount of resistance

Sprinting

Little body weight is placed on the heel in sprinting. For most track runners, even those who run the longer distances, landing and propulsion are carried out on the ball and middle part of the foot. For this reason, track shoes used in the faster and shorter races have just enough padding at the heel to prevent a contusion.

Tennis

Tennis requires body control with quick side-to-side movement, sprinting, jumping, and stretching (Fig. 3-2). Running heel-to-toe is a frequent movement in tennis. Landing on the forefoot is very common in good players. Lateral movements are important, and supination is required during lateral movement and changes in direction. The body must be moved with control in all directions. The sport is played on lawn, clay, asphalt, synthetic, and rubberized courts. The selection of an appropriate shoe must be

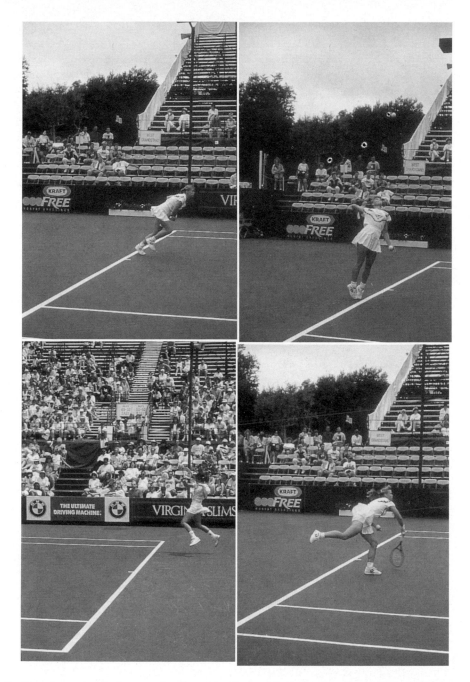

Fig. 3-2 Tennis requires body control with quick side-to-side movement. **A,** Sprinting. **B,** Toe dragging. **C,** Jumping. **D,** Stretching. In the elite player, running and sideslipping are seen more frequently.

made for each surface; however, not all surfaces react equally to the shoes.

The function of the foot and ankle in tennis includes a variety of movements that are not cyclical as in running. The difference between the motions of an average player and an elite level player is that walking is the primary motion in the average player, followed by forward running and sideslipping. In the elite player, running and sideslipping are seen more frequently. The playing surface seems to have little effect on the frequency of specific movements among average players and those at an elite level, the only exception being sliding, which occurs only on clay surfaces.[21]

In Nigg's study, the average recreational player most frequently made ground contact on the heel of the foot, contact on the ball of the foot occurring 50% less often. In contrast, the elite level player made more frequent contact on the ball of the foot. It was also noted that contact with the inner or outer edge of the shoe occurred frequently in both players. The direction of movement of the average player is usually forward, occurring in more than 60% of all plays. The elite player showed more lateral movements compared to the average player. With baseline play and the volley, lateral and forward movements occurred with equal frequency. Lateral movements frequently require landing on the forefoot.

The greatest strains in tennis seem to be generated with braking and/or rotatory motions while the foot is planted on the ground. If the strain is great enough in this situation, the foot and ankle can undergo considerable structural distortion.

Manufacturers of tennis shoes recommend more cushioning in the ball of the foot for the serve-and-volley player. For the baseline player, a solid heel counter, strong reinforcement in the heel and midfoot area, and good rear foot stability are recommended.

Basketball

Basketball requires backward, forward, and vertical accelerations, quick stops, and side-to-side movements. The playing surface is usually wood but may be synthetic or rubberized material. The predominant motion in basketball is running. The sport requires lateral, backward, forward, rotational, and jumping movements. The playing surface properties can compound these demands significantly. With indoor courts, there is a relatively firm resistance to rotatory and lateral momentum, which can lead to consider-

able stress on the ankle and subtalar joint (Fig. 3-3).

Jumping is possible only if there is good mobility of the ankle and the subtalar joints. The landing forces are captured, for the most part, by the previously contracted muscles. Well-conditioned ligaments and muscles contribute to a stable, safe landing.

The landing from a jump can be either on the forefoot or with the foot in a less typical horizontal position. Landing in the horizontal position can generate forces up to six times the body weight.[26]

Landing on the forefoot is more frequent, with the foot eventually being levered into dorsiflexion and pronation. After about 50 ms the heel makes contact with the ground, and the calf muscles have enough time to act as antagonists to this motion. The forces generated with this landing are 3.5 to 4.3 times the body weight.[18,26]

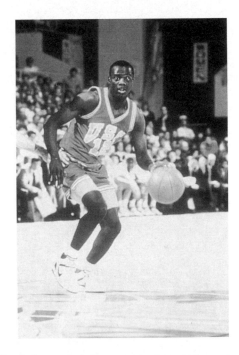

Fig. 3-3 Basketball requires backward, forward, and vertical accelerations, quick stops, and side-to-side movements. With indoor basketball courts, there is a relatively firm resistance to rotatory and lateral momentum, which can lead to considerable stress on the ankle and subtalar joint.

Anatomy and Physiology

A forefoot landing occurs with internal rotation of the tibia and adduction of the foot. Loose lateral ligaments, fatigue, or muscular imbalance can increase supination and the risk of injury. During a landing, it is not uncommon to land on the foot of another player. If the impact occurs on the medial side of the sole of the landing player, there is rapid supination and considerable load placed on the lateral collateral ligaments of the ankle.

Friction is an important force in lateral movements. Elite players often prefer greater friction between the shoe and the playing surface, which provides more grip and permits rapid braking and takeoff.

Ankle sprains are the most common, traumatic injury at all levels of play in basketball.[1,7,28] Ankle sprains most often occur with a cutting or turning maneuver when the player is pushing off with the foot in plantarflexion and inversion.[12]

The ankle can also be everted and externally rotated. This occurs when a planted leg receives a blow from the lateral side or when a player is coming down and lands on another player's foot.

The emphasis of recent design research in basketball shoes has been on the reduction of inversion injuries to the ankle. Studies have shown that shoes with increasing amounts of ankle restriction in the upper significantly reduce ankle joint inversion. However, it was also shown that with increasing amounts of ankle restriction,[24] movements were restricted not only in the sagittal plane but also the frontal plane, which leads to reduced agility. Therefore, a design compromise must be made between performance and protection of the athlete from injury.

Soccer

Field sports combine many types of movement and a variable degree of body contact. Running is basic to all field sports. Soccer involves mainly running, kicking, jumping, sliding, stretching, and multidirectional movements. The playing surfaces are natural grass and artificial turf. Soccer is played almost entirely by the feet, with the ball being kicked off the medial, lateral, and dorsal aspects of the foot. With soccer-style kicking, the nonkicking foot is planted even with or just behind the ball. The kicking leg is raised in back and swung in an arc, pivoting through the hip. Extension at the knee and a stiff foot position are present at the moment of ball contact so that the dorsal, medial, or lateral aspect of the foot can make the contact. The foot is in the direct line of the ball, and the body's center of gravity moves from backward to forward in position with the follow-through.

When evaluating foot and ankle function in this sport, the ball, shoe, and playing surface must be considered together. The ball can reach velocities of 120 to 140 km/hr, with the generation of collision energy of 250 to 300 kPa. If the ball is wet, collision energy may come close to 600 kPa.[14] Considerable distortion of the ball and the foot can occur at impact, which can lead to repetitive microtrauma to the foot. When spikes are solidly anchored to the playing surface, large forces can be generated. These contact forces are often combined with rotation and flexion.

Football

Football requires a maximal amount of motion: running, jumping, walking, throwing, kicking, and stance. The sport requires muscular strength, balance, endurance, speed, agility, coordination, alertness, timing, rhythm, reaction time, motivation, flexibility, steadiness, accuracy, and discipline.

Running is the primary motion in football, along with quick lateral movements and the production of great forces secondary to blocking and hitting. In football, even running requires adjustments such as jogging, sprinting, right-angle pivots, outside-inside cuts, reverse or cross-over steps, stop and go, diagonal circles backward, lateral zigzag steps, run to jump, and jump to run. The unpredictable forces of contact and collision can be added to these movements. Studies have shown that injuries may be caused by wearing fewer, longer cleats, which produce excessive pressure beneath the cleats from increased foot fixation.[25] More specifically, it is the excessive resistance to rotation that causes knee injuries during the twisting motions of football. As a result of these studies it has been determined that the maximum diameter of a cleat tip should be $\frac{7}{16}$ inch with a maximum overall length of $\frac{1}{2}$ inch. A 7-stud pattern is preferred on natural grass.

Skating

Skating mechanics are similar for all skating events, although footwear and blades are specialized. Ankle movement and support are essential to skating performance. However, the subtalar joint must be free to allow positioning of the blade on the ice.

Figure Skating

Figure skating requires the athlete to jump, skate, balance, spin, dance, and lift. The performing surface is the ice on artificial and natural rinks. A snug-fitting, high-cut boot is used to stabilize the ankle and subtalar joints in order to prevent excessive transverse or frontal movements below the ankle. Movement of the foot, which largely maintains a pronated position, is required during pushoff.

Strong lever action is exerted on the boot by the blade. The lever force depends on the distance between the boot and the ice. The boot should offer some protection to the ankle against supination and pronation but should not have as much effect on dorsiflexion and plantar flexion. The loads placed on the foot and ankle can vary with solo and pair skating, ice dancing, and compulsory exercises. Boot design is specific for each activity.

Pressure points commonly develop from skating boots, which can affect foot function in figure skating. Montag reported that almost 50% of German master-class skaters had required surgery on their medial or lateral malleolus because of pressure sores, inflammatory bursitis, and significant tissue damage of the malleoli due to boot pressure.[15]

A triple jump is an expected technique today, even from junior level skaters. This maneuver can produce large loads not only on the foot and ankle but also on the boot. In the past, these types of loads were expected only from master-class skaters.

Skating maneuvers take place on the inner or outer edge of the blade. The inner edge is being used more aggressively today. If there is a varus or valgus deformity of the foot or ankle, this affects the position of the boot and can determine weight distribution on the edges of the skate. The position of the blade can be shifted slightly anteriorly or posteriorly, medially or laterally, to accommodate for this.

Ice Hockey

Ice hockey requires skating, quick stops, quick turns, and balance on the ice of artificial and natural rinks. Ice hockey demands that the boots be maneuverable and allow rapid starts and stops. The runner of the blade is considerably thinner than that of figure skates. The length of the blade runner in contact with the ice is approximately 8 cm. Skaters who demand maximal maneuverability hone their blades down to a smaller contact area. Overall, this reduces the maximum skating speed, since speed depends on the contact area of the blade. If the edge is too sharp, maneuverability can be lost.

Strong lateral stability should be provided by the boot and by conditioning in order to prevent serious ankle injuries. Elite level skaters depend less on support provided by rigid boot construction, their musculature being better able to play a major role in the maintenance of foot and ankle position. Professional skaters often prefer to have reinforced nylon mesh used in the construction of their top-quality boots, which provides sufficient stability and a form f it.

Speed Skating

Speed skating requires balanced skating with a low center of gravity in the lunge position. Skaters often compete with bare feet in skates. The skating surface is ice on artificial or natural ice tracks.

Alpine Skiing

Alpine skiing requires ankle and knee flexion, forward lean, and balance on snow-covered surfaces. The biomechanics of the foot inside the ski boot are affected by shell construction, shaft height, design of the sole, entry, closure, and design of the inner boot. The edges of the skis must act as extensions of the leg and the foot. The feet are basically anchored to the skis for maximum control accomplished through a rigid ski boot that greatly limits ankle and foot motion. The ankle and the foot are for the most part locked in dorsiflexion with a pronated heel and act as extensions of the upper leg.

The boot is the connecting link between the foot and the binding with its complex safety release mechanism. Extreme rotational momentum on the ankle can be prevented for the most part by the automatic release of the safety bindings during a fall. The high shaft construction of the shell reduces the pronation and supination allowed by the foot and ankle.

During dorsiflexion and plantar flexion, the motion of the shaft should correspond to the motion the ankle and tibia. Appropriate adjustments must be made to ensure that the relative lever lengths of the shaft of the boot correspond to that of the tibia (Fig. 3-4). If the lever-length ratios are unfavorable and the shaft is rigid, the skier is at high risk of shearing the tibia off at the upper edge of the shaft during a fall.

Furthermore, if the axis of ankle joint flexion is not in line with the axis of shaft flexion, an unfavorable lever ratio will result and any advantages of flexibility will be overshadowed. Most boots must be safely locked at a forward angle of no more than 40 to 45 degrees. Dorsiflexion of the ankle must be assured for the entire range necessary in skiing. Boot manufacturers realize that although the shaft and the tibia may be parallel in the upright position, they may not be parallel during forward flexion, a common skiing position. The anterosuperior edge of the shaft can produce pressure or braking points that can cause severe pain and injury. Ideally, the tibia should be parallel to the shaft in all ranges of flexion, and the forces should be distributed equally along the entire shaft. If these criteria are followed, an inner boot can be used to prevent the development of pressure points.

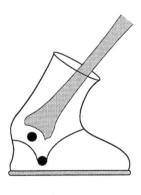

Unfavorable lever relationships

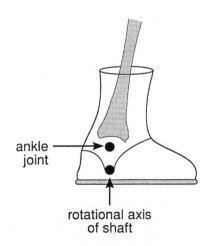

ankle joint

rotational axis of shaft

Favorable lever relationships

Fig. 3-4 During dorsiflexion and plantar flexion, the motion of the shaft of the boot should correspond to the motion of the ankle and the tibia. Appropriate adjustments must be made to ensure that the relative lever lengths of the shaft correspond to that of the tibia.

The appearance of pressure points is often unpredictable due to ongoing change in the areas of contact in the boot. While the original fixed position of the foot is lost once skiing maneuvers begin, levering of the entire foot and its components occur at different times. Depending on the angle of the shaft, continuous changes occur in the spatial and pressure relationships between the foot and the shell. The axis of flexion of the ankle joint may deviate from that of the boot. Traction from the Achilles tendon will cause the calcaneus to displace from the exact heel position in the boot. Even the normal shifting of load from the hindfoot to the forefoot through the arch can be lost through the effects of shell compression.

The relationship of the shell to the foot will vary considerably depending on the boot model and on whether the situation is one of normal skiing or falling.[23] Forward sliding of the foot should not be possible, and the sole of the foot should not lose contact with the boot. The foot should be in the correct position and should not be constrained or squeezed.

Since foot and ankle function may be affected by fit, it is important to keep in mind that there are variations in total foot volume, forefoot volume, and forefoot width. For a more custom fit, orthopedic inserts, polyurethane foam, special inner shoes, and air cushions may be used. The function of the foot and ankle should not be affected by external temperature or moisture, so the boot should be well insulated.

Cross-Country Skiing

Cross-country skiing requires fast walking movements, running, jogging, downhill skiing, and balance on snow-covered terrain. Although the ski edges are used when ascending and descending slopes, the basic motion in cross-country skiing involves a forward movement. Boot and bindings act together as a hinge between the foot and the ski and must be compatible. Good forefoot flexion is essential. The foot together with the boot, binding, and ski makes contact with the ground as it does in walking.

In fact, this sport has more in common with walking and jogging than with alpine skiing.

During cross-country skiing, the muscles of the lower extremity work much as they do in jogging and walking, but the foot has different demands placed on it. The weight-bearing foot maintains pronation, with the heel down to act as a platform. This maintains balance during the glide-through motions. The ski slides, and the foot goes from a supinated to a pronated position. The full body weight is supported by the foot and the ski, and the cycle is repeated. As with walking, one foot maintains contact with the ground while the other goes through a swing cycle. Poles are used for balance and propulsion.

The most common technique in cross-country skiing is the diagonal step, which has a dynamic pushoff and swing phase. Aspects of the diagonal step are incorporated into other cross-country moves, including the two-pole pushoff, the herringbone step, the circling step, and the gliding step. Basically, the skier achieves forward motion by shifting weight from ski to ski. The greatest possible distance should be covered from the resultant glide before another pushoff is necessary.

The cross-country ski boot must help perform required motions by transmitting the necessary forces for every phase of the exercise. Flexibility in the front part of the boot and enough rigidity to provide torsional and lateral stability are important boot requirements. The great forces generated during pushoff cause those parts of the sole extending beyond the surface of the ski to bend downward. Adequate rigidity is also important to prevent displacement of the foot from the ski during maneuvers such as the herringbone step. The greatest sole flexibility must be under the ball of the foot to allow the toes adequate motion during the step. This also helps to maintain the position of the sole firmly on the surface of the ski during pressure phases. A boot that has a stable anchor should help maintain proper orientation of the skis and keep them firmly pressed onto the snow surface.

At the end of the step, the rear end of the ski is usually elevated, with the maximum boot-to-ski angle rarely exceeding 70 degrees. For the skating technique and the herringbone step, smaller angles are required but with increased momentum.

Aerobic Dancing

Aerobic dancing requires stationary running, skipping, jumping, stretching, dancing, and stair climbing. The dance surface is carpet or other covered surfaces. Flexibility in the forefoot is important.

Korzick[9] made measurements of ground reaction forces developed during aerobic dance movements with two distinct styles of landing: forefoot landing followed by rearfoot contact and forefoot landing alone. He concluded that the risk of injury and force peaks generated were reduced when heel contact was emphasized. Heel contact could also reduce the incidence of sore shins in aerobic dancers by reducing the load on muscles that control stability and the rate of dorsiflexion of the hindfoot, such as the tibialis posterior.

Recently there has been a trend toward low-impact aerobic exercises, in which, unlike conventional aerobic exercise, at least one foot is touching the floor at all times. Rather than the ballistic impacts that result from high-impact jumping, the low-impact classes encourage increased range of motion and lateral movements.

Bicycling

Bicycling involves use of the gluteus, quadriceps, hamstrings, and calf muscles to generate the power necessary to perform upward and downward thrusts through the forefoot. The foot is often placed in a valgus or varus position on the pedal, causing pressure to develop on the lateral or medial sides of the foot. Cleat and pedal placements can be changed to prevent this canting. The foot should be clamped onto the pedal, with the forefoot placed at the correct angle and longitudinal position. The foot is usually flat or at a right angle to the shin when the pedal is at the 12 o'clock position. As the foot moves into the 6 o'clock position, the heel is pulled up. The foot assumes a slightly plantarflexed position as it moves into the 9 o'clock position and returns to the 12 o'clock position (Fig. 3-5).

Golf

The principal movement in golf occurs during the swing and involves a lateral move in a frontal plane and a rotational motion along a longitudinal axis. These motions are more pronounced than in most other sports. A relatively minor motion of the sole of the foot is seen in relation to the ground during most of the swing phase, except for the final maneuvers. Interaction between the golf shoes and the ground should allow the golfer to perform these necessary body movements during the swing, which result in contact between the club head and the ball. Golf shoes should make foot and ankle function easier and provide a solid base of support (Fig. 3-6).

Ground reaction forces have been studied for each foot during the golf swing.[2,4] At the precise moment when the head of the club makes contact with the ball, approximately 75% of the maximum vertical force was acting on the leading foot (the foot closest to the green). This ranged from 150% of body weight when a wood was used to 133% of the body weight when a 7 iron was used. The peak vertical forces were created just before contact with the ball when a wood was used but right after the contact when an iron was used. The least vertical force, representing 80% of the body weight, was seen shortly after impact and was thought to be secondary to the force of the club, which pulls the player's body upward. The rotational momentum (in right-handed players) was determined for both feet using a measuring plate and indicated an initial clockwise motion peak during the early phase of the swing. This changed to a contrary, counterclockwise motion just before impact, with a peak reported at the beginning of the second phase of the swing.

Kinematic data show that there may be functional and biomechanical differences in the golf

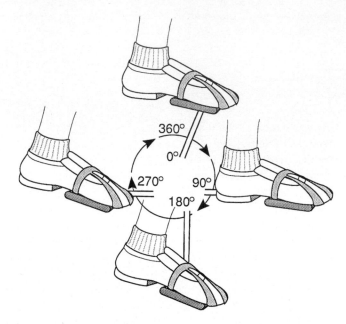

Fig. 3-5 The foot is usually flat or at a right angle to the shin when the pedal is at the 12 o'clock position. As the foot moves into the 6 o'clock position, the heel is pulled up. The foot assumes a slightly plantarflexed position as it moves into the 9 o'clock position and returns to the 12 o'clock position.

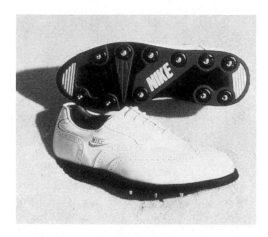

Fig. 3-6 The principal movement in golf occurs during the swing and involves a lateral move in a frontal plane and a rotational motion along a longitudinal axis. Golf shoes should make foot and ankle function easier and provide a solid base of support.

swing when different clubs are used. The greatest club-head velocity is seen with the woods and the lowest with the 7 iron. The velocity of the club head continues to increase at the moment of contact when a wood or 3 iron is used but decreases at the moment of contact when a 7 iron is used.[27]

Williams and Cavanagh[27] felt there was no symmetry in the motion of the two feet and that the motion of the two feet had to be studied independently. With the sport of golf, one cannot overlook the fact that there is a large amount of straight walking covering the distances between strokes. Spikelike projections on the sole improve ground contact and help in the aeration of the greens.

The phase of the swing places very different demands on the right and left golf shoe. The right foot of the golfer must provide for a rocking movement during and at the end the swing. The golfer first rests on the anterolateral edge of the big toe and finally on the tip of the toe. Meanwhile the left foot shows a weight shift from the medial to the lateral edge and a supination through the ankle and the subtalar joints. If carried to the extreme, this motion can terminate with a bending of the foot to almost 90 degrees, coming to rest on the lateral side. All the toes will be pressed up against the toe cap, almost as in a braking maneuver.

Anatomy and Physiology

The function of the toes during a golf swing has been analyzed during a barefoot swing, where there is no shoe upper to oppose the movement of the toes.[27] In this situation the toes assume a clawing or grasping position to gain a toe hold. The motion of the feet inside golf shoes has also been analyzed by motion picture and pressure-sensitive plate studies. The results were studied as graphic displays of the pressure distribution and as mathematical patterns to obtain an absolute pressure value. At the moment of swing, the right shoe has little demand placed on it, although it should be able to rock without much force generated and provide some support with appropriate flexibility in the sole. The demands on the left shoe are much greater. At the time of the swing and just before club-ball contact, the left foot assumes a very insecure stance with a simultaneous shifting of forces from the medial to the lateral edge.

Bibliography

1. Apple DF, O'Toole J, Annis C: Professional basketball injuries, *Physician Sports Med* 10:81, 1982.
2. Carlsoo SA: A kinetic analysis of the golf swing, *J Sports Med Phys Fitness* 7:76, 1967
3. Cavanagh PR: The biomechanics of running and running shoe problems. In Segesser B, Pforringer W, editors: *The shoe in sports,* Chicago, 1989, Year Book Medical Publishers.
4. Cooper et al: Kinematic and kinetic analysis of the golf swing. In Nelson RC, Morehouse CA, editors: *Biomechanics IV,* Baltimore, 1974, University Park Press.
5. Frederick EC, Hagy JL: Double impact peaks in vertical force while running. Presentation at the 11th International Congress of Biomechanics, Amsterdam, July 2, 1987.
6. Frederick EC, Hagy JL, Mann RA: The prediction of vertical impact force during running, *J Biomech* 14:498, 1987.
7. Henry JH, Lareau B, Neigut D: The injury rate in professional basketball, *Am J Sports Med* 10:16, 1982.
8. Holden JP et al: Foot angles during walking and running. In *Biomechanics IX,* Champaign, Ill, Human Kinetics, in press.
9. Korzick DH: Ground reaction forces in aerobic dance, *Med Sci Sports Exerc* 19(Suppl):S90, 1987.
10. Kuo CY, Louie JK, Mote CD Jr: Field measurements in snow skiing injury research, *J Biomech* 16:609, 1983.
11. Luethi SM et al: The influence of shoe construction on lower extremity kinematics and load during lateral movement in tennis, *Int J Sport Biomech* 3:166, 1986.
12. Mack RP: Ankle injuries in athletics, *Clin Sports Med* 1:71, 1982.
13. Mann RA: Biomechanics of running. In Nicholas JA, Hershman EB, editors: *The lower extremity and spine in sports medicine,* St Louis, The CV Mosby Co, 1986.
14. Masson M, Hess H: Typical soccer injuries—effects on the design of the athletic shoe. In Segesser B, Pforringer W, editors: *The shoe in sport,* Chicago, 1989, Year Book Medical Publishers.
15. Montag W-D: The figure skating boot. In Segesser B, Pforringer W, editors: *The shoe in sport,* Chicago, 1989, Year Book Medical Publishers.
16. Moritz A, Grana WA: High school basketball injuries, *Physician Sports Med* 6:91, 1978.
17. Nicholas JA, Grossman RB, Hershman EB: The importance of a simplified classification of motion in sports in relation to performance, *Orthop Clin North Am* 8:499, 1977.
18. Nigg BM, Denoth J: *Sportplatzbelage,* Zurich, 1980, Juris.
19. Nigg BM, Segesser B: The influence of playing surfaces on the load on the locomotor system and on football and tennis injuries, *Sports Med* 5:375, 1986.
20. Nigg BM et al: Factors influencing short-term pain and injuries in tennis, *Int J Sport Biomech* 2:156, 1986.
21. Nigg BM, Luethi SM, Bahlsen A: Influence of shoe construction on the supination during sidewards movements in tennis. In Perren SM, Schneider E, editors: *Biomechanics: current interdisciplinary research,* Dordrecht, 1985, Martinus Nijhoff.
22. Nigg BM, Luethi SM, Bahlsen HA: The tennis shoe: biomechanical design criteria. In Segesser B, Pforringer W, editors: *The shoe in sport,* Chicago, 1989, Year Book Medical Publishers.
23. Pfeiffer M: Kinematics of the foot in the ski boot. In Segesser B, Pforringer W, editors: *The shoe in sport,* Chicago, 1989, Year Book Medical Publishers.
24. Robinson
25. Torg J, Conrad W, Kalen V: Clinical diagnosis of anterior cruciate ligament instability in the athlete, *Am J Sports Med* 4:84, 1976.
26. Valiant GA, Cavanagh PR: A study of landing from a jump: implication for the design of a basketball shoe. In Winter DA, editor: *Biomechanics IX,* Champaign, Ill, 1983, Human Kinetics.
27. Williams KR, Cavanagh PR: The mechanics of foot action during the golf swing and implications for shoe design, *Med Sci Sports Exerc* 15:247, 1983.
28. Zelisko JA, Noble HB, Porter M: A comparison of men's and women's professional basketball injuries, *Am J Sports Med* 10:297, 1982.

4

Functional Examination of the Foot and Ankle

J. Christopher Reynolds

In the functional evaluation of the foot and ankle, it is essential to remember that there is a linkage and integration between all the bones, joints, muscles, and connective soft tissues to allow coordinated flexibility in the function of these structures during the gait cycle. All abnormalities discovered during the examination must be consistently measured and evaluated. A constant attempt must be made to assess what abnormalities may be rehabilitated and by what means rehabilitation can be accomplished.

For a complete functional evaluation of the foot and ankle, one must have an examination room with sufficient space for the patient to stand and take at least a few steps. The examination table must allow room for the evaluation of the range of motion of all the joints of the lower extremity including the hip. There should be adequate room at the end of the examination table for the patient to lie prone with the feet hanging over the end of the table and for the examiner to stand and examine the feet.

The scope of the examination may be all-encompassing, while the examiner searches for some subtle abnormality, or limited, if the history indicates a rather localized abnormality. The examination must be adaptable to these extremes. It is important for the examiner to have and use some type of record sheet for recording the findings, which include range of motion, and other functional measurements. With a chronically injured patient, one will expect to see some abnormalities in the examination. Normal gait, function, and posture are not to be expected. Using the normal extremity, if one is available, the examiner relates abnormal to normal by comparison, concentrating on the abnormal while reporting and evaluating the differences. The history can be as detailed as necessary, but one needs to determine the patient's chief complaints, duration of symptoms, and mechanism of injury or cause for the complaints. Previous treatments, laboratory results, X rays, and so forth may be reviewed at this time. I find it more relaxing to elicit the history while the patient is sitting in a comfortable chair rather than on the examination table. Once an adequate history is obtained from the patient, one should be able to ascertain the complexity of the problem and determine what aspects of the physical examination are necessary.

The examination begins with observation of the patient's gait and standing foot and leg posture. It continues with the patient sitting as each important element is examined in a systematic fashion, evaluating each component that is significantly different from the expected normal. The neurological and vascular status are examined. The patient is then examined in the supine position and in the prone position for biomechanical abnormalities. Finally, the patient is re-examined, if necessary, in the sitting position, standing, and walking, confirming any previously noted abnormality.

Gait Examination

The patient has usually been told to remove his shoes and stockings prior to the examination. Therefore, the examination can begin by asking the patient to walk to and fro and observing the barefooted gait. It may be necessary to take the patient into an adjacent hall for better observation. The patient can be observed while walking with shoes on, if necessary, at this time or later. An obvious limp, lurch, Trendelenburg gait, steppage gait, dragging the feet, in-toeing, and out-toeing are observed. In normal gait, one expects to see an equal stride length and equal in-toeing and out-toeing in the two legs.

At heel strike the heel everts and the ankle plantarflexes. The weight transfers along the lateral side of the foot. The foot, which was rigid at heel strike to resist impact, becomes increasingly flexible as the forces at impact are absorbed. Pronation occurs in the foot, with dorsiflexion occurring at the ankle, and internal rotation occurring in the leg, knee, and hip. An abnormality in the joints above the ankle, which limit internal and external rotation of the legs, can limit motion of the foot and ankle during gait. As the body and leg pass forward, supination begins with plantarflexion of the ankle. Inversion of the heel and adduction of the forefoot occur as the foot regains stability prior to toe-off, during

which time the leg externally rotates. Subtle gait differences or abnormalities between the two limbs may be difficult to perceive in this type of examination, but more obvious abnormalities should be noted. A significant external rotation deformity of the femur or leg is frequently accompanied by increased pronation of the foot with weight-bearing and walking. One should try to evaluate the various components of this complex linkage system to determine any weak link. Abnormalities of arm swing and position are important to observe, such as in a patient with cerebral palsy. The affected patient may be able to walk very slowly with a relatively normal-appearing gait but holding the extremity in a rigid, nonswinging, position. With the nonambulatory or semiambulatory patient, one can at least observe what functions, if any, the patient is able to perform with each foot as he or she stands facing the examining table or tries to sit up on the examining table.

Standing Evaluation

The examiner next has the patient stand facing away and notes general body symmetry. The patient should be asked to bend forward and backward, and any spinal curvature should be noted. One palpates the posterior superior iliac spine for symmetry and evidence of clinical leg length discrepancy. Blocks of varying thickness can be used under the foot to eliminate pelvic tilt while trying to estimate any leg length inequality.

Patients are asked to stand barefooted on a low stool in a relaxed position, not looking at their feet, because this changes the alignment of the feet. The overall aspect of the legs in standing is noted with particular regard to in-toeing and out-toeing. The general configuration of the arch is estimated at this point. Any obvious high arched or cavus foot or markedly flat foot with loss of the longitudinal arch is noted. The patient is next asked to internally and externally rotate the leg. With internal rotation of the leg, the arch flattens, and additional pronation of the foot from the amount present with normal standing

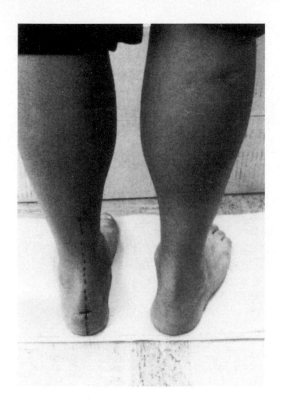

Fig. 4-1 The "too many toes" sign visible on the left foot.

is noted. With external rotation, the foot supinates with increase in the longitudinal arch. This is done with the patient standing facing toward and away from the examiner. Heel position, motion, and leg alignment are noted, as well as the changes occuring in the arch. With a swollen, chronically injured foot, testing these mechanisms may reveal that there are few adaptive qualities in the affected foot, or result in little change in the appearance of the foot. Viewing the foot from behind, with collapse of the longitudinal arch, the examiner may see that more of the toes are visible on the lateral side, the "too many toes" sign (Fig. 4-1).

At this point, if the patient is able to do so, he or she is asked to stand on the toes of each foot, one foot at a time, with normal toe rise on that foot alone. The patient should have enough strength to stand on the toes with full weight-bearing, and as this occurs the heel normally inverts. Inability to do this, with or without pain, indicates that instability is present in the foot, or there is weakness of the posterior tibial muscle. The posterior tibial muscle acts as a supinator, and adducts, inverts the foot, and plantarflexes the ankle. With insufficiency of this muscle, the calcaneus goes into valgus with the calcaneus subluxing under the talus. Pain may be what prevents the patient from performing this maneuver, and the weakness may or may not be due

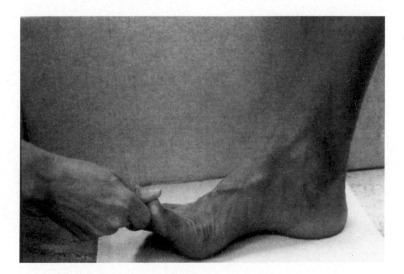

Fig. 4-2 A normal toe extension test with elevation of the arch and external rotation of the tibia.

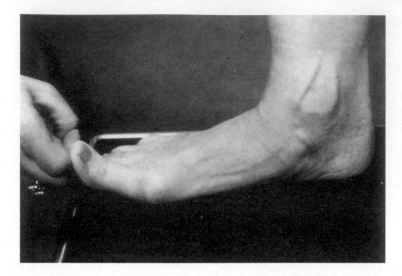

Fig. 4-3 An abnormal toe extension test with no elevation of the arch on dorsiflexion of the great toe.

to actual tendon rupture.

Facing the patient, the basic toe extension test can be easily performed. With the patient standing and relaxed, the great toe is passively dorsiflexed by the examiner, causing the arch to rise and the leg to externally rotate (Fig. 4-2). Both these effects should be present for the test to be considered normal. With no arch rise, one is looking at an abnormal foot with abnormal function (Fig. 4-3). If only arch rise occurs, one should suspect an abnormal foot. These tests are brief and simple and give the examiner some idea of the quality of the stability, adaptability, and function of the legs and feet, directing one's attention in the subsequent examination. Obvious genu valgus or genu varus should be noted with the patient standing and facing away from the examiner.

Sitting Examination

The sitting examination is performed with the patient facing the examiner with the knees hanging over the edge of the table. Internal and external hip rotation and symmetry are checked (Fig. 4-4). A sitting straight leg-raising test is performed. It may be helpful in evaluating this subjectively to add an element of "confusion" by

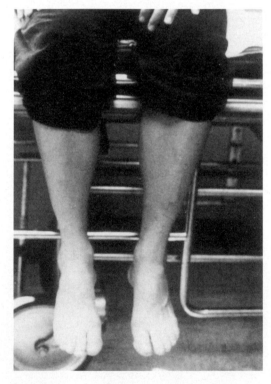

Fig. 4-4 Alignment of legs and feet in the sitting examination.

questioning the patient while holding the foot and distracting the patient from any back complaints. Many industrial patients with a long history of one lower extremity injury, with the use of a cast or brace, will have complaints of low back pain that may or may not be functional and may result in secondary gain. Complaints of leg, back, or hip pain are noted and whether or not they are accompanied by consistent abnormal guarding of the extremities. These tests are later repeated with the patient supine. The knees can be quickly examined for a normal range of motion, effusion, contracture, swelling, tenderness, and instability at this time. Patellofemoral crepitus or tenderness should be noted. Patellofemoral alignment is noted. Quadriceps insufficiency and obvious thigh atrophy should be noted and can be objectively measured.

In-toeing or out-toeing in relation to the rest of the extremity should be noted by placing a finger on the medial and lateral malleoli. The axis of the ankle joint is thus relatively determined and should lie at approximately an 18- to 20-degree angle externally rotated in relation to the axis of the knee joint. Internal or external tibial torsion and variance from the norm may be significant, and this may be easily measured with the knee extended.

Obvious injury to joints and structures above the foot and ankle with deformity or limitation of motion will affect normal foot and ankle motion in gait. An attempt should be made by the examiner to determine in which of the joints the pathology lies. One tries to determine if soft tissue contracture is interfering with motion or if there is a fixed bony deformity.

At this point it is convenient to assess the general appearance of the leg, foot, and ankle. The calf should be checked for any tenderness suggestive of phlebitis, and the tibia and fibula palpated throughout their lengths for tenderness. Obvious deformities, scars, swelling, atrophy, color, rash, telangiectasia, skin texture, scales, discoloration, hair distribution, or signs of chronic venous insufficiency are noted. In many patients with chronic injury, there may some swelling and discoloration of the leg, as well as some brawny edema present in the lower extremity (Fig. 4-5). These findings may be absent in the other extremity. Significant edema of this type can result in pericapsular fibrosis with scarring and limitation of motion. The girth of the calf is then measured at a point equidistant below each patella. The girth of the midfoot below the ankle should be measured and recorded.

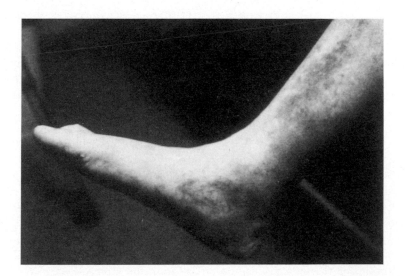

Fig. 4-5 A chronically injured extremity with brawny edema, clawing of toes, and skin changes (hyperpigmentation) of chronic venous stasis.

Functional Examination of the Foot and Ankle

Chapter 4

Examination of the Ankle Joint

The axis of this joint has already been observed, lying between the malleoli. The ankle is palpated for subjective tenderness, swelling, and range of motion. Normal dorsiflexion is approximately 20 degrees, and any dorsiflexion of less than 10 degrees raises suspicions of ankle pathology or tightness of the heel cord.

With tightness of the heel cord, a relative ankle joint equinus exists with decreased dorsiflexion of the foot. Contracture of the Achilles tendon may be accompanied by increased foot pronation or, in the more extreme cases, midfoot and subtalar subluxation and instability with dorsiflexion occurring through the foot and not the ankle. Plantarflexion of the ankle should be 40 degrees or more. In a patient with a history of regularly wearing high-heeled shoes, any decrease in dorsiflexion may reflect this type of shoe wear and be normal for the patient. The degrees of dorsiflexion and plantarflexion should be measured with a goniometer and noted. Because of the obliquity of the axis of the ankle joint, dorsiflexion is accompanied by some lateral deviation of the foot, and plantarflexion is accompanied by some medial deviation of the foot. Tightness of the heel cord is tested by holding the heel in inversion and dorsiflexing the foot. This should be measured both with the knee extended and with the knee flexed. Tightness of the heel cord with the knee extended, but not flexed, indicates contraction of the gastrocnemius portion of the gastrocnemius soleus complex. Tightness with the knee flexed indicates a tightness of the soleus muscle. In the foot with obvious midtarsal and subtalar instability and breakdown, with the appearance of having fallen in a "half-hemisphere appearance," dorsiflexion and plantarflexion may occur only through the midfoot and not through the ankle.[7] In this instance, the tightness of the Achilles tendon may be secondary to the abnormal foot. Inverting the heel to stabilize the subtalar joint and restore some of the normal foot alignment and subsequently dorsiflexing the foot will demonstrate this tightness of the heel cord.

Motion of the ankle joint occurs in the sagittal body plane. Subjective quality and ease of motion are observed. A large and tender subfibular fat deposit may be present. The anterior talofibular and calcaneofibular ligaments are next tested by stressing these ligaments. The anterior talofibular ligament is tested by an inversion stress with the foot maximally plantarflexed, placing the ligament in a position perpendicular to the stress applied. The calcaneofibular ligament is tested by inversion stresses with the ankle in neutral dorsiflexion. By holding the tibia in one hand and the foot in the other, one can pull the foot forward to assess an anterior drawer sign and abnormal laxity as compared with the opposite side. Pain may accompany these movements. If the patient has significant pain and guarding, the reliability of these findings will be questionable. In my experience, one can assess anterior and lateral instability by moderately plantarflexing the ankle, pulling the foot forward, and inverting the relaxed foot. Lateral laxity can be detected as the foot shifts forward with this maneuver. This is often accompanied by a grinding sensation, which, if noted by the patient, can be painful. If both ankles seem lax, one can check the general ligamentous condition of the patient by the laxity of the metacarpophalangeal joints of the fingers, as well as the ligamentous tightness present in the knees. One can see if general joint laxity exists. If the wrist can be flexed so that the fingers almost touch the side of the forearm, this demonstrates a general ligamentous laxity. In these cases, a positive ankle stress test may not be diagnostic. Laxity in the ankle joint can be documented with an inversion talar tilt test and anterior drawer sign stress test on X-ray evaluation.

The patient may have had clinical complaints of weakness, or giving out of the ankle joint. Clinical instability on one side, in the absence of guarding, may be more functionally significant than an X-ray evaluation. It is essential in trying to determine normal ligament strength that the patient be in a relaxed position. In the chronically swollen and painful ankle joint, it may be impossible to get enough soft tissue relaxation for a reliable test. After recording the range of motion of the ankle joint, the examination continues to the remainder of the foot.

Examination of the Hindfoot and Subtalar Joints

In palpating the foot, it is essential to palpate the sinus tarsi region, where not infrequently, with a chronic injury, the patient may note subjective tenderness. Over the subtalar joint, one finds the extensor digitorum brevis muscle belly and within the tarsal sinus the interosseus ligaments that help control motion of the heel relative to the talus. An injury to the interosseus ligaments may allow increased heel eversion and valgus position of the hindfoot. An attempt can be made to test the stability of the subtalar joint and the interosseus ligaments by stabilizing the talus in the ankle mortis and trying to invert and evert the heel. Again, lack of symmetrical movement is most important. In this maneuver, one hopes to get a relative assessment of stability. In my experience, based on magnetic resonance imaging evaluation, the patient with a so-called sinus tarsi syndrome may exhibit an interstitial tear of the interosseus ligaments in the sinus tarsi. Injury and chronic contracture of these ligaments may limit subtalar excursion.

The function of the subtalar joint is to convert the motion of the ankle, which occurs in the sagittal plane, to motion of the foot in the frontal and transverse planes. In evaluating the function of the foot and ankle, it is essential to think of motion in these planes and to describe the motion and performance consistently and in a reproduceable fashion, as described by Bordelon and McConnell.[1,9] The joints of the foot and ankle function essentially as hinge joints, with the motion perpendicular to their axes. A hinged joint provides freedom of motion in only one plane. Table 4-1 summarizes the planes of motion, axis of motion, motion occurring, position after motion, and the deformities as described in the abnormal position. This allows adequate and reliable recording of the position of the foot and ankle.

As noted, motion of the ankle joint occurs primarily in the sagittal plane and less in other planes. Motion of the subtalar joint occurs in all three planes. This is a triplane motion. The axis of the subtalar joint lies approximately 42 degrees from the horizontal and 23 degrees from the midline. Subtalar motion is initially tested in the sitting position by grasping the heel in one hand and the leg in the other, moving the heel in inversion/eversion, and noting the range of motion, subjective discomfort, crepitus, guarding, and tightness. One may evaluate voluntary and involuntary guarding. Is any contracture rigid, or can it be overcome by repetitive attempts at moving the joint?

Motion of the calcaneus in inversion and eversion is partially governed by restriction of the calcaneal ligaments, joint congruency, abutment of the talus against the calcaneus at the posterior facet, the surrounding medial and lateral

Table 4-1 Movements and Planes of Motion of the Foot

Planes of Motion	Axis of Motion	Motion Occurring	Position after Motion	Abnormality (Deformed Position)
Transverse plane	Vertical	Adduction	Adducted	Adductus
		Abduction	Abducted	Abductus
Frontal plane	Longitudinal	Inversion	Inverted	Varus
		Eversion	Everted	Valgus
Saggital plane	Horizontal	Dorsiflexion	Dorsiflexed	Calcaneus equinus
		Plantar flexion	Plantar-flexed	
Three planes	Combination	Pronation	Pronated	Pronatus supinatus
		Supination	Supinated	

ligaments, and peroneal and posterior tibial muscles.[2] Therefore, any bony incongruency, abnormal tightness, or laxity of any of the soft tissue structures secondary to injury can result in an abnormal increase or decrease of subtalar motion. For example, in a chronic peroneal tendon injury with some limitation of its excursion, this initial limited foot and ankle restriction of motion may progress to permanent secondary contracture of other related tissues, muscles, ligaments, and joints.

Pronation is a combination of abduction, eversion, and dorsiflexion, whereas supination is a combination of adduction, inversion, and plantarflexion. In trying to objectively measure and evaluate subtalar and other foot motion in a chronically injured patient, it is essential to keep in mind the various components of motion and try to isolate each in order to determine during which motion, and in which plane, loss of function is occurring.

Heel inversion and eversion are measured by moving the heel in and out while stabilizing the leg. Normally, twice as much inversion as eversion is present, with approximately 20 degrees of inversion and 10 degrees of eversion normally found. What is significant is asymmetrical motion from the opposite side, or grossly limited or lax motion. In the "peroneal spastic flat foot," motion of the heel into inversion is resisted by spasm, the foot is held everted at the heel, and the forefoot is abducted. With these findings present, one should have a high suspicion of some significant subtalar complex abnormality, coalition, or injury.

Examination of the Transverse Tarsal Joints

The transverse tarsal joint motion is through the talonavicular and calcaneocuboid joints. Motion occurs in these joints during pronation and supination. The transverse tarsal joints play a significant role in the rigidity, suppleness, and support of the foot in different phases of stance. With pronation, there is a relative parallelism of the axes in these two joints, allowing laxity of

motion. As the stance continues, with supination, the axes of these joints lose their parallelism, and they become rigid, adding to the stiffness in the foot at toe-off. The motions of abduction and adduction that are taking place in these joints are measured in the transverse plane. Normally, checking the abduction and adduction of the foot in the transverse plane with the foot in neutral, one expects to find twice as much adduction as abduction. Neutral position is defined as the most congruent position of the talonavicular joint. This position can be determined in the sitting position or in the prone position.

In evaluating these motions, the heel can be stabilized by holding it into inversion, and any loss of flexibility in the transverse tarsal joints is noted. Similarly, holding the heel in eversion is accompanied by some degree of increased suppleness in the transverse tarsal joints. In the chronically injured foot, one can usually expect to see some injury to and limitation of motion in one or both of these joints. These joints are palpated for laxity, rigidity, crepitus, swelling, and tenderness. Abnormal motion may be accompanied by subjective discomfort. It is important to palpate in the area under the talonavicular joint and to assess the condition and integrity of the spring ligament. Decreased support of the spring ligament with weak support of the talus on the calcaneus produces some plantar and medial deviation of the talus and pronation, with the calcaneus going into increased eversion.

Examination of the Tarsometatarsal Joints and the Forefoot

At this point the tarsometatarsal joints and the rest of the forefoot are analyzed. Passive inversion of the forefoot yields twice as much inversion as eversion from the neutral position. Pain, deformity, crepitus, and tenderness are evaluated in the tarsometatarsal joints. One must remain aware of the possible disruption of these joints by an acute or chronic Lisfranc type of injury to the tarsometatarsal joints. A subtle abduction of

Anatomy and Physiology

the forefoot may be seen in these injuries and should make the examiner highly suspicious of pathology at the tarsometatarsal joints and midfoot. In my experience, this may be missed by other treating orthopedic surgeons familiar with this type of injury. In fact, the initial X-ray evaluation and examination may have been reported as normal. In these injuries with tarsometatarsal or cuneiform disruption, even if minimal, the foot "just doesn't look right," with some medial prominence present, as well as subtle or gross abduction of the forefoot.

Plantarflexion and dorsiflexion at the first tarsometatarsal joint are normally about equal. The joint should be free and mobile without crepitus or subjective pain. The plantar aspect of the first tarsometatarsal joint should be palpated for tenderness or other abnormality. Loss of dorsiflexion or plantarflexion from the position of normal alignment may be significant at all the tarsometatarsal joints. Normally, there should be very limited dorsiflexion or plantarflexion of the second and, to a lesser degree, the third tarsometatarsal joints. Increased mobility of the fourth and fifth tarsometatarsal joints is present, allowing some dorsiflexion, plantarflexion, and rotation More mobility is present in the first, fourth, and fifth tarsometatarsal joints and accompanying rays. With chronic edema after trauma, the range of motion of the metatarsals at the tarsometatarsal joints can be expected to be significantly reduced.

All the metatarsal shafts are palpated with care, especially the base of the fifth metatarsal, for subjective pain to try to rule out a chronic stress reaction or fracture. With arthritis, and after a fracture, the dorsal surface of the metatarsal may be prominent. A painful cuneiform exostosis, unrelated to trauma or a recent injury, may be present.

Fixed deformities of the forefoot may occur, such as forefoot varus. The forefoot is held in inversion with the first metatarsal elevated relative to the lesser metatarsals. With the hindfoot held firm in the rigid deformity, the first ray cannot be passively pronated to the horizontal plane. In a more normal, flexible foot, one can bring the first ray and forefoot down to the foot flat position. With a fixed deformity, this may well

result in increased pronation with weight-bearing. Any fixed deformity of the forefoot with inability of the metatarsals and phalanges to passively reach a foot flat position in relation to the hindfoot will result in compensatory changes in the hindfoot. As the great toe meets the floor, the hindfoot compensates through the subtalar joints and everts. The increased pronation present can cause pain in the foot, ankle, or the leg because with increased pronation, there is increased internal rotation of the tibia. Increased pronatory forces in motion of the hindfoot can eventually result in collapse of the subtalar and midtarsal joints. If the subtalar joints are unable to compensate for this deformity, there may be some increased forefoot mobility, resulting in subluxation of the talonavicular and navicular cuneiform joints with medial arch tenderness, pain, and arthritis.[3]

For the great toe to dorsiflex at the first metatarsophalangeal joint, there must be some degree of plantarflexion of the first metatarsal at the tarsometatarsal joint. Less obvious is the dorsiflexion needed at the first tarsometatarsal joints for plantarflexion of this toe. This can be demonstrated to the patient by pressing up on the first metatarsal from below, which effectively eliminates passive dorsiflexion of the toes.

With any abnormal elevation of the metatarsals following surgery or fracture, abnormal metatarsophalangeal motion is expected. Loss of motion at the first tarsometatarsal joint may significantly limit motion in the great toe. Normal range of motion of the metatarsophalangeal joints is about 90 degrees dorsiflexion and 40 degrees plantarflexion. Painful loss of motion in the first metatarsophalangeal joint, hallux rigidus or hallux limitus, is normally accompanied by palpable dorsal osteophytes, which restrict motion.

A foot with increased pronation accompanied by lack of first ray stability will be manifested by a depressed medial side. With the first metatarsal maximally dorsiflexed in this position, any additional plantarflexion of the first ray is impossible, and no passive dorsiflexion of the first metatarsophalangeal joint is possible when walking. Abnormal metatarsophalangeal laxity, swelling, erythema, or tenderness may be present. Abnormal deviation of the toes, especially the second toe at the metatarsophalangeal joint, may be noted.

Passive dorsiflexion and plantarflexion of the metatarsophalangeal joints of all the toes should be pain-free. Pain in these motions may accompany metatarsophalangeal synovitis or other pathological processes in the joints. It may be possible to dorsally or plantarly sublux the metatarsophalangeal joints or even dislocate the joints with abnormal laxity present. Abnormal medial or lateral deviation of the second toe at the metatarsophalangeal joint may occur, known as the "crossover toe." Abnormal lateral deviation of the toes relative to the metatarsals affects both the plantar aponeurosis as it inserts into the toes, and both the intrinsic and extrinsic muscles acting on the toes.

The joints of the phalanges are checked for alignment, swelling, range of motion, and flexible or rigid deformities such as hammertoes or mallet toes. A flexible hammertoe deformity can be eliminated by passively pushing up on the metatarsal heads from below, whereas rigid hammertoes will not be passively straightened by this measure. The presence of a painful interdigital clavus should be noted.

The submetatarsal areas are done next, palpating for any bony prominence under the sesamoids or under a metatarsal head. A localized plantar lesion, such as an intractable plantar keratosis, may be present. This lesion may be discrete, localizing under a bony prominence of a metatarsal head, or of a diffuse variety, which may accompany abnormal plantarflexion of ametatarsal or abnormal length of a metatarsal. Pain between the metatarsal heads, which may be associated with a clicking sensation (Mulder's click), may cause suspicion of an entrapped interdigital nerve (Morton's neuroma). This is especially true between the second and third or third and fourth metatarsal heads. Additional restriction of motion of the metatarsophalangeal joints may be secondary to trauma and pericapsular fibrosis around the joints. The joints and toes themselves can be stiffened secondary to trauma involving the calf muscles with muscle contracture of the extrinsic muscles going into the toes. In a patient with extrinsic muscle contracture, passive dorsiflexion of the foot results in hammering of the toes, and plantarflexing the foot eliminates this hammertoe contracture. If dorsiflexion and plantarflexion do not influence the toe posture, intrinsic contracture or problems in the joints themselves may be the cause of the impairment and limitation of motion.

Metatarsophalangeal Joint Break

Because the respective distal ends of the metatarsals lie at different levels relative to the rest of the foot, with the first and second metatarsal heads lying more distally than the others, there results a functional obliquity of these joints. Mann described this obliquity as the metatarsophalangeal joint break.[8] As the foot supinates and thrusts laterally at toe-off, when there is decreased metatarsophalangeal joint dorsiflexion present, as with a hallux rigidus, and decreased range of motion of the great toe, there is an increased "break" noted functionally to allow greater motion of the lesser metatarsophalangeal joints. This protects the painful, stiff first metatarsophalangeal joint. This may be appreciated by looking at the patient's foot, as well as looking at the patient's shoes. In the patient's shoes, there is an increased obliquity at the distal crease reflecting the abnormal lateral motion; in a shoe with a normal break, the shoe crease is more transverse. Restrictions of metatarsophalangeal joint motion in the chronically injured patient result in an abnormal "break" and a change in foot function at toe-off that results in increased stress on the metatarsophalangeal joints and tarsometatarsal articulations laterally. In a chronically injured foot with gross edema of the forefoot, as well as pericapsular fibrosis, some limitation of motion at the metatarsophalangeal joints is to be expected. The toes may dorsiflex or plantarflex little, either actively or passively. In the presence of fixed deformities, such limitations, which interfere with normal gait, may be amenable to rehabilitative techniques.

Cavus and Flat Feet

One obvious variant from what one normally expects to see is the flat foot with a depressed longitudinal arch. Some of the various causes of a flat foot have already been discussed, namely insufficiency of the posterior tibial tendon, peroneal spastic flat foot associated with subtalar pathology, a flat foot with midtarsal and subtalar breakdown, and secondary to tightness of the Achilles tendon. A flat foot, namely a foot with little arch present in the weight-bearing position, is a foot that appears grossly abnormal. In the asymptomatic flexible flat foot deformity, a general ligamentous laxity is noted with absence of the normal arch.

Another variant from normal is the high arched, cavus foot, which may or may not have been symptomatic prior to injury. Additional symptoms or deformities may be present after an injury. Abnormalities present from a slight elevation of the arch to marked calcaneus of the hindfoot and equinus of the forefoot with rigid claw and hammertoe deformities. Inversion of the heel may be fixed. One may note on the plantar aspect of the foot that the weight-bearing pattern is located primarily on the lateral aspect of the sole. With the high arched foot, a contracture of the plantar fascia (plantar aponeurosis) is almost always present. The cavus foot has a relative elevation of the arch arising either from the posterior portion of the foot with increased inclination of the calcaneus or anteriorly with depression of the metarsals and forefoot relative to the calcaneus, or from a combination of both.[3] In these patients, dorsiflexion of the ankle is usually reduced when the patients wears a low-heeled shoe for walking. With a flat shoe and anterior depression of the forefoot, for the foot to be flat on the floor, some of the ankle dorsiflexion range of motion is "used up" in dorsiflexion of the forefoot from the equinus position to a foot-flat position. True ankle motion may be checked by examining range of motion with the forefoot plantarflexed.

In general there is poor shock-absorbing ability in the supinated, cavus type of foot. In this type of foot, any type of injury may be slow to resolve, and rehabilitation can be expected to be more difficult.

In the cavovarus foot, plantarflexion of the first metatarsal and first ray relative to the lesser metatarsals is found. This condition results in a relative valgus position of the forefoot with the plantar aspect of the forefoot facing outward. Weight-bearing results in forefoot supination as the lateral toes rotate to touch the ground leading to an inversion torque and inversion of the calcaneus. In the presence of weak peroneals or a chronically sprained ankle with ligament laxity, "instability" may be noted by the patient, and the patient may give a history of falling.

In this type of foot, it is essential to note if there is a fixed varus deformity of the hindfoot. The Coleman and Chestnut test for cavovarus foot (the Sherman Coleman test for heel flexibility) is performed. In these patients, there is plantarflexion of the first metatarsal. The patient stands with a 1- to 1½-inch block under the heel and under the lateral third, fourth, and fifth metatarsals, allowing the first metatarsal and forefoot to drop down, eliminating the action of the forefoot on the hindfoot. A flexible hindfoot in this position will go into a normal valgus position with weight-bearing.[11]

In patients with decreased heel eversion with the calcaneus secondarily fixed in varus, there is a decrease in the pronatory ability of the hindfoot, and the patient is susceptible to ankle sprains. The patient may have an ankle sprain that is resistant to treatment or have an increased number of subsequent sprains. An example would be a gymnast who, landing on the heel, has repetitive inversion of the heel, lateral ankle pain, and recurrent sprains.

Muscle Strength Evaluation

The function of the extrinsic muscles of the foot is summarized in Table 4–2. These muscles should be tested against resistance at this point in the examination. The results should be graded and recorded.[5] Also recorded is the relative strength of each muscle and group. Functional

Table 4-2 Muscle Function

Muscle	Function
Tibialis anterior	Dorsiflexion, inversion
Flexor hallucis longus, flexor digitorum longus, posterior tibial muscle, gastrocnemius, soleus	Plantarflexion, inversion
Peroneus longus	Plantarflexion, eversion, depression of the longitudinal arch
Peroneus brevis	Plantarflexion, eversion
Extensor hallucis longus, extensor digitorum longus	Dorsiflexion, eversion

range of motion and functional length should be assessed. In chronic injury, a contracture of the muscles of the calf may be present secondary to disuse or injury of the muscles themselves. Palpation of the muscle, especially the deep muscles, for tenderness, is performed. A functional restriction due to a deep myofascial contraction will result in some abnormal muscle function and length. This will ultimately cause some restriction in the normal gait and stance sequence. It is important to assess the quality of muscles in the calf as a source of loss of motion noted in a joint more distally. To check for posterior tibial tendon function (a tendon commonly involved in the chronically injured foot) one places the muscle in a relatively disadvantaged position, namely slight abduction, to begin the test. This eliminates some force of the anterior tibial muscle, and the forces of inversion in this instance should be due largely to the posterior tibial muscle.

Next, one should palpate along the tendon course to feel passive motion, pain, and crepitus and to see if any restrictions can be overcome passively or if there is a fixed contracture present. It is not uncommon in the injuries, tendinitis, or disruption to the posterior tibial tendon that the tendon is most painful at a point proximal to the medial malleolus. The peroneal tendons can also be palpated distally behind the lateral malleolus and along the lateral side of the foot. Partial ruptures or longitudinal splits in situ of the peroneal tendons have been noted on the lateral aspect of the foot below the sinus tarsi. To check the function of the peroneus longus, one must push up on the medial arch because one major function of the peroneus longus is to depress the medial column in addition to everting the foot, whereas the peroneus brevis primarily acts to evert the foot. The other tendons on the dorsum of the foot are more easily palpated for evidence of tenderness, contracture, crepitus, and normal excursion.

The intrinsic muscles are more difficult to evaluate because their function is primarily to aid in maintaining positions of stability of the toes and metatarsophalangeal joints and help to support the longitudinal arch. These muscles primarily flex the toes at the metatarsophalangeal joints and extend the interphalangeal joints. With denervation of the intrinsics, one may see some atrophy of the dorsal muscles of the foot, cock-up deformities with hyperextension of the metatarsophalangeal joints, and flexion of the toes at the interphalangeal joints. As noted earlier, with muscle contracture in the calf, dorsiflexion of the ankle may result in hammertoe contractures of the toes, which are relieved by plantarflexion of the ankle.

A rigid cock-up deformity of the metatarsophalangeal joints may be isolated as part of the cavus deformity, and one must be aware of the possibility of congenital neurological problems or chronic muscle disease in these cases. With chronic injury, the etiology of muscle imbalance is more likely to be a residual of a compartment syndrome, secondary to crush of muscles, after burns, or following a foot or leg fracture (Fig. 4-6). The evaluation of a more subtle myofascial contracture, as discussed earlier, is important. One must assess the calf musculature, its quality and its potential for rehabilitation.

Vascular Evaluation

In general, in evaluation of the foot, one notes the skin texture, color, and temperature at the

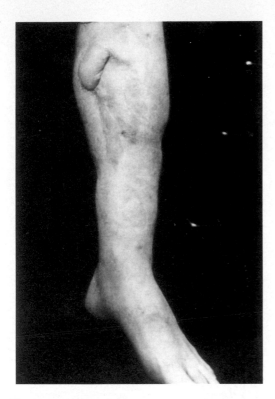

Fig. 4-6 A chronically injured leg after fracture and crush injury with little motion of the extrinsic muscles into the foot.

same time. It is important to palpate and try to grade the arteries, particularly the posterior tibial artery and dorsalis pedis artery, which are palpated as the foot is examined. Capillary filling is easily noted in the toes, with a normal refill of about 1 second to be expected after squeezing and blanching the toe. The presence or absence of hair and its distribution are also important. Asymmetry between the two feet is important. Another test, which is to be performed later when the patient is supine, namely, the venous filling time test, is brief and simple. In this condition, the patient is placed supine on the table and the extremity elevated to 90 degrees for 1 minute. The leg is then placed in a dependent position, and the superficial veins should begin to fill within 10 to 20 seconds. A positive test indicates the presence of enough good or collateral circulation for most wound healing.[10]

Neurologic Evaluation

Sensation, reflexes, and motor function should be evaluated in respect to the nerve roots, which may be involved, as well as individual sensory or motor nerves. A crush injury, laceration, or chronic edema and scarring can interrupt nerve function, resulting in a deformity that may or may not be amenable to surgery or rehabilitation. The major branches include the following:

1. The sural nerve, which supplies innervation to the lateral aspect of the foot and ankle.
2. The superficial peroneal nerve, which in the calf innervates the peroneus longus and peroneus brevis muscles before dividing into medial and lateral branches, which supply sensation to the medial side of the great toe on the dorsum, as well as to the dorsum of the third, fourth, and fifth toes.
3. The deep peroneal nerve, which supplies, in the calf, the extensor hallucis longus, tibialis anterior, and extensor digitorum longus muscles, and the extensor digitorum brevis muscle in the foot. It also provides sensation to the lateral side of the great toe and the medial side of the second toe.
4. The tibial nerve, which innervates the muscles in the posterior aspect of the leg, including the gastrocnemius, soleus, posterior tibial muscle, flexor hallucis longus, and flexor digitorum longus, as well as the rest of the intrinsic muscles of the foot, with the exception of the extensor digitorum brevis. The tibial nerve divides below the medial malleolus into the medial and lateral plantar branches, which supply the intrinsics and provide sensation to the plantar aspect of the foot, toes, and heel.
5. The nerve branch to the abductor digiti quinti (a mixed motor and sensory nerve), which divides from the tibial nerve just proximal to the medial malleolus, passes underneath the abductor hallucis muscle, and travels to the lateral side of the foot. This provides sensation to the lateral side of the heel posteriorly. Injury to the posterior, or medial, side of the foot can result in entrapment of

this nerve with symptoms of heel pain medially, as well as laterally. A positive Tinel's sign may be elicited at the tarsal tunnel but also from over the nerve branch to the abductor digiti quinti.

Relative to nerve root distribution, L4 provides sensation to the dorsal medial side of the leg, foot, ankle, and great toe. L5 provides sensation to the dorsal and medial aspects of the ankle and foot and the medial distal aspect of the plantar surface of the foot. S1 supplies the dorsal and plantar-lateral aspect of the foot including the sole.[5] It is important in sensory and motor defects to determine nerve root as opposed to individual nerve injuries. The knee jerk and ankle jerk are tested and compared. Vibratory sense is checked with a tuning fork. A sensory evaluation is performed using light touch or, for a more sensitive evaluation, using various calibrated monofilaments.

Examination of the Skin

In the chronically injured foot or extremity, skin changes are frequently found, with signs of chronic venous insufficiency, temperature changes, loss of hair, scarring, and edema. Skin adjacent to and underneath the toes is inspected for tinea pedis, an interdigital clavus, or bacterial infection. Nail changes, with discoloration, flaking or thickening, infection, and deformity, are also frequently found in a chronically injured extremity. A chronic fungal infection may be present. Poor hygiene may be noted. Small blisters filled with clear liquid (dyshidriosis) may affect the interdigital skin or soles of the feet.

The skin on the sole of the foot is checked for calluses and for small hyperkeratotic plugs (porokeratosis or seed corns) and warts. Warts normally bleed when trimmed and hurt when squeezed from side to side, whereas a callus or intractible plantar keratosis is avascular, hurts to direct pressure on the lesion, and does not bleed when trimmed. The thickness, character, and location of the skin underlying the metatarsal heads

is important. With chronic injury and muscle imbalance after blunt trauma or with rheumatoid arthritis, a cock-up or hammertoe deformity of the toes may be present, and normal skin may be pulled distally by the toes, leaving relatively poor skin underneath the metatarsal heads. This skin may be less resistent to trauma. The predisposing lack of motion may be improved by rehabilitation, which eliminates fixed contractures in the metatarsophalangeal joints. Injury to the heel may result in rupture of the septa dividing the fatty tissues in the sole of the heel. This results in poor shock–absorbing ability of the heel. The plantar heel pad can actually be displaced medially and laterally following heel fracture with very little skin underlying the heel itself. The heel may be widened and deformed.

The plantar fascia is inspected for integrity as it passes from its origin on the calcaneus into the insertion on the base of the proximal phalanges of the toes. Diffuse nodules (plantar fibromatosis) may be present, palpated and measured in the plantar fascia. These may or may not be painful to palpation. Trauma to the plantar fascia (plantar aponeurosis) may precede development of these nodules, but they do not usually result from trauma. At toe-off, the toes are dorsiflexed and the plantar aponeurosis is tightened as it is wrapped around the metatarsophalangeal joints acting as a windlass.[5]

Excess laxity or contracture of the plantar aponeurosis affects its ability to stabilize the foot. For example, if the amount of dorsiflexion needed for the great toe to function normally is absent (as with hallux rigidus), then excessive pressure may be noted under the great toe, and at toe-off, the foot may lift off earlier. The great toe may actually plantarflex to resist dorsiflexion and to prevent discomfort at the first metatarsophalangeal joint. Dorsiflexion of the great toe will help one to estimate the functional integrity of the plantar aponeurosis, as noted earlier. The toe extension tests while standing demonstrated the same function. Excessive laxity of the plantar aponeurosis results in decreased stability of the arch at toe-off (see Figs. 4-2 and 4-3).

Supine Examination

The patient is next placed in a supine position on the examining table. The straight leg raising tests are performed, and subjective complaints are noted. Hamstring tightness is checked by extending the leg with hips flexed 90 degrees. Internal and external rotation of the hips in extension is noted. Complaints of back pain frequently accompany a chronic foot injury and emphasize the need for a thorough neurologic examination. The presence or absence of true sciatica is important to evaluate. At this point, leg length can be more objectively measured by using a tape measure, measuring from the anterior superior iliac spine to the medial malleolus on the ipsilateral side. Patients with a leg length deformity may develop biomechanical compensation of the subtalar joints. This occurs with the long leg side pronating to decrease leg height, while on the short side the foot supinates to increase the relative height of the foot.

Prone Examination

The patient is placed on the examination table with the feet hanging over the end. In this position, the feet usually lie rotated and are difficult to visualize from above (Fig. 4-7). To eliminate this problem, the leg opposite the one being evaluated is flexed at the knee and bent over the extremity, forming almost a number 4 configuration (Fig 4-8). This removes some of the rotation of the examined leg and places it more in a straight up and down position for evaluation. A line drawn down the back of the tibia should be continuous with a line dividing the calcaneus in this position. These lines may be marked on the tibia and the heel for more objective measurement of the angles (Fig. 4-9). A fixed, inverted (varus) or everted (valgus) position of the calcaneus and the relative position of the tibia are noted (Figs. 4-10 and 4-11). In these instances, the line bisecting the calcaneus does not align with the line down the back of the tibia.

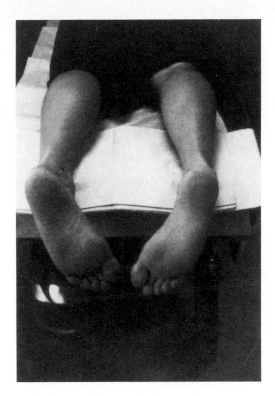

Fig. 4-7 In the prone position the legs rotate, making a straight-on examination of legs and feet difficult.

The above positions, and other positions of the foot, are determined from the foot in "neutral." Neutral position of the foot is defined as the position where the talonavicular joint is most congruent. This position is located by placing one hand over the fifth metatarsal and gently rocking the foot while the other hand palpates the talonavicular joint for the position of maximum joint congruity (Fig. 4-12). At the neutral position, a line bisecting the heel and leg should be perpendicular to a line drawn through the metatarsal heads. A line down the front of the leg should normally pass through the foot in the area of the second metatarsal. The alignment of the heel relative to the tibia and to the position of the forefoot is noted. The forefoot may be inverted in varus or everted in valgus.

Normally, 20 degrees of inversion and 10 degrees of eversion of the heel are noted. The po-

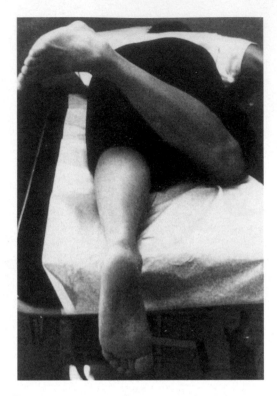

Fig. 4-8 Moving the opposite leg into the 4 position eliminates rotation in the examined leg, allowing easier examination.

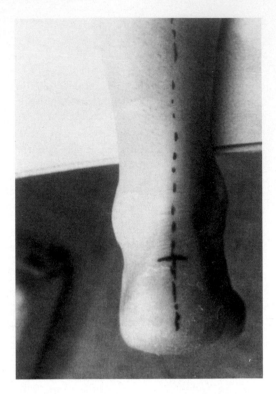

Fig. 4-9 Hindfoot (calcaneus) aligned with axis of tibia.

sitions are described in the frontal plane and are the position of varus or valgus. Adduction and abduction of the forefoot can be measured as well and their motion in the transverse plane. In neutral position the normal axis for motion of abduction and adduction of the foot should pass through the second metatarsal. In neutral, the relative position of the forefoot and heel must be noted, with limitations and asymmetries suspected with chronic injury, particularly following trauma. From neutral position, the foot is pronated and supinated, and symmetry, character of motion, and limitation are noted relative to the combination of inversion/eversion, adduction/abduction of the forefoot and inversion/eversion of the heel, and dorsiflexion/plantarflexion of the ankle. Lack of heel eversion is frequent in subtalar injuries. In neutral position with the foot visualized from behind, the examiner has the best opportunity

to check and record foot alignment in the nonweight-bearing position. As noted earlier, with a position such as fixed forefoot valgus, the position of plantarflexion of the first metatarsal can easily be detected. Similarly, fixed hindfoot varus with loss of eversion is best evaluated in this position.

With the patient prone, the heel cord insertion into the calcaneus is examined. A painful, erythematous, bony mass may be noted under the tendon insertion or more commonly on the lateral side of the heel. Nodular thickening or a defect may be found in the tendon. Retrocalcaneal thickening or tenderness may be present. The integrity of the Achilles tendon can be checked by the Thompson test. In this test, one squeezes the muscle belly of the gastrocnemius soleus complex, and such a squeeze results in plantar flexion of the foot if the Achilles tendon is in continuity.

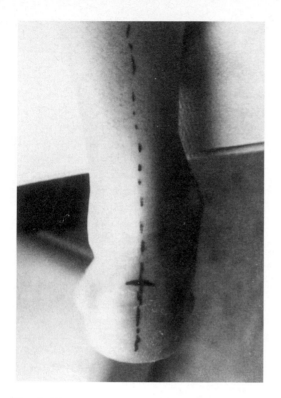

Fig. 4-10 Hindfoot in valgus position.

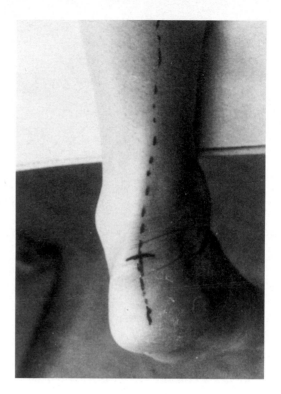

Fig. 4-11 Hindfoot in varus position.

Conclusion of the Examination

With the prone examination completed, the patient again sits and faces the examiner, and the positional findings can be reevaluated and demonstrated to the patient. It is particularly useful at this point to explain the position of the forefoot relative to pronation and supination, if abnormal. With the patient sitting in a nonweight-bearing position, the various aspects of the pronation (with the ankle dorsiflexing and foot abducting and everting) and supination (with the ankle plantarflexing and the foot adducting and inverting) can be demonstrated. These interrelated activities, which are triplane motions, are performed as an open kinetic chain in the nonweight-bearing position. Having initially evaluated the foot standing, then evaluating the individual components of the foot and ankle in the open kinetic chain, it may be necessary to reobserve the patient standing and walking barefooted and with shoes on to decide how any isolated abnormalities affect the gait sequence. In weight-bearing, there is a closed kinetic chain formed and some motions are eliminated by the presence of the foot against the floor. With early stance, the tibia internally rotates, but the calcaneus is fixed on the floor and cannot dorsiflex, plantarflex, abduct, or adduct. Eversion of the calcaneus occurs in pronation. Adduction and plantarflexion occur in the talus. Conversely, at toe-off, the tibia externally rotates, the foot supinates, inversion takes place in the calcaneus, and the actions of abduction and dorsiflexion occur in the talus.[2] Pericapsular fibrosis in and about the ankle joint and around the talus can limit normal talar excursion, preventing normal foot biomechanics.

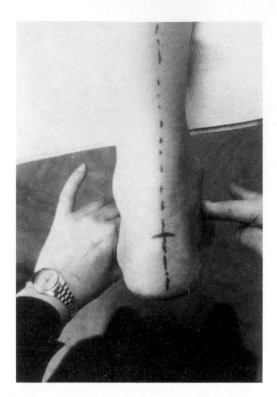

Fig. 4-12 Neutral position. The right hand palpates congruency of the talonavicular joint, while the left hand on the fifth metatarsal manipulates the forefoot.

Reflex Sympathetic Dystrophy

With a history of injury to a lower extremity and symptoms of severe, burning pain and hyperpathia/allodynia that seem out of proportion and more prolonged than one would expect after such an injury, one should have a high index of suspicion that reflex sympathetic dystrophy exists in the affected extremity. Abnormalities may have been noted throughout the exam earlier, such as abnormalities of temperature, edema, skin and hair changes, nail growth change, stiffness, muscle atrophy, sweating, and extreme sensitivity to touch. Where extreme sensitivity is present, the other aspect of the functional examination may be impossible to perform or evaluate.

Summary

The functional analysis of the foot and ankle is now completed, and abnormal and normal values recorded in an orderly fashion. The AMA Guide to the Evaluation of Permanent Impairment may serve as a guide for proper data recording.[4a] Deformities, rigid or flexible, should be noted. One has to concentrate on the key elements of motion and their restrictions, keeping in mind the mechanism of injury that may have created such an abnormality. As the exam procedes, one must constantly keep in mind what may be corrected and by what means, nonsurgical or surgical, make a fair estimate of the particular body function relative to rehabilitation potential, and note which modalities may help each of the involved areas. See the following Bibliography for excellent texts on foot examination by other authors.[1,2,5,6]

Bibliography

1. Bordelon L: *Foot care,* Thorofare, NJ, 1988, Slack.
2. Donatelli RA: Normal anatomy and biomechanics. In Donatelli RA, editor: *The biomechanics of the foot and ankle,* Philadelphia, 1990, FA Davis.
3. Donatelli RA: Abnormal biomechanics. In Donatelli RA, editor: *The biomechanics of the foot and ankle,* Philadelphia, 1990, FA Davis.
4. Huson A: Functional anatomy of the foot. In Jahss MH, editor: *Disorders of the foot and ankle,* ed 2, vol I, Philadelphia, 1990, WB Saunders.
4a. Doege TC, Houston TP, eds: *Guide to the evaluation of permanent impairment,* ed 4, 1993, American Medical Association.
5. Jaffe WL, Gannon PJ, Laitman JT: Paleontology, embryology, and anatomy of the foot. In Jahss MH, editor: *Disorders of the foot and ankle,* ed 2, vol I, Philadelphia, 1991, WB Saunders.
6. Jahss MH: Examination. In Jahss JH, editor: *Disorders of the foot and ankle,* ed 2, vol I, Philadelphia, 1990, WB Saunders.
7. Mann RA: Principles of examination of the foot and ankle. In Mann RA, Coughlin MJ, editors: *Surgery of the foot and ankle,* ed 6, vol I, St Louis, 1992, Mosby.
8. Mann RA: Principles of examination of the foot and ankle. In Mann RA, Coughlin MJ, editors: *Biomechanics of the foot and ankle,* ed 6, vol I, St Louis, 1992, Mosby.
9. McConnell B: Motions, positions, and abnormalities of the foot, personal communication to the Orthopaedic Foot Club, 1990.

10. Rowbotham JL, Gibbons GW, Kozak GP: Guidelines in examination of the diabetic foot and leg. In Kozak GP et al, editors: *Management of diabetic foot problems,* Philadelphia, 1984, WB Saunders.
11. Tachdjian MO: Pes cavus and claw toes. In Tachdjian MO, editor: *The childs foot,* Philadelphia, 1985, WB Saunders.

SUGGESTED ADDITIONAL REFERENCES

1. Engelberg AL, editor: *Guides to the evaluation of permanent impairment,* ed 3, Chicago, 1988, American Medical Association.
2. Sarrafian SK: *Anatomy of the foot and ankle,* Philadelphia, 1983, JB Lippincott.

5

Normal and Abnormal Muscle and Ligament Physiology

Rafael F. Escamilla

The foot, which is designed in such a way as to provide both stability and mobility, functions primarily to support and propel the body. It is comprised of a forefoot, midfoot, and hindfoot. The forefoot consists of the metatarsals and phalanges; the midfoot consists of the cuneiform, navicular, and cuboid bones; and the hindfoot includes the talus and calcaneus. These structures are controlled by both extrinsic and intrinsic ligaments and muscles. Ligaments largely provide stability and structure to the foot, especially in static positions. For example, during normal sitting and standing, the muscles of the foot do very little work; it is the ligaments of the foot that maintain the longitudinal and transverse arch structures. However, during dynamic movements, the muscles of the foot become much more active. They not only help propel the body by increasing ground reaction forces but also play a major role in maintaining normal arch structures. This latter role is paramount, since ground reaction forces applied to the foot can be several times body weight during many dynamic activities, such as running. Muscle and ligament im-

balances can produce joint deformation and discomfort; furthermore, as the mechanical axes of the foot are altered, movement patterns become inefficient. This chapter discusses normal and abnormal functions of the muscles and ligaments that act on the foot, as well as specific pathologies that occur as a result of muscle and ligament abnormalities.

Muscle Physiology

Extrinsic Muscles

There are 12 extrinsic muscles that control the foot. These muscles originate in the leg but insert and act upon the foot. Visualization of the origins, insertions, and anatomical locations of these muscles is helpful in understanding normal and abnormal muscle function. This helps clinicians diagnose foot disorders due to paralysis of specific muscle groups and also determine which muscles may be substituted to help correct muscle imbalances.

In general, muscles anterior to the axis of the ankle joint produce dorsiflexion, while muscles posterior to this axis produce plantarflexion. Similarly, muscles medial to the axis of the subtalar joint produce inversion, while muscles lateral to this axis produce eversion. When the ankle and subtalar axes are considered collectively, muscles posterior and medial to these axes produce plantarflexion and inversion, while muscles anterior and lateral to these axes produce dorsiflexion and eversion. It is important for clinicians to realize that the greater the moment arm and the stronger the muscle, the greater the action (i.e., torque output) at that joint. For example, the tibialis anterior muscle is located along or just medial to the axis of the subtalar joint; consequently, it is an ineffective invertor of the foot when in a neutral position. However, as the foot inverts, its moment arm medial to the subtalar joint increases, thus increasing its inversion action at this joint. Conversely, as the foot progresses in eversion, its moment arm may eventually (e.g., in severe pronation) become lateral to the subtalar joint, thus acting to evert the foot. Steindler believes that although the tibialis anterior is normally a weak invertor and evertor of the foot at the subtalar joint, it acts as a strong foot invertor relative to the transverse tarsal axis, which lies more in the sagittal plane.[15] The same may be true of the extensor hallucis longus. The moment arm of a muscle is determined by the perpendicular distance from the line of action of the muscle to the axis of rotation, while the strength of a muscle is proportional to its physiological cross-sectional area (PCSA). The PCSA of a muscle can be expressed numerically as the ratio between its volume and its true fiber length. Muscle architecture can greatly affect this quantity. As muscle pennation increases within a muscle, its PCSA also increases; therefore, two muscles may have identical anatomical cross-sectional areas (ACSAs) but differ greatly in their PCSAs and force-generating potentials. For this reason it is very important to differentiate between ACSA and PCSA, especially when constructing a mathematical physiological model of the foot. While this type of modeling can be quite helpful to clinicians, it is outside the scope of this chapter.

In addition to PCSA, muscle force is also a function of its length, contraction velocity, and contraction type (i.e., eccentric, concentric, or isometric). In general, as a muscle deviates from its normal resting length, muscle tension decreases. Similarly, the faster a muscle shortens (concentric contraction), the less tension it is able to generate; conversely, the faster a muscle lengthens (eccentric contraction), the more tension it is able to generate.

The extrinsic muscles of the foot, which are divided into *anterior, posterior,* and *lateral* compartments, are as follows.

Anterior Compartment

Comprised of muscles that cause dorsiflexion, eversion, inversion, and toe extension, this compartment contains the *tibialis anterior, extensor digitorum longus, extensor hallucis longus,* and *peroneus tertius.* During normal gait, electromyographic studies have shown that these pretibial muscles are active during the first 25% of the stance phase (from heel contact to shortly after the foot becomes flat) and throughout the entire swing phase.[9] It is during this period that the ground reaction resultant force vector acting on the foot, which is much greater than the weight of the foot, is posterior to the ankle joint; therefore, a plantarflexion torque (moment) is produced. This torque peaks at about the time the foot becomes flat. To counteract this effect, the pretibial muscles must contract eccentrically (dorsiflexion torque) to slow down the plantarflexing foot. During the swing phase, the primary external force acting on the foot is gravity. This force acts anterior to the ankle joint through the foot's center of mass and also produces a plantarflexion torque. To resist this effect, the pretibial muscles must now produce a concentric dorsiflexion torque and thus permit the toes to clear the floor and prepare for heel contact.

The role of the anterior compartment muscles in supporting the longitudinal arch of the foot has long been debated. All these muscles are innervated by the deep peroneal nerve, which is a branch of the common peroneal nerve. Due to its superficial location around the fibular head, the common peroneal nerve is the most commonly injured nerve in the lower limb. If this nerve is severed (e.g., fibular fracture), local paralysis occurs, which severely hinders dorsiflexion, inversion, eversion, and toe extension. These are also symptoms of what is commonly referred to as *anterior compartment syndrome*. When the leg is injured (e.g., fractured tibia) or chronically stressed (e.g., excessive exercise), compartmental muscles swell and stretch the elastic limit of the surrounding fascia. Pressure increases within the compartment and impedes normal circulation. Critical pressure levels are thought to occur when the capillary hydrostatic pressure exceeds 30 mmHg.[6] Consequently, perfusion of the muscle capillaries is limited, resulting in ischemia. This ischemic condition can only continue for several hours before muscle and nerve necrosis begins. Subsequent scarring within the necrotic muscle only exacerbates the problem. There are two primary conditions that result from anterior compartment syndrome. First, since normal dorsiflexion of the toes and ankle cannot occur, a *drop foot* condition occurs. Consequently, the muscles of this compartment may assume a stretched position. This stretching effect is adversely influenced by prone or supine sleeping positions since in both cases gravity and reactive forces tend to cause the foot to assume a position of plantarflexion. Clawing of the toes can also occur. Second, the muscles within this compartment may form a contracture, thus leaving the muscles in a permanently shortened position of dorsiflexion. The former condition is more common and often develops in conjunction with posterior compartment syndrome, which will be explained later. Orthotic devices are often not required in the latter condition.

Tibialis Anterior

This muscle functions to dorsiflex the ankle and invert the foot. It has been estimated that two thirds of dorsiflexion power is generated by this muscle.[10] In inversion, this muscle supports the medial longitudinal arch of the foot. However, since the line of action of this muscle lies along the subtalar axis, its effectiveness in inverting the foot is minimal. When it is paralyzed, dorsiflexion is severely limited and the integrity of the medial longitudinal arch may be compro-

mised. Support to the transverse arch is also provided by this muscle. Flaccid paralysis from peroneal nerve palsy can cause the foot to drop into plantarflexion when raised from the ground (drop foot). With this condition, during the swing phase in gait the foot must be raised higher than usual; furthermore, at heel contact the foot is brought down suddenly, producing a "clop" sound when it hits the floor. This is described as a steppage gait.

Extensor Digitorum Longus

This muscle functions to dorsiflex the ankle, evert and abduct the foot, and extend the phalanges of the lesser toes. Its tendons insert into the middle and distal phalanges of the four lesser toes, and an extensor sling anchors these tendons at the metatarsophalangeal (MTP) joints. Consequently, it is able to also extend the MTP joints by this mechanism. This muscle, along with the tibialis anterior and the extensor hallucis longus, contracts concentrically to dorsiflex the ankle during the swing phase in gait and contracts eccentrically just after heel strike to slow down the foot. Since this muscle is inserted into the convexity of the lateral longitudinal arch, abnormal muscle function can cause the lateral arch to be flattened, resulting in a flat foot condition. This can occur when there is too strong a pull from this muscle, as well as from the peroneus tertius and the triceps surae, which also insert on the convexity of the arch.

Extensor Hallucis Longus

This muscle functions to dorsiflex the ankle, extend and adduct the great toe, and invert the foot. Since this muscle is inserted into the convexity of the medial longitudinal arch, abnormal muscle function (e.g., too strong a pull by both this muscle and the tibialis anterior) can cause the medial arch to be flattened, resulting in a flat foot condition.

Peroneus Tertius

Sometimes described as the fifth tendon of the extensor digitorum longus, this muscle functions with the extensor digitorum longus to dorsiflex and evert the foot. It also plays a supportive role in maintaining the lateral longitudinal arch.

Posterior Compartment

This compartment is subdivided into superficial and deep muscles, which plantarflex and invert the foot. All these muscles are innervated by the tibial nerve. Since this nerve is deep and well protected, it is not commonly injured. However, posterior knee joint dislocations or tears in the popliteal fossa may injure the tibial nerve, producing paralysis in all the muscles of the posterior compartment. *Posterior compartment syndrome* occurs in a manner similar to that described in anterior compartment syndrome. This syndrome is rare in the superficial compartment since this compartment does not contain nerve bundles passing to the foot and is not tightly bound by fascia. The deep compartment, however, has the greatest occurrence of compartmental syndrome. This is especially true following tibia fractures. The most common result of this syndrome is severe contracture of the muscles in this compartment. As is the case with anterior compartment syndrome, sleeping positions tend to exacerbate this condition. While sleeping, the anterior leg muscles are constantly stretched, while the necrotic posterior leg muscles scar and place the foot in a semirigid position of plantarflexion. Combinations of varus, cavus, and toe clawing may also occur. The intrinsic muscles in the sole of the foot may also be adversely affected. When this happens, the patient is unable to curl the toes and stand on them, and pressure sores may occur due to a loss of sensory perception in the sole of the foot.

Superficial Layer

The *triceps surae (gastrocnemius* and *soleus)* and *plantaris* comprise the superficial layer, otherwise known as the calf muscles. These muscles collectively are the *primary* plantarflexors of the foot. This is true for two reasons. First, the triceps surae can produce over twice the force output of all the other plantarflexors of the foot combined (i.e., the muscles of the lateral compartment and the deep layer muscles of the posterior compartment). This is because the cross-sectional area of the triceps surae is over twice that of all the other plantarflexors of the foot combined. Second, the moment arm of the triceps surae is greater than the moment arms of the other plantarflexors,

which all pass very close to the ankle joint. The triceps surae strongly acts during the middle and latter portions of the stance phase during gait. In fact, normal gait electromyographic studies have shown that these muscles are active during the last three fourths of the stance phase.[9] It is at this time that the ground reaction force vector is anterior to the ankle joint, thus producing a dorsiflexion torque about this joint. Consequently, the calf muscles contract eccentrically to control the rate of dorsiflexion due to the forward rotation of the leg with respect to the foot. At about two thirds of the way through the stance phase, just before heel-off, the calf muscles begin contracting concentrically, thus helping to propel the body forward.

Since the gastrocnemius also crosses the knee joint, it is more effective as a plantarflexor when the knee is extended. This is due to the length-tension relationship of muscles mentioned previously. Thus as the gastrocnemius muscle shortens (i.e., knee flexion), its ability to produce force diminishes. The soleus, however, only crosses the ankle joint so the position of the knee does not affect its ability to plantarflex the foot. Consequently, the soleus is a more effective plantarflexor when the knee is flexed since the force output of the gastrocnemius is less.

Deep Layer

The deep layer is composed of the *tibialis posterior, flexor digitorum longus,* and *flexor hallucis longus.* Since all these muscles pass posterior to the ankle and under the medial malleolus, they function to supinate (plantarflex, invert, and adduct) the foot and steady the leg on the foot while standing. Like the triceps surae, these muscles are also active during the mid and late stages of the stance phase in gait. In addition, they all function as tighteners and stabilizers for the medial arch of the foot. The flexor digitorum longus and the flexor hallucis longus also flex the lesser toes and the great toe, respectively.

Tibialis Posterior This large muscle lies between and deep to the flexor digitorum longus and the flexor hallucis. Since this muscle inserts into the medial longitudinal arch and spans several tarsal bones, it serves a supportive role to this arch. When it contracts, the navicular is pulled back posteriorly and inferiorly under the head of the talus, thus lowering the anterior portion of the medial arch. In addition, the arch is further supported since its plantar attachments blend with the plantar ligaments, which act on the proximal portion of the three middle metatarsals. The fibrous expansions of this muscle run obliquely, anteriorly, and laterally and insert into the cuneiform and cuboid bones, as well as in the base of the second, third, and fourth metatarsals. Therefore, these fibers function as a tightener to the transverse arch. Acquired flat foot can occur when this muscle is injured or in a state of paralysis because the loss of this muscle may be responsible for a collapsed arch.

Flexor Digitorum Longus This muscle actively elevates the medial longitudinal arch of the foot. Since its tendon inserts into the distal phalanx of the four lesser toes, it has greater flexion capability at the distal interphalangeal (DIP) joints than it does at the proximal interphalangeal (PIP) or MTP joints. If the MTP joint is not hyperextended, this muscle assists in flexing that joint.

Flexor Hallucis Longus This long, powerful muscle, which is the largest of the three deep muscles, helps elevate the medial longitudinal arch of the foot. It functions as the "pushoff" muscle during running and walking and provides much of the spring during each step. Its tendon occupies two grooves within the foot—first a shallow groove on the posterior surface of the talus, and second a groove below the sustentaculum tali. Consequently, its tendon helps stabilize both the talus and calcaneus. It does this in two ways, analogous to the way a bowstring exerts a greater force on an arrow the further it's pulled back. First, it resists posterior translation of the talus caused by a posterior force exerted on it by the navicular bone. In a similar manner, it reelevates the anterior medial portion of the calcaneus in response to the downward vertical force the talus exerts on the calcaneus (e.g., going from stance phase to swing phase in gait).

Lateral Compartment

This compartment is composed of the *peroneus longus* and *peroneus brevis* muscles. Since these muscles pass posterior to the ankle and under the lateral malleolus, they function to cause plantarflexion and eversion of the foot along with abduction. Like the other plantarflexors of the foot, these muscles are also active during the mid and late stages of the stance phase in gait. These muscles are innervated by the superficial peroneal nerve, which is a branch of the common peroneal nerve. Like the common peroneal nerve, the superficial peroneal nerve is also vulnerable to injury due to its superficial location in the distal third of the leg. Foot eversion and lateral ankle stability are severely hindered if either the common or superficial nerve is damaged, thus resulting in an inverted foot.

Peroneus Longus

This long, slender muscle is the more superficial of the two peroneal muscles. Since the peroneus longus passes under the apex of the medial longitudinal arch, it functions as a "sling" to help support this arch. By its plantar insertion on the first metatarsal and medial cuneiform, it accentuates the curvature of the arch by flexing the first metatarsal on the medial cuneiform, and the medial cuneiform on the navicular. This muscle also runs obliquely across the transverse arch to the medial border of the foot. By its posterior and lateral pull on the medial cuneiform, the medial border of the foot is pulled toward the lateral border. Consequently, the transverse arch, which bridges between the two longitudinal arches, is supported. Since the peroneus longus tendon runs under the peroneal tubercle of the calcaneus, its own elasticity helps elevate the anterior lateral calcaneus, similar to the way the bowstring effect of the flexor hallucis longus elevates the anterior medial calcaneus. The peroneus longus also plays a supportive role in actively tightening the lateral arch. Its primary functions are plantarflexion, abduction, and eversion of the foot.

Peroneus Brevis

This muscle is shorter and smaller and lies deep to the peroneus longus. In fact, it is only about half as strong as the much larger peroneus longus. Like the peroneus longus, this muscle aids in plantarflexion, abduction, and eversion of the foot. It also helps maintain the lateral longitudinal arch as it depresses the foot by actively tightening the arch; however, it appears less important in this supportive role since it only spans part of the arch, and its tendon does not pass through the sole of the foot.

Intrinsic Muscles

There are 19 intrinsic muscles that help control and stabilize the foot. These muscles originate, insert, and function within the foot. These muscles primarily function as elevators and stabilizers of the arches of the foot, as well as stabilizers of the toes at the MTP joints. Their contractions are primarily along anterior-posterior axes. During normal gait, electromyographic studies have shown that these muscles are inactive during the first 25% of the stance and throughout the entire swing phase.[9] Therefore, the foot articulations are most unstable and vulnerable during this initial weight-bearing phase. There are 18 muscles (four layers) in the plantar surface of the foot, while the dorsum of the foot has only one muscle. All the plantar surface muscles are innervated by the medial and lateral plantar branches of the posterior tibial nerve, while the single muscle of the dorsum is innervated by the lateral branch of the deep peroneal nerve. The abductor hallucis, adductor hallucis, flexor digitorum brevis, flexor hallucis brevis, and abductor digiti quinti make up the primary intrinsic muscle mass.

Dorsal Surface
Extensor Digitorum Brevis

This small, thin muscle is located in the lateral portion of the dorsum. Since its only function is to assist the extensor hallucis longus and extensor digitorum longus muscles in extending toes one through four, it is functionally unimportant. The medial portion of this muscle is often called the extensor hallucis brevis since its tendon inserts into the proximal phalanx of the great toe. Its three lateral tendons insert into the tendons of the extensor digitorum longus for toes two through four.

Plantar Surface

These muscles have gross functions rather than the individual functions of the intrinsic muscles of the hand.

First Layer

The three muscles that make up the first layer all originate from the posterior calcaneus and insert on the proximal phalanges. The superficial position of these muscles allows for support of the arches of the foot, thus supporting the foot's concavity.

Abductor Hallucis This muscle abducts and flexes the proximal phalanx of the great toe. Since this muscle spans the whole medial arch, it also helps support the medial longitudinal arch of the foot during weight-bearing. It is an efficient tightener and accentuates the curvature of the arch.

Abductor Digiti Minimi The most lateral muscle of the first layer, this muscle abducts and flexes the small toe. Since it spans the entire length of the lateral longitudinal arch of the foot, it also helps maintain the integrity of this arch, especially during weight-bearing.

Flexor Digitorum Brevis This short muscle, which lies between the abductor hallucis and abductor digiti minimi, inserts into the middle phalanx of the four lesser toes. Therefore, it functions to flex the PIP joints of the four lateral toes. It also helps support the medial and lateral longitudinal arches of the foot, especially during weight-bearing.

Second Layer

The muscles of the second layer, which control toe motion, are located deep with respect to the muscles of the first layer. The tendons of the flexor hallucis longus and the flexor digitorum longus are also located in this layer.

Quadratus Plantae (Flexor Digitorum Accessorius) This small, flat muscle assists the flexor digitorum longus muscle in flexing the lateral four toes. Since its line of action is along the longitudinal axis of the lateral toes, it partially straightens the oblique pull of the flexor digitorum longus.

Lumbricales By their origin in the tendons of the flexor digitorum longus muscle and their plantar passing to the MTP joint axis, these four worm-shaped muscles (Latin *lumbricus,* earthworm) flex the proximal phalanges of the second through fifth toes. The lumbricales produce flexion at the MTP joints by exerting tension on the extensor sling; therefore, their ability to flex this joint decreases as the MTP joints extend. Since these muscles also insert into the extensor digitorum longus tendons and pass dorsal to the axis of the PIP and DIP joints, they also extend the middle and distal phalanges of the second through fifth toes. Since all its terminal fibers insert into the extensor sling, the lumbricales, unlike the interossei, produce strong extension at the interphalangeal (IP) joints. Their absence or abnormal function may result in claw toes.

Third Layer

These muscles all reside in the anterior portion of the sole of the foot and are made up of the short muscles of the great and small toes. Except for the interosseus muscles, these are the deepest of the intrinsic muscles.

Flexor Hallucis Brevis This two-headed muscle flexes, adducts, and stabilizes the MTP joint of the great toe. Its medial head inserts into the inner base of the proximal phalanx of the great toe, blending with the abductor hallucis. Its lateral head inserts into the outer base of the proximal phalanx of the great toe, blending with the adductor hallucis. Two sesamoid bones, one contained in each tendon, protect the tendons at the metatarsal head during weight-bearing. The lateral portion of this muscle blends with the adductor hallucis muscle and passes obliquely from the posterior lateral foot to its insertion in the proximal phalanx of the great toe. Consequently, it aids in supporting the integrity of the transverse arch.

Adductor Hallucis This muscle, the abductor hallucis, and the flexor hallucis brevis are the three intrinsic flexors of the big toe; consequently, they all play an important role in stabilizing the big toe in weight-bearing, especially during the final phases of gait leading up to push-off. Paralysis of these muscles can cause a claw deformity of the big toe. The adductor hallucis has both oblique and transverse heads. Its oblique

portion both adducts and flexes the great toe. Its transverse portion helps maintain the transverse arch of the metatarsus. This muscle is fairly weak and gives way easily, thus flattening the arch.

Flexor Digiti Minimi This small muscle flexes the proximal phalanx of the small toe.

Fourth Layer

The fourth and deepest layer is composed of three plantar and four dorsal *interosseus* muscles, as well as the tendons of insertion of the tibialis posterior and peroneus longus muscles. These muscles are important in helping to maintain the integrity of the metatarsus, as well as helping to stabilize the toes. It has been suggested that the interossei generate forces that are transferred across the tarsometatarsal joints.[11] These authors further state that the interossei might function as stabilizers of the foot, causing the metatarsal joints to become rigid during weight-bearing. As was the case with the lumbrical muscles, paralysis of these muscles can result in claw foot or claw toes. The dorsal (abductor) interossei are located between each adjacent pair of metatarsals, while the plantar (adductor) interossei are positioned more inferiorly to each of the three lateral metatarsals. The abductor and adductor function of the interossei is with respect to the second metatarsal.

Plantar Interossei Due to their medial insertion on the proximal phalanges, these muscles adduct and assist in flexing the proximal phalanges of the three lateral toes. Since these muscles insert directly into the proximal phalanges, they exert a stronger flexion at this joint than do the lumbricales. By their insertion into the aponeurosis of the common extensor tendon, these muscles also extend the IP joints of the three lateral toes. However, since only a few fibers reach the extensor sling, they are relatively weak extensors of the IP joints.

Dorsal Interossei By its medial insertion on the second proximal phalanx, the first interosseus muscle both abducts and flexes the second proximal phalanx. Due to lateral insertions into the second through fourth proximal phalanges, the remaining three interossei abduct and flex the second, third, and fourth proximal phalanges.

Like the plantar interossei, these muscles insert directly into the proximal phalanges. Therefore, they also exert a stronger flexion at this joint than do the lumbricales. These muscles also extend the IP joints of their respective toes. Like the plantar interossei, since only a few fibers reach the extensor sling, these muscles are relatively weak extensors of the IP joints.

Ligament Physiology

Extrinsic Ligaments

As is the case with extrinsic muscles, these ligaments originate in the leg but insert and act upon the foot. All seven extrinsic ligaments, which insert in the hindfoot, span and provide stability to the *talocrural (ankle) joint*. The ankle joint allows for both dorsiflexion (extension) and plantarflexion (flexion). These terms anatomically describe movement occurring at the ankle. Consequently, they are often the preferred terms for referring to this joint instead of flexion and extension, which are often erroneously interchanged. The ankle joint is injured more frequently than any other major joint in the body. These seven ligaments collectively make up the *medial collateral (deltoid) ligaments* and the *lateral collateral ligaments*. Abnormal function of these ligaments can cause rotary instability and increased supination and pronation tilt.

Medial Collateral Ligaments

These powerful ligaments limit foot pronation, thus providing medial stability of the ankle joint and the medial longitudinal arch. They hold the calcaneus and navicular bones snugly against the talus. Less than 10% of all ligament injuries to the ankle involve these ligaments.[14] In fact these ligaments are so strong that often an avulsion of the medial malleolus will occur instead of the ligament tearing. Three superficial ligaments and one deep ligament comprise the medial collateral ligaments; the *tibionavicular, tibiocalcanean, posterior tibiotalar,* and *anterior tibiotalar* ligaments, respectively.

Tibionavicular Ligament

This ligament functions to stabilize the anterior portion of the ankle and subtalar joint, as well as to limit plantarflexion and pronation.

Tibiocalcanean Ligament

In addition to stabilizing the anterior ankle and subtalar joints, this ligament also functions in limiting pronation.

Posterior Tibiotalar Ligament

This ligament primarily limits dorsiflexion.

Anterior Tibiotalar Ligament

This two-part deep ligament functions in keeping the medial talus close to the medial malleolus, thus increasing medial stability of the ankle joint. Plantarflexion and pronation are also limited.

Lateral Collateral Ligaments

The lateral ligaments are not as strong as the medial ligaments and are injured much more frequently. They are the *anterior talofibular, posterior talofibular,* and *calcaneofibular* ligaments. Most injuries are to the anterior talofibular and calcaneofibular ligaments and occur during excessive supination of the foot. These ligaments become even more vulnerable to injury during paralysis or muscle weakness of the peroneal muscles.

Anterior Talofibular Ligament

In the majority of ligamentous injuries of the ankle joint, this ligament alone is injured. Excessive or forceful supination and inward rotation are usually the mechanisms of injury. This ligament limits plantarflexion and adduction, resists excessive inversion, and prevents the foot from moving forward relative to the tibia. The so-called anterior drawer test can be used to test for instability in cases of partial and total ligament tears.

Posterior Talofibular Ligament

Dorsiflexion and adduction are both limited by this ligament. It also resists excessive medial rotation and translation of the talus.

Calcaneofibular Ligament

This ligament provides resistance against extreme inversion, thus providing stability at the subtalar joint. It is sometimes injured along with the anterior talofibular ligament. Adduction is also limited by this ligament.

Intrinsic Ligaments

These ligaments originate, insert, and function within the foot. They function to provide stability and structure to the foot. Along with the aforementioned muscles and the *plantar aponeurosis* (arch ligament), these ligaments also help maintain the arches of the foot. Intrinsic ligaments form several articulations in the hindfoot, midfoot, and forefoot. The single articulation in the hindfoot is the *subtalar (talocalcaneal) joint*. The *talocalcaneonavicular, calcaneocuboid, cuboideonavicular, cuneonavicular, intercuneiform,* and *cuneocuboid* joints are the articulations of the midfoot (midtarsal joints). Lastly, the articulations of the forefoot are the *tarsometatarsal, intermetatarsal, MTP,* and *IP* joints.

Subtalar Joint

This multiaxial synovial joint, which involves primarily supination (inversion, adduction, and plantarflexion) and pronation (eversion, abduction, and dorsiflexion) movements, forms the articulation of the inferior talus with the superior calcaneus. It contains both anterior and posterior facets. As the foot progresses in inversion, the anterior calcaneus slightly adducts and plantarflexes on the fixed talus; conversely, during eversion, both abduction and dorsiflexion of the calcaneus occur. The movements at this joint have been compared to the movements of a ship at sea, for the calcaneus pitches, turns, and rolls under the talus. Powerful *medial, lateral, posterior,* and *interosseous talocalcaneal* ligaments provide stability during the supination and pronation movements that occur at this joint, as well as strengthen the medial arch of the foot. These ligaments resist violent short-term stresses imposed upon the foot. The medial, lateral, and posterior talocalcaneal ligaments provide stability and thickening of the joint capsule. Functionally, the interosseous talocalcaneal ligament is the most important. It is composed of anterior and posterior bands, which tightly bind the talus to the calcaneus. The anterior portion of this ligament limits eversion, while inversion is limited by the powerful posterior bands. The interosseous talocalcaneal ligament is primarily responsible for limiting supination and pronation movements of the foot. In addition, the posterior talocalcaneal ligament aids in limiting inversion, while the lateral talocalcaneal ligament helps limit eversion.

Talocalcaneonavicular Joint

This joint, which is closely related to the subtalar joint, allows for supination and pronation movements. Ligaments supporting this joint are the *dorsal talonavicular, bifurcated (Y-shaped),* and *plantar calcaneonavicular (spring)* ligaments.

Dorsal Talonavicular Ligament

This ligament reinforces the joint dorsally. Since the tibialis posterior displaces the navicular medially and inferiorly relative to the talus, this ligament is responsible for limiting that translation. Even though it is fairly weak, it is considered a major ligament in limiting inversion.

Bifurcated (Y-shaped) Ligament

This ligament is composed of a medial (lateral calcaneonavicular) and lateral (medial calcaneocuboid) band, which form a solid right angle superiorly and laterally. It is considered a principal support to the midtarsal joints; consequently, abnormal stretching of this ligament can cause laxity and instability at these joints. It is primarily the function of the medial band to support this joint. Since the medial band is under tension in eversion, it helps to limit this movement. The medial band also provides lateral support for this joint and aids in limiting dorsiflexion.

Plantar Calcaneonavicular (Spring) Ligament

This ligament is called the spring ligament because of its abundant supply of elastic fibers. It functions as a bond between the calcaneus and navicular bones, preventing the medial longitudinal arch from collapsing. This ligament and the talocalcaneal ligament are the most important ligaments in providing elasticity and spring to the medial arch of the foot. As this arch yields, which occurs during gait, the talar head is pressed inferiorly, medially, and anteriorly. Consequently, the foot is flattened, expanded, and turned outward. Under normal conditions, the resilient foot will once again assume a normal arch. However, if these ligaments are abnormally stretched, the foot may permanently assume the flat foot position. Like the medial band of the bifurcated ligament, the spring ligament is under tension in eversion; therefore, this movement and dorsiflexion are limited. Since the deltoid ligament is attached to the medial border of this ligament, medial displacement of the talus is limited. Abnormal stretching of this ligament may result in medial and inferior deviation of the talar head.

Calcaneocuboid Joint

The articulation between the anterior calcaneus and the posterior cuboid occurs at this saddle-shaped joint. It is supported by the *bifurcated, dorsal calcaneocuboid,* and *plantar calcaneocuboid (long* and *short plantar)* ligaments. This joint provides limited supination and pronation movements, primarily during inversion and eversion. The calcaneocuboid and talocalcaneonavicular joints are collectively referred to as the *transverse tarsal joint (Chopart's joint).* The transverse tarsal joint usually moves in conjunction with the subtalar joint, and together they make up the *subtalar complex.* The axes of the subtalar complex run in an anterior, medial, and inferior direction. When the foot pronates, the talocalcaneonavicular and calcaneocuboid axes parallel each other, thus allowing greater range of motion (i.e., the foot becomes unstable). Conversely, as the foot supinates, these axes diverge, thus decreasing range of motion and increasing stability. During gait, the subtalar complex receives the body weight and transmits it to the longitudinal lateral arch before it is accepted by the medial arch.

Bifurcated Ligament

It is the lateral band of this ligament (the medial calcaneocuboid ligament) that limits inferior translation of the cuboid as it moves over the convex facet of the calcaneus. This ligament also aids in limiting inversion.

Dorsal Calcaneocuboid Ligament

This ligament, in addition to thickening and strengthening the capsule of this joint, is responsible for limiting medial translation of the cuboid and also aids in limiting inversion.

Plantar Calcaneocuboid Ligament

This ligament is composed of deep *(short plantar ligament)* and superficial *(long plantar ligament)* layers. Proper functioning of this ligament (especially the long plantar ligament) is very important in maintaining the lateral longitudinal arch of the foot. It functions as a bond between the calcaneal tubercle and the plantar surface of the cuboid. In addition, it spans nearly the entire length of the lateral longitudinal arch. Comparatively, the medial longitudinal arch is much more flexible than the lateral arch due to the increased mobility of the talus on the calcaneus. A rigid lateral arch is necessary because it is this arch that first receives the propulsive thrust generated by the triceps surae during gait. The powerful plantar calcaneocuboid ligament helps maintain the rigidity of this arch by preventing the interspaces of the calcaneocuboid and cubometatarsal joints from opening out inferiorly. Lastly, this ligament acts powerfully in limiting both inversion and dorsiflexion.

Cuboideonavicular Joint

The cuboid and navicular bones are held together by the *plantar, dorsal,* and *interosseous* ligaments. These strong ligaments limit this fibrous joint to slight gliding and rotational movements, especially the strong transverse fibers of the interosseous ligament.

Cuneonavicular, Intercuneiform, and Cuneocuboid Joints

These plane synovial joints, which collectively form the distal intertarsal joints, all share a common capsule and synovial cavity. There are three bundles each of *plantar* and *dorsal cuneonavicular ligaments,* which connect the navicular bone to the three cuneiform bones. Multiple *dorsal, plantar,* and *interosseous intercuneiform ligaments* connect the cuneiform bones together. Lastly, *dorsal, plantar,* and *interosseous cuneocuboid ligaments* provides stability between the lateral cuneiform and the cuboid. While the dorsal ligaments of these joints are fairly weak, the plantar and interosseous ligaments are quite strong. The slight gliding and rotational movements provided at each of these joints enhance foot flexibility and mobility. Since the dorsal and plantar cuneonavicular ligaments are longitudinal bands, slight displacements of the three cuneiform bones relative to the navicular take place along the long axis of the foot. Consequently, the curvature of the longitudinal medial arch is enhanced.

Tarsometatarsal Joints (Joint of Lisfranc)

These plane synovial joints, which are formed by articulations of the cuneiform and cuboid bones with the proximal metatarsal bones, consist of *medial, intermediate,* and *lateral* tarsometatarsal joints. The medial (cuneometatarsal) joint is formed by the articulation between the medial cuneiform and the first metatarsal; the intermediate (cuneometatarsal) joint is formed by articulations between the intermediate and lateral cuneiforms and the second and third metatarsals; the lateral (cubometatarsal) joint is formed between the cuboid and the fourth and fifth metatarsals. These articulations allow slight gliding and sliding movements, with most of the movement occurring at the medial and lateral joints. This arrangement allows the foot to be more flexible at these joints while providing stability to the transverse arch in the middle section of the foot (intermediate joint). All the tarsometatarsal joints except the first have a continuous articular capsule. These cuneometatarsal and cubometatarsal joints are held together by powerful *dorsal, plantar,* and *interosseous* ligaments, which give stability to the medial and lateral longitudinal arches, as well as to the transverse arch.

Plantar Ligaments

Plantar Cuneometatarsal Ligaments These ligaments, which generally are quite strong, provide stability between the cuneiforms and first through third metatarsals. Collectively they help support the medial longitudinal arch of the foot. They are composed of both longitudinal and oblique fibrous bands. Since the first metatarsal has

long been accepted as an important stabilizer during weight-bearing, normal function of the first cuneometatarsal ligament (medial joint) is essential. It has been shown that this ligament alone, independent of the removal of plantar skin, fascia, and intrinsic musculature, can affect stability during weight-bearing.[13] If this ligament is injured and functions abnormally, the distal first metatarsal tends to displace dorsally during weight-bearing. Consequently a lateral shifting of weight occurs, often followed by metatarsal pain.

Plantar Cubometatarsal Ligaments These ligaments provide stability between the cuboid and the fourth and fifth metatarsal bones. In addition, they assist the plantar calcaneocuboid (long plantar) ligament in preventing the interspace of the cubometatarsal joint from opening out inferiorly.

Dorsal Ligaments

Dorsal Cuneometatarsal Ligaments While a single fibrous band enhances stability at the first, third, and fourth cuneometatarsal joints, the second cuneometatarsal is composed of three dorsal ligaments—one from each cuneiform. Consequently, this is the most stable of the tarsometatarsal joints.

Dorsal Cubometatarsal Ligament One strong fibrous band provides stability at the fourth and fifth cubometatarsal joints.

Interosseous Ligaments

Interosseous Cuneometatarsal Ligaments The intermediate cuneiform is the cornerstone of the transverse arch, and the three interosseous cuneometatarsal ligaments help maintain the rigidity of this arch. Two of the ligaments provide stability at the second cuneometatarsal joint, while the final ligament helps maintain the integrity of the third cuneometatarsal joint.

Intermetatarsal Joints

These four plane synovial joints, which are formed by articulations between the lateral four metatarsals, permit slight gliding movements. The base of the first metatarsal resembles the thumb in that no ligaments connect it to the second metatarsal. The bases of the second through fifth metatarsal bones are tightly bound together by *dorsal, plantar,* and *interosseous ligaments.* The transverse fibrous bands of the dorsal and plantar ligaments, although relatively weak, provide some support to the transverse arch; however, the much stronger transverse fibers of the interosseous ligaments provide much more support to the transverse arch. This arch is further supported by the *deep transverse metatarsal ligament,* whose transverse fibers connect the heads of all the metatarsal bones. Since the first and fifth metatarsals are not tightly bound together with their respective adjacent metatarsals, increased flexibility of the forefoot is permitted.

Metatarsophalangeal Joints

These five condyloid synovial joints permit flexion, extension, abduction, and adduction. Due to the size of the first metatarsal bone and the presence of two sesamoid bones (medial and lateral), the first MTP joint is the largest of these joints. These medial and lateral sesamoid bones articulate with the plantar surface of the first metatarsal head. They are connected to each other by an *intersesamoidal ligament* and connected to the metatarsal head by *medial* and *lateral metatarsal sesamoid ligaments.* These ligaments aid in stability during weight-bearing (e.g., during the end of the stance phase in gait) since both sesamoid bones and the first metatarsal head must absorb large forces during this phase. Each of the MTP joints is stabilized by strong, thick *medial* and *lateral collateral ligaments.* The plantar portion of the joint capsules is strengthened by thick, dense *plantar ligaments.* These fibrocartilaginous plates are firmly attached to the articular surfaces of the proximal phalanges, thus helping to limit joint dorsiflexion. They are also attached to the collateral ligaments and are interconnected by the deep transverse metatarsal ligament. This arrangement assists in transferring forces between the flexor tendons, plantar fascia, and metatarsal heads.

Interphalangeal Joints

These synovial hinge joints allow only dorsiflexion and plantarflexion, and are formed by the head and base of adjacent phalanges. The arrangement of these joints is quite similar to that of the MTP joints. Stability of these joints is provided by *medial* and *lateral collateral ligaments,* as well as *plantar ligaments* composed of fibrocartilaginous plates. These ligaments aid in limiting dorsiflexion by tightening as these joints dorsiflex. Greater plantarflexion is permitted at the PIP joints than at the DIP joints.

Common Foot Disorders

This section discusses several common foot disorders influenced by or causing abnormal muscle and ligament function. There are many factors that adversely affect each of the following disorders, but only abnormal muscle and ligament function relative to each disorder are addressed here.

Pes Calcaneus

This deformity occurs when the anterior foot is held in a dorsiflexed position, thus causing a person to walk on their heels. This occurs primarily because of muscle imbalance and weakness, especially between the triceps surae and tibialis anterior, rather than structural abnormality. This condition worsens as the plantarflexing muscles of the posterior compartment weaken, and the anterior compartment muscles, which dorsiflex, become stronger. Not only is foot stability compromised due to having the anterior foot off the ground, but there is also an inability to push off with the toe during gait. In this dorsiflexed position, the muscles of the deep posterior (primarily the tibialis posterior) and lateral (peroneals) compartments are stretched; consequently, the tension exerted by these muscles helps depress the metatarsus and the distal tarsus. This effect causes a cavus deformity, in which the flexors of the plantar surface of the foot now have a shortened excursion range and the extensors on the dorsal surface have an increased excursion range. A muscle imbalance resulting in toe clawing occurs between the toe extensors and flexors, with the flexors being at an advantage. With the metatarsal heads depressed, hyperextension occurs at the MTP joints, while flexion occurs at the IP joints. This deformity is called claw toes.

Anatomy and Physiology

Pes Cavus (Claw Foot)

Pes cavus is a foot with an excessively high longitudinal arch (Fig. 5-1). The foot is supported primarily by the heel and the metatarsal heads. The failure of the arch to flatten, though not well understood, is thought to be due to combinations of the following mechanisms: (1) muscle and ligament contractures on the plantar surface, (2) muscle imbalances among extrinsic muscles, (3) muscle imbalances among intrinsic muscles, and (4) muscle imbalances between intrinsic and extrinsic muscles.

As mentioned previously, ligaments provide foot integrity (especially between tarsal bones) primarily under static loading (e.g., normal standing) or nonweight-bearing conditions. There are five primary ligamentous structures that provide integrity to the medial and lateral longitudinal arches of the foot: (1) the short and long plantar ligaments (lateral longitudinal arch), (2) the talocalcaneal and plantar calcaneonavicular ligaments (medial longitudinal arch), and (3) the plantar aponeurosis (both medial and lateral arches). If these plantar ligaments incur a state of contracture, a cavus deformity may follow. Secondarily, the heel may be tilted into a slight varus position due to contractures of these ligaments. Contractures of muscles on the plantar surface can also help create a cavus condition. Although this is uncommon, it can occur when wearing shoes with too rigid soles or when the plantar aponeurosis shortens. Contracture of the plantar aponeurosis alone has been thought to cause a cavus disorder.[5] This shortening causes the forefoot to move inferiorly and medially, causing both a cavus and a varus deformity.

The mechanism of extrinsic muscle imbalance involves several theories. In general, a simple muscle mechanical model can explain how muscle function affects the arch. The longitudinal arch is flattened due to the weight of the body as well as contractions from muscles inserted into the convex dorsal surface of the foot. These are the triceps surae, tibialis anterior, peroneus tertius, extensor digitorum longus, and extensor hallucis longus. The last two muscles are effective only if stabilized by the interosseous muscles. If these muscle are underactive, a cavus deformity may result. Similarly, the longitudinal arch is hollowed by contractions of muscles inserted into the concave plantar surface of the foot. These muscles are the tibialis posterior,

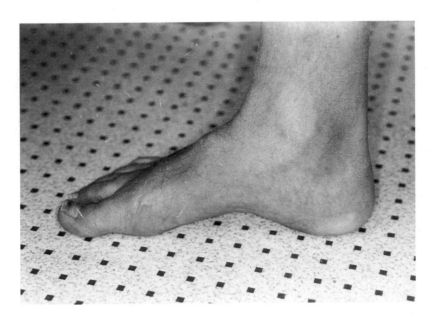

Fig. 5-1 Pes cavus (claw foot). (Courtesy of Kenneth W. Bramlett, Alabama Sports Medicine and Orthopaedic Center, Birmingham, Ala.)

peroneus longus, peroneus brevis, flexor digitorum longus, and flexor hallucis longus. Overactivity of these muscles can result in a cavus deformity. It should be clear by now that there are many combinations of extrinsic muscle dysfunction that can lead to the pes cavus condition.

More specifically, one theory suggests that a strong peroneus longus and a weak tibialis anterior cause the first metatarsal and medial cuneiform to plantarflex and abduct.[1] The extensor digitorum longus attempts to compensate for the weak tibialis anterior; however, because its function is to slightly evert and abduct the foot, it collaborates with the peroneus longus in creating a slight valgus deformity. A weak peroneus brevis has been thought to exacerbate this problem by causing the peroneus longus to hypertrophy, thus overpowering the tibialis anterior.[8]

Another theory involves overactivity or contracture of the posterior tibialis and peroneal muscles functioning against a weak triceps surae.[12] It has been shown that both the peroneal and posterior tibialis muscles actively increase the height of the arch. In particular, the peroneal longus powerfully depresses the medial border of the forefoot by turning it laterally. Consequently, the plantar arch is narrowed and its curvature increased.

Garceau and Brahms proposed that there are four intrinsic muscles that may cause a cavus deformity.[7] They are the adductor hallucis, flexor digitorum brevis, flexor hallucis brevis, and quadratus plantae muscles. All of these muscles are flexors of the foot and may shorten the foot and elevate the arch.

Combined extrinsic and intrinsic muscle imbalances can also lead to a cavus deformity as well as secondary claw toes and varus heel deformities. Chuinard and Baskin proposed that the extrinsic and intrinsic muscles of the foot and ankle form a right triangle; consequently, imbalances within this triangle may lead to a cavus deformity.[2] Claw toes can occur either mechanically or due to muscle imbalances between the long and short extensors and the interossei and lumbricales. Mechanically, a cavus deformity causes the anterior foot to drop. It has been postulated that this causes the long extensors to shorten, thus causing hyperextension at the MTP joints.[3]

Subsequently, the flexor tendons shorten, causing flexion at the IP joints. Another mechanical possibility assumes that during a cavus condition the toes need to be hyperextended to clear the ground during the swing phase in gait. The extensor hallucis longus and the extensor digitorum longus then have to work harder; therefore, these muscles hypertrophy and become stronger. The combination of a stronger pull by the toe extensor muscles and an already abnormally high arch causes hyperextension at the MTP joints. This causes the bases of the proximal phalanges to sublux dorsally over already depressed metatarsal heads. The lumbricales and interossei muscles now contract dorsal to their flexor axis at the MTP joints. Consequently, these muscles now reverse their function; they become extensors at the MTP joints and flexors at the IP joints.

Claw toe of the hallux can also occur due to an underactive tibialis anterior and an overactive peroneus longus. The tibialis anterior functions to elevate the first metatarsal, while the peroneus longus acts to depress it. These antagonistic actions may produce a depressed metatarsal head.

Duchenne stated that a claw toe deformity was due to muscle imbalances rather than mechanical abnormalities.[4] He implied that claw toe was a primary cause of pes cavus rather than vice versa. His reasoning was as follows: The primary functions of the long extensors and flexors are to extend the proximal phalanges and flex the distal phalanges, respectively. The long extensors have a secondary role of extending the middle and distal phalanges; similarly, the long flexors have a secondary role in flexing the proximal phalanges. These primary and secondary functions are opposed by the interossei and lumbricales, which flex the proximal phalanges and extend the IP joints. Due to the primary function of the long extensors to powerfully extend the proximal phalanges, any dysfunction of these intrinsic muscles can quickly lead to a claw toe disorder. Consequently, the proximal phalanges assume a state of hyperextension, while the middle and distal phalanges are hyperflexed. Duchenne deduced from this that the extreme hyperextended position of the proximal phalanges exerted forces onto the metatarsal heads, thus depressing them and creating a cavus deformity.

Anatomy and Physiology

Pes Equinus (Drop Foot)

Drop foot is a condition where the foot is fixed in a plantarflexed position. This position is usually due to muscle imbalances between the muscles of the anterior (dorsiflexors), lateral (plantarflexors), and posterior (plantarflexors) compartments. Muscle imbalances between extrinsic and intrinsic muscles can also produce an equinus deformity. Weak or inactive dorsiflexors (e.g., due to paresis or paralysis of the common peroneal nerve) can cause the foot to drop, as can overactive plantarflexors. Contractures occurring in plantarflexor muscles (e.g., injured triceps surae) can also lead to drop foot. Usually a varus or valgus component accompanies drop foot. These deformities are known as *equinovarus (clubfoot)* or *equinovalgus (convex pes valgus* or *vertical talus),* respectively. They may occur due to abnormal function of the extrinsic muscles of the three compartments. Most of these extrinsic muscles produce other movements in addition to dorsiflexion and plantarflexion. This is true because these muscles traverse more than one joint. All the long tendons of the foot insert distal to the subtalar and transverse tarsal joints, thus causing movements at multiple joints. An equinovarus deformity can occur when the peroneal and toe extensor muscles are weak or nonfunctional since these muscles help position the foot in a valgus position. An overactive or contractured posterior tibialis, triceps surae, or flexor digitorum longus—as well as laxity in lateral ankle ligaments or contractures in medial ankle ligaments—can exacerbate equinovarus. The posterior tibialis muscle further worsens this deformity by its tendency to elevate the medial longitudinal arch of the foot. In general, overactive foot supinators and underactive foot pronators can produce equinovarus. Paralysis of the intrinsic muscles may play a role in producing a convex sole.

Congenital vertical talus is largely due to soft tissue contractures. Contractures of the tibionavicular portion of the deltoid ligament, the bifurcated ligament, the dorsal capsule ligament of the talonavicular joint, and the calcaneofibular ligament tightly bind the navicular to the upper surface of the talar head. Muscle contractures deform the foot in a equinovalgus position. The muscles involved are primarily the triceps surae, long toe extensors, and peroneal muscles.

A weak tibialis anterior, which ineffectively adducts the foot as it dorsiflexes, and overpowering peroneals, which abduct the foot as they aid in plantarflexion, can cause a equinovalgus condition. In addition, an inactive tibialis posterior and an overactive triceps surae can also produce this deformity. Laxity in the medial ankle ligaments or contractures in lateral ankle ligaments may worsen equinovalgus. The primary factor in causing convex pes valgus seems to be muscle imbalances between the foot invertors and evertors. In addition, paralysis or weakness in the intrinsic muscles may play a role in the convex shape of the plantar surface of the foot.

Pes Planus (Flat Foot)

Flat foot occurs when the arches of the foot (the medial longitudinal arch primarily) are no longer able to maintain their normal curvatures (Fig. 5-2). The extent of this disorder can be determined visually by comparing the patient's footprint with a normal footprint. Using this method, flat foot can be effectively diagnosed if the medial border of the foot is gradually filled out. Flat foot is usually due to muscle insufficiency. The primary muscles involved are also the main muscles that provide support to the medial longitudinal and transverse arches of the foot; namely, the tibialis posterior and the peroneus longus muscles. However, the tibialis anterior may also contribute to the deformity. A more lateral insertion on the first metatarsal would increase its eversion tendencies at the subtalar joint while concurrently decreasing its ability to invert at the transverse tarsal joint. This may exacerbate an evolving flat foot condition.

Paralysis, chronic stress due to overuse, or general weakness due to underuse are common etiologies of abnormal function in these muscles. In the absence of normal muscular function, the plantar ligaments and plantar aponeurosis incur abnormal stresses, which eventually cause them to become abnormally stretched. Stretching of these and other midtarsal ligaments produces ligamentous laxity within the midtarsal joints. Consequently, there is an increased parallelism between the axes of the talocalcaneal and trans-

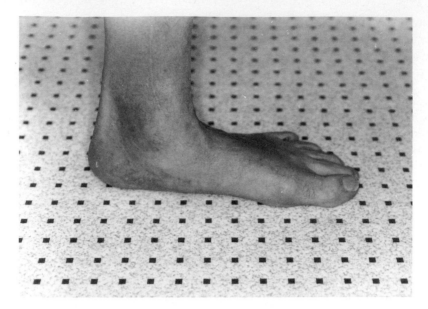

Fig. 5-2 Pes planus (flat foot). (Courtesy of Kenneth W. Bramlett, Alabama Sports Medicine and Orthopaedic Center, Birmingham, Ala.)

verse tarsal joints and between the axes of the talocalcaneonavicular and calcaneocuboid joints. This causes increased transverse motion and instability of the talus. Muscles not normally recruited become active to compensate for the abnormally functioning ligaments.

During gait or other weight-bearing activity, the plantar aponeurosis plays a very important role in helping to prevent the longitudinal arches of the foot from flattening excessively. When the MTP joints are extended, the windlass of the plantar aponeurosis tightens, thus raising the longitudinal arch. With abnormal stress the spring ligament can no longer adequately support the talar head, causing the medial longitudinal arch to flatten. Due to stretched or strained plantar muscles, plantar aponeurosis, and plantar ligaments, pain often accompanies this disorder.

During gait, there is increased time for foot inversion during the toe-off phase, thus allowing the longitudinal arch to be raised. This is often accompanied by greater activity from the intrinsic muscles. Over time, this can produce a chronic fatigue condition of these muscles.

During weight-bearing with a collapsed medial arch, a valgus deformity can occur. This oc-

curs for two primary reasons. First, since the aforementioned muscles all support the transverse arch, their dysfunction results in a flattening of this arch. This, coupled with a flattened medial arch, causes the forefoot to rotate medially along its longitudinal axis. A slight lateral displacement of the forefoot results. Second, the calcaneus rotates medially along its long axis as the foot pronates and tends to lie on its medial surface. As this valgus deformity increases, the interosseous talocalcaneal ligament may be abnormally stretched, thus adversely affecting the function of this ligament in limiting pronation. The effects of this valgus deformity are increased stress on the medial aspect of the foot, and a talar head that is displaced medially and inferiorly.

Hallux Valgus (Bunion)

This deformity occurs when the great toe is laterally displaced and pronated (i.e., rotated medially) in a valgus position and the first metatarsal is displaced medially in a varus position (Fig. 5-3). Consequently, several mechanical changes occur within the extrinsic and intrinsic musculature. First, the abductor hallucis longus is displaced inferiorly and bowstringed, while the

Anatomy and Physiology

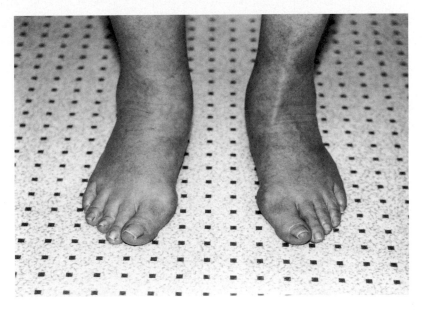

Fig. 5-3 Hallux valgus (bunion). (Courtesy of Kenneth W. Bramlett, Alabama Sports Medicine and Orthopaedic Center, Birmingham, Ala.)

flexor and extensor hallucis longus and flexor hallucis brevis muscles are displaced laterally and bowstringed. These changes cause the abductor hallucis to change from an abductor of the great toe to a flexor, and the flexor hallucis longus, extensor hallucis longus, and flexor hallucis brevis muscles to increase their mechanical advantage for adduction of the great toe. Collectively, these changes produce an increased valgus force on the great toe, thus exacerbating the already lateral displaced phalanx. As the valgus deformity progresses, the hallux often underlaps the second toe. This causes hammering or clawing of the second toe, as well as medial displacement. Dorsal subluxation at the second MTP joint also occurs. This can cause the base of the second proximal phalanx to be displaced superiorly and permanently fixed over the metatarsal head. As a result, the line of pull by the lumbricales and dorsal interossei changes, and they may now act as extensors of the second MTP joint and flexors of the PIP and DIP joints. This causes hyperextension of the MTP joint and flexion at the PIP and DIP joints; therefore, a claw or hammer toe condition occurs.

If extension occurs at the MTP joint, flexion at the PIP joint, and slight flexion or a neutral position at the DIP joint, the condition is referred to as hammer toe. Hammer toe, which is a type of claw toe, usually occurs in the second digit in conjunction with hallux valgus. Because of the extensor sling mechanism mentioned previously, only when the proximal phalanx is in a neutral or flexed position can the extensor digitorum extend the PIP joints. This is important to understand in hammer or toe claw deformities because the hyperextension of the MTP joints that normally occurs during these conditions inhibits PIP joint extension. Since the tendons of the flexor digitorum longus and brevis insert on the middle and distal phalanges, flexor influence at the MTP joints is minimal. This is especially true when the MTP is hyperextended. It is the plantar plate and capsule under the MTP joint that primarily resists hyperextension of this joint. As these structures are abnormally stretched, their ability to restore the joint to its normal function is lost.

Clearly this anatomical arrangement of toe flexors and extensors favors flexion at the PIP and DIP joints when the MTP joint is extended. As previously mentioned, hyperextension at the

MTP joint and flexion at the PIP and DIP joints describes a claw toe condition. Over time, contractures at the second MTP, PIP, and DIP joints can occur in the lumbricales, dorsal interossei, flexors, and extensor muscles, as well as in the collateral ligaments. A once flexible claw or hammer toe now becomes rigid.

Articular changes also occur at the first tarso-metatarsal and MTP joints, which are subluxed laterally. Consequently, the medial collateral ligament and medial capsule of the first MTP joint may be stretched, thus causing an inflammation to occur over the soft tissue of the medial metatarsal head. This painful condition is referred to as a bunion. A bunion may also be partially formed by the uncovering of the medial metatarsal head, as well as by exostotic formations and bursal thickening. The lateral subluxation of the first MTP joint may also sublux the two sesamoid bones laterally, causing the medial sesamoid ligament to stretch and the lateral sesamoid ligament to shorten. This new position of the sesamoids under the metatarsal head can cause abnormal stress to these bones during weight-bearing.

In summary, the diagnosis and treatment of muscle and ligament foot disorders can be quite complicated because numerous intricacies are involved. Nevertheless, understanding normal and abnormal muscle and ligament function can greatly help clinicians in their rehabilitative endeavors. The majestic design of the foot mandates careful study and analysis with respect to both structure and function. The importance of visually anatomizing the ligamentous and muscle structures of the foot cannot be overstressed, for it is at the anatomical level that one's understanding of muscle and ligament physiology begins.

Acknowledgement

The author would like to extend a special thanks to Julie Jinkins, P.T., A.T.,C., and Yvonne Satterwhite, M.D., for their critical review of this manuscript. Miss Jinkins is currently employed as a physical therapist at HealthSouth Medical Center, Birmingham, Ala. Dr. Satterwhite is presently an orthopedic surgeon at Kentucky Sports Medicine, Lexington, Ky. The author would also like to recognize the American Sports Medicine Institute, Birmingham for their support. A special thanks is also extended to Dr. Kenneth W. Bramlett, who supplied the pes planus, pes cavus, and hallux valgus figures. Dr. Bramlett is employed by Alabama Sports Medicine and Orthopaedic Center, Birmingham, Ala. Finally, a special thanks to my family for all their love, support, and encouragement throughout the writing of this manuscript. I love them dearly.

Bibliography

1. Bentzon PGK: Pes cavus and the medial peroneus longus, *Acta Orthop Scand* 4:50, 1933.
2. Chuinard EG, Baskin M: Claw-foot deformity: treatment by transfer of the long extensors into the metatarsals and fusion of the interphalangeal joints, *J Bone Joint Surg* 55A:351, 1973.
3. Daw SW: Clawfoot, *Clin J* 61:13, 1932.
4. Duchenne GB: *The physiology of motion,* Philadelphia, 1959, WB Saunders (Translated by EB Kaplan).
5. Dwyer FC: The present status of the problem of pes cavus, *Clin Orthop* 106:254, 1975.
6. Evarts CM, editor: *Surgery of the musculoskeletal system,* vol 4, New York, 1990, Churchill Livingstone, p 3965.
7. Garceau GJ, Brahms MA: A preliminary study of selective plantar muscle denervation for pes cavus, *J Bone Joint Surg* 38A:553, 1956.
8. Hallgrimsson S: Studies on reconstructive and stabilizing operations on the skeleton of the foot with special reference to subastragalar arthrodesis in treatment of foot deformities following infantile paralysis, *Acta Chir Scand* 88(suppl 78):1, 1943.
9. Jahss MH: *Disorders of the foot and ankle,* vol 1, Philadelphia, 1991, WB Saunders, p 400.
10. Jahss MH: *Disorders of the foot and ankle,* vol 2, Philadelphia, 1991, WB Saunders, p 1287.
11. Kalin PJ, Hirsh BE: The origins and functions of the interosseous muscles of the foot, *J Anat* 152:83, 1987.
12. Karlholm B, Nilsonne U: Operative treatment of the foot deformity in Charcot-Marie-Tooth disease, *Acta Orthop Scand* 39:101, 1968.
13. Mizel MS: The role of the plantar first metatarsal first cuneiform ligament in weightbearing on the first metatarsal, *Foot Ankle* 14:82, 1993.
14. Peterson L, Renstrom P: *Sports injuries,* St Louis, 1986, Mosby Year Book, p 345.
15. Steindler A: *Mechanics of normal and pathological locomotion in man,* Springfield, Ill, 1935, Charles C Thomas, pp 260, 265, 267.

Anatomy and Physiology

6

Proprioception in Injury Prevention and Rehabilitation of Ankle Sprains

Paul S. Cooper

Ankle sprains are currently the most common specific injury in most sports. Jackson et al, in a 1974 study at the U.S. Military Academy at West Point, reported that approximately one third of the cadet population had sustained one or more inversion sprains over the 4-year period.[38] Similarly, a study conducted at the U.S. Naval Academy indicated that 17% of athletes selected at random reported a history of ankle instability.[6] Garrick reported that over a 6-year period no less than one sixth of time lost to injuries involved ankle sprains.[26] Basketball was involved in 38% of all ankle injuries reported in men and 45% in women. Football, followed by women's cross-country, had the next highest frequency of ankle injuries. Mack, in 1975, reported that ankle sprains made up approximately 25% of all time-loss injuries in every running to jumping sport.[50]

While the majority of ankle sprains are isolated events that resolve uneventfully, a significant number of sprains result in chronic instability. Chronic instability due to mechanical instability consists of laxity of the lateral ankle ligaments in restraining both anterior and varus forces to the

ankle. More often, however, subjective sensations of "giving way" have been described in the weight-bearing ankle following injury. In the absence of defined mechanical instability, this is termed *residual functional instability*. Functional instability has been reported as a sequela in 20% to 40% of ankle sprains in various series.[5,20,21,62] Bosien et al are generally credited with first identifying and approaching the problem of residual symptoms.[5] A study at Dartmouth College of 148 patients with 177 ankle sprains after a mean follow-up of 29 months revealed that 43% had residual changes. The single causative factor identified with statistical significance was an associated peroneal weakness in 66% of the individuals with residual changes and ankle symptoms. Bosien et al concluded that early peroneal muscle strengthening through resistive exercises was crucial to correct such disabilities.

Freeman et al, in 1965, have been acknowledged as providing the definitive work attributing functional instability to a proprioceptive deficit.[20,21] At a 1-year follow-up of 42 ankle sprains, they noted that 17 patients had no clinical or radiographic evidence of instability but still complained of functional instability. By using a modified Romberg test to assess for a proprioception deficit, the authors found some degree of proprioceptive disturbance in 34% to 84% of the groups studied. They postulated that a partial "deafferentiation" occurs from damage to the afferent joint receptors sustained with a lateral ankle ligament injury. They concluded that "mechanical instability rarely, if ever is responsible for initiating this disability." Staples, in 1972, reported residual symptoms in 51 ankles (42% of those studied) after an average follow-up of 9.4 years, with 18% of the ankles having no evidence of instability.[62] He summarized that "lateral ligament defects, either early or late, are not the essential basis of annoying residual symptoms so frequently found in these patients; and that motor weakness or a proprioceptive defect or some other abnormality is the crucial matter." In a follow-up study in 1975, he outlined four possible causes for functional complaints, including mechanical instability, peroneal weakness, distal tibia-fibula sprains, and proprioceptive deficits. Brand et al, in 1981, having reviewed the literature on nonsurgical management of lateral ankle injuries, noted that 20% to 40% of sprains in all series had residual functional instability and therefore advocated early repair of the ligaments.[7]

The role of proprioception in contributing to residual functional instability extends to the risk for recurrent ankle injuries. Garrick and Requa noted that in individuals with a history of a previous ankle sprains there was a twofold likelihood of reinjury compared to their uninjured counterparts.[27] The likelihood increased to three times in athletes with a history of "frequent" previous ankle sprains. The relationship of chronic ankle instability to articular damage was examined by Harrington, who documented degenerative arthrosis in 28 of 36 individuals (78%) with chronic instability and symptomatic ankles as seen on standing ankle films; 12 patients were confirmed by arthroscopy.[36] He concluded that restoration of lateral ankle stability could potentially arrest progression of the degenerative changes seen.

Surprisingly, the role of proprioception in ankle injury rehabilitation and injury prevention has been either poorly understood or not generally accepted by physicians. Kay reported that 48% of physicians and paramedical specialists responding to a questionnaire on management of Grade II and III ankle sprains had prescribed range of motion and muscle strengthening exercises in the rehabilitation program.[42] In contrast, only 11% of those questioned had similarly prescribed a proprioception reeducation program. Kay noted that only 3% of family practitioners, 2% of emergency room physicians, and 24% of orthopedic surgeons had advocated proprioception training as part of the rehabilitation program.

Ankle Joint Neurophysiology

Sensations originating about joints yield information to the body on proprioception. While no accepted definition of proprioception exists, Beard et al summarize proprioception as consisting of three components: (1) a static awareness of joint position, (2) kinesthetic awareness (the detection of movement and acceleration), and (3) a closed loop efferent reflex response required for regulation of muscle tone and activity.[3] The specialized end organs capable of converting the mechanical energy of physical deformation into action nerve potentials to yield information on proprioception are referred to as mechanoreceptors. Common to all receptors is the extinction phenomenon, with each specific type of receptor varying in the pattern and duration of response after stimulus application. The receptors most frequently found in joint capsules and their associated ligaments include Pacinian corpuscles, Ruffini end organs, Golgi tendon apparatus, and free pain nerve endings. Pacinian corpuscles are examples of rapidly adaptive or phasic receptors, which exhibit extinction quickly from the time of stimulus application. They are sensitive to the onset of sudden changes and pressure movements and are therefore stimulated by the initiation or termination of joint motion, rapid acceleration or directional change, or a rapid loading or change in tension applied to the capsuloligamentous complex. These receptors are located at ligamentous insertions of associated joint capsules and serve to initiate protective reflexes. Golgi tendon capsules and Ruffini end organs are examples of slow-adapting or tonic receptors, which decline to a constant steady state of impulse generation with continued stimulation. They respond to constant pressures and slow changes and best yield information about body position as well as sensing motion and changes in the angle of rotation.[22] These receptors are sensitive to capsular stretching and serve to signal the proximity of a joint to the limits of motion.[65] Golgi and Ruffini receptors can be selectively stimulated and measured clinically through threshold of detection using a slow passive motion. At an angular velocity of .5 degrees per second, motion within 2 to 4 degrees can normally be detected. Muscle spindle fibers have been postulated to have a possible role in position sense through mediation of muscle tension from subcortical reflexes and therefore not under conscious level of control. Halata has isolated Ruffini corpuscle type mechanoreceptors in the skin surrounding the feline knee joint and found the receptors intimately associated with hair follicles (Pilo/Ruffini complex).[34] This similarity between cutaneous and joint receptors creates the potential to restore the loss of afferent proprioceptive input of the joint through cutaneous stimulation from a variety of external support devices. The afferent pathway of the mechanoreceptors is along the posterior column of the central nervous system and is carried on large myelinated fibers representing high conduction velocities. These fibers terminate on the cerebral cortex with a high degree of spatial orientation disproportionate for representation of the lower limb.[2] Freeman et al confirmed in feline knees that the afferent nerve pathway follows Hilton's law, where joints innervated by articular branches of nerves supply the muscles crossing the joint by eliciting a reflex contraction of the gastrocnemius muscle with ankle motion even after the division of all tendonous attachments, skin, and other sources of stimuli.[2,20,22,23]

Testing of Proprioception and Kinesthesia

Several theories have arisen concerning the etiology for dysfunction that causes recurrent ankle sprains. Insufficient protection of passive joint structures, exposing the lateral ligaments to excessive loads at high strain rates, has been a long popular theory.[37,53] Others advocate that recurrent sprains result from altered position sense and loss of postural reflexes from the initial trauma, as initially proposed by Freeman et al.[20,21,33] A third body of evidence emphasizes the importance of muscle receptors in signaling joint position and their subsequent damage with ankle sprains.[1,5,22] The clinical testing of proprioception and kinesthesia often utilizes passive movement testing, including kinesthesiometry, one-legged standing balance, and posturography. Threshold to detection measurements at slow passive angular velocities of .3 to .5 degrees per second are a common form of testing. This form of testing, however, does not recreate active the angular velocities often seen with vigorous activity. Another common test is repositioning of a joint to a predetermined angle established either actively or passively. Gross felt that passive positioning was superior to active in judging joint position.[33] A modified Rhomberg balance test to assess impaired stability while the individual stood on a single limb with eyes closed was advocated by Freeman et al and later Garn and Newton to discriminate for a proprioceptive deficit.[21,25] Gordon devised a simple pedal goniometer to assess ankle proprioception.[30] This consisted of a mobile uniaxial platform whereby the ankle joint would be moved passively without visual clues. Gordon states that the test was sensitive to detection within 1 degree of motion but was not able to accommodate for either velocity or angular changes.

Freeman et al noted in several studies that when testing individuals with ankle sprains using a modified Romberg test, proprioceptive disturbances were evident to some degree in 34% to 84% of patients studied.[20,21] None of these patients, however, had clinical evidence of mechanical instability, although stress radiography was not used. Based on previous work on the innervation of feline knee joints, Freeman and Wyke postulated that afferent nerve fibers of the joint capsule and ligaments surrounding the ankle subserve reflexes that help to stabilize the foot during locomotion.[23] They further proposed that a sprained ankle led to "deafferentiation" of the joint, and therefore protective reflex stabilization of the foot and ankle was impaired, leading to the subjective sensation of "giving way." Coordination exercises to reeducate the "central process" would compensate for the deafferentiation.[21]

Glencross and Thornton expanded on these observations and proposed that degree of proprioception loss was related to the severity of the ankle injury.[28] They evaluated 24 subjects after a minimum of 8 months' follow-up from injury, and classified them based on degree of severity and functional loss from injury. Ankles were passively repositioned from a starting angle of 110 degrees of plantarflexion into various degrees of plantarflexion, and the subject was then asked to replicate the target position. The authors noted that while significant errors in active replication of the target joint position were made in the injured group, no significant difference was noted among the three groups with regard to degree of ankle sprain. They also noted, however, that the greatest degree of error with active testing was noted at large angles of 130 to 140 degrees plantarflexion on the injured side. The finding of a specific angle yielding the greatest error on active replication of a target joint position has also been supported in studies of the knee joint, where near terminal extension has yielded the greatest discrepancy between sides.[11,48] Garn and Newton evaluated 30 athletes at the U.S. Naval Academy who had sustained multiple ankle sprains, the average being 5.7 sprains per ankle.[25] Using a one-legged balance test to detect passive plantarflexion movements on a tilt platform moving at .3 degrees per second, the authors found that subjects had significantly greater difficulty detecting passive motion in the injured ankle as compared to the uninjured side. The authors also noted that 67% of subjects had experienced either subjective or objective balance deficits using the modified Rhomberg test, which is higher than the 42% deficit Freeman et al noted with single sprain injuries.[21]

Increasing research has been directed at electromyographic (EMG) activity of ankle musculature in reflex stabilization responses to postural sway in the frontal coronal and sagittal planes. Deitz and Berger demonstrated the role of spinal stretch reflexes in equilibrium by measuring EMG responses of the anterior tibial tendon when individuals were subjected to an anterior sway on a balance board.[12] They noted coordinated right to left leg muscle activation at a spinal level to provide a symmetric leg muscle EMG during balancing. The authors felt that this was not a result of supraspinal motor involvement, due to the short latencies in the EMG studies. Diener et al examined latency responses to ankle joint displacements in patients with cortical or spinal cord lesions.[13] With use of a toe up tilt platform to evoke activity of the triceps surae, EMG responses were measured in 27 patients with spinal cord lesions, 20 with central and 18 with frontal lesions, compared with 50 normal subjects. They found median latencies absent in 47% of patients with spinal lesions and believed that muscle activity at the ankle joint level was secondary to segmental reflexes but that the amplitude was modulated by supraspinal structures. DeFabio contradicted prior findings that muscle patterns were preprogrammed and centrally driven.[15] He tested subjects using a forward body sway test and a hand-held response key pad to signal the onset of postural disturbance. EMG measurements were simultaneously obtained of the gastrocnemius muscles. The authors felt that surface orientation information obtained from the ankle contributed to an "online" correction of a wide range of postural disturbances. They proposed that balance was an automatic neuromuscular response that was peripherally driven and occurred on a subconscious level. Tropp et al found a predictive relationship between postural sway amplitude and risk for joint injury in both the uninjured and chronic ankle injury subjects.[64] The authors examined the unilateral postural sway in soccer players and found that abnormally large sway amplitudes were linked to a delay in muscle force generation at the ankle, thereby increasing the risk of injury.

Not all studies have correlated a latency of peroneal muscle activity with proprioceptive deficits in injured ankles. Isakov et al found no significant difference in peroneal EMG activity with sudden inversion displacement in both previously sprained and unsprained ankles.[37] The authors concluded that contraction of peroneal musculature was due to an arc stretch reflex and played no role in ankle joint protection; mechanical damage was felt to occur before recruitment. This was supported by Nawoczenski et al, who noted a trend in delay of peroneus longus motor response that was not statistically significant when compared to that in uninjured ankles using an inversion stress test.[53] Johnson and Johnson evaluated postoperative ankles using a 35-degree inversion drop platform test.[39] They found no statistically significant difference in latency times between groups of nonoperative, operative, and normal ankles. The authors refuted the concept of permanent deafferentiation proposed by Freeman and suggested that joint proprioceptors could in fact be reeducated to a level comparable to that of the uninjured ankle. Gross tested 14 subjects with a history of recurrent ankle sprains for active and passive replication of predetermined ankle joint positions using a Cybex II dynometer at .5 degree per second inversion and eversion speeds.[33] He found that ankle sprain injuries have no substantial effect on judgments of joint position and was unable to substantiate the findings of Glencross and Thornton. Gross concluded that while joint receptors have a dominant role in angular detection, muscle receptors yield the perception of joint motion. The muscle spindle receptors through both afferent and efferent intrafusal muscle fibers have been reported to measure muscle tension over a wide range of lengths.[48]

Identifying the Ankle at Risk

Factors placing the ankle at risk for initial or recurrent ankle sprains can be determined based on the history and physical examination of the athlete. A history of previous ankle injuries, especially in athletes with recurrent sprains during the childhood or adolescent period, has been strongly correlated with weaker ankles prone to injuries in the third and fourth decades.[56] Fiore and Leard noted that certain footwear and playing surfaces may add increased traction and rotation to prevent early foot release and may therefore potentiate ankle ligament injuries.[19] Findings on physical examination contributing to ankle sprains include peroneal muscle weakness, lateral ligament deficiency, generalized ligamentous laxity, joint adhesions, bony malalignment of the ankle joint, and a cavus or cavovarus foot.[5,62] Kaumeyer and Malone noted that loss of flexibility of the gastrocnemius muscle may limit dorsiflexion, thereby increasing subtalar supination and placing the ankle at high risk for injury.[41]

Treatment

Treatment of ankle sprains with proprioceptive deficits consists of a progressive series of coordination exercises to reeducate the ankle, the use of external support devices, and possibly surgical intervention. The ideal external support device provides for mechanical stability, swelling control, and proprioceptive feedback without limiting the normal range of motion or function of the ankle. Garrick noted that the use of either high-top athletic shoes or prophylactic ankle taping decreased the frequency of sprains most notably in those individuals with a history of prior sprains.[26] The normal frequency of 22 ankle sprains per 1000 player games was reduced to 6.5 sprains per 1000 games when a high-top sneaker and taping was used. A fivefold higher rate was noted when using a low-top athletic shoe and no taping support. Glick et al studied peroneus brevis activity in taped ankles.[29] They noted that the peroneus brevis activity was prolonged during the end of swing phase and felt that taping stimulated the peroneal tendons without decreasing muscle tone, thus serving a dynamic action in addition to a mechanical one.

Karlsson and Andreasson evaluated 20 patients with isolated chronic unilateral ankle instability with ankle taping applied.[40] Evaluation of mechanical stability with stress radiographs found little difference in the anterior drawer and talar tilt, either with or without taping. Peroneal muscle reaction time, with simulation of a sprain using a trap door tilting mechanism, was significantly shorter but did not reach that of the uninjured side. The greatest improvement was noted in those individuals with the greatest degree of instability.

Adhesive taping has been a popular form of external support for athletes for many years. Recent studies, however, have questioned the effectiveness of the taping over time with vigorous activity. Rarick et al found that 40% of the net support strength conferred by ankle taping was lost after 10 minutes of vigorous exercise.[55] Myburgh et al reported no significant restriction of ankle motion after 1 hour of athletic activity with ankle taping.[52] Although mechanical stability obtained by the taping may drop off quickly, taping may continue to serve a role in cutaneous proprioceptive feedback throughout the athletic event.

Stover advocated the use of a removable air stirrup spint to supplement afferent stimuli at the site of ankle injury while the reparative process takes place[63] (Fig. 6-1). The air cells attached to the stirrup splint could reach pressures of up to 75 mmHg weight-bearing, thus creating a milking effect on edematous tissue. Kimura et al postulated that these air cells conform to the skin and thus enhance cutaneous proprioceptive feedback.[44] The author's experience supports this theory, where individuals with cruciate-deficient knees and an initial marked proprioceptive deficit approached that of the cruciate intact knee while using a neoprene sleeve.[11] Greene and Hillman evaluated 7 female volleyball players before, during, and after 3 hours of play and com-

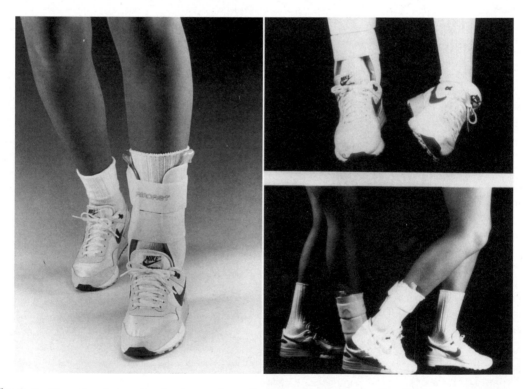

Fig. 6-1 Example of a popular air stirrup splint utilized for ankle sprains. It offers the advantages of mechanical stability to inversion stress without restriction of ankle plantarflexion and dorsiflexion new line. The stirrup splints may also serve to stimulate cutaneous mechanoreceptors. (Courtesy of Aircast, Inc., Summit, NJ.)

pared taping with an external support device.[32] While neither treatment restricted vertical jumping ability, the maximum loss of restriction with taping was seen at 20 minutes and was reduced from 41% to 15% of total inversion-eversion motion. The external support device was noted to maintain almost all of the initial restriction and only decreased from 42% to 37% of total restrictive inversion-eversion motion. Feuerback et al studied the effect of the air cast external support on unilateral postural sway in the coronal and sagittal planes.[18] Unilateral stability was enhanced in both static and dynamic testing in 15 volunteers. The authors also concluded that the air cast enhanced afferent feedback between the air cast and the cutaneous receptors and so improved postural stabilization.

Central to the return of proprioception in ankle sprains is the integration of balancing and coordination exercises into the rehabilitation protocol. Freeman advocated an early mobilization and coordination exercise program using balance board exercises, with a notable reduction in proprioception deficit.[20,21] Tropp et al found a significant improvement in ability to balance on the injured ankle after a 6-week regimen of balance board exercises.[64] Patients studied also reported a decrease in subjective "giving-way" sensations after completion of the training program. Glencross and Thornton summarized that rehabilitation was as much of a relearning process as it was a physical recovery from the sprain.[28] The outcome of improved proprioception is to improve the dynamic stability of the ankle joint, which then plays a protective role against future sprains. Beard et al noted that with autoconditioning of the cruciate-deficient knee, the faster contraction of hamstring muscles occurred.[3] This process can be applied to the ankle, and retraining of the peroneal muscles to contract faster may be achieved. Fiore and Leard described a protocol involving coordination exercises with unilateral balance boards, uniaxial and multiaxial teeter boards, and jumping rope.[19]

Strengthening, agility, and endurance were the final phase of the rehabilitation program. Kisner and Colby outline a protocol for proprioceptive rehabilitation of the sprained ankle in their text.[45] They emphasize weight-bearing training in order to stimulate proper functioning and balance of the extremity. Lattanza et al found a closed chain program in rehabilitation superior for range of motion in the subtalar joint as well as proprioceptive feedback.[47] The authors conclude that rehabilitation in traditional open kinetic chain positions yields suboptimal results in range of motion, function, strengthening, and proprioceptive return. A rocker or balance board is used with weight-shifting from side to side and front to back positions to enhance balance and timing of muscle contraction.[45] The balance board is first used in a sitting position, then in a standing position while supported on bilateral feet, and finally on a single foot with the goal of controlling motion in the prescribed direction at all times. Increased motion is achieved through successively larger spheres and balancing without hand support[1] (Fig. 6-2). Weight-bearing activities are increased to walking on uneven surfaces with side to side weight shifting, or on a low balance beam. Kareokas, agility drills, and obstacle maneuvering are incorporated in the program, with a support-specific program as the final phase. The Star Station Model #460 (Spectrum Therapy Products, Inc., Jasper, Mich) offers the latest in technology applied to proprioceptive rehabilitation (Fig. 6-3). This system utilizes computer-assisted assessment and rehabilitation with closed chain kinetic exercises. Conscious motor activity is combined with simultaneous proprioceptive reactive responses in a dynamic triplane environment. A video screen allows for instantaneous biofeedback in the functional rehabilitation of hip, knee, or ankle injuries.

A reduction in ankle joint swelling is prerequisite for the optimal return of kinesthetic awareness and peroneal muscle conditioning. This is supported by previous studies on effusion in knee joints. Kennedy et al noted that an infusion of 60 ml of fluid into the knee joint inhibited quadriceps function by 30% to 50%.[43] When 10 ml of 1% lidocaine were first infused, this blocked the inhibition of the iatrogenic effusion. Electrical stimulation was noted to bypass the inhibitory effect of the joint afferent to the quadriceps muscle and to prevent subsequent wasting. Transposing these findings to ankle sprains, the potential for delayed rehabilitation of the pe-

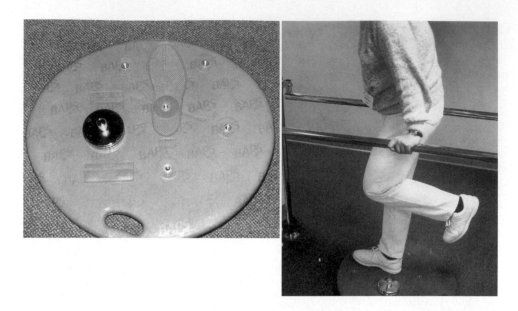

Fig. 6-2 Use of a multiaxial teter board such as the BAPS board is an integral part of the rehabilitation program for proprioception and neuromuscular coordination.

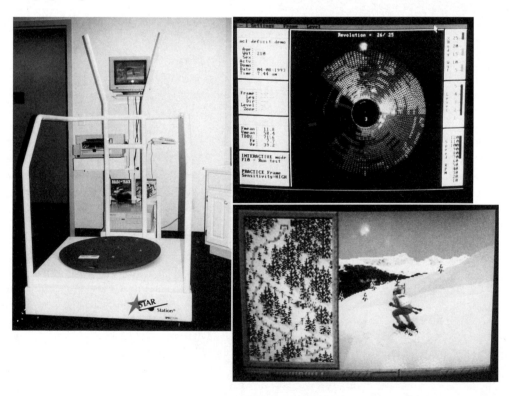

Fig. 6-3 The STAR Station combines the use of a multiaxial tilt board with computer-assisted assessment to facilitate conscious motor activity with simultaneous proprioceptive reactive response in a dynamic triplane environment. Sports-specific video game programs are available to recreate realistic proprioceptive requirements. (Courtesy of Spectrum Therapy Products, Inc. Jasper, Mich.)

Anatomy and Physiology

roneal muscles with swelling exists. Swelling control should therefore be an important component to muscular and proprioceptive rehabilitation, and certainly no athlete should return to full unrestricted sports until the effusion subsides.

The use of biofeedback has been effective in retraining the vastus medialis obliquus in athletes with patellofemoral dysfunction, and it may be of benefit in ankle rehabilitation. Koheil and Mandel demonstrated superior results in rehabilitation of stroke patients with the use of joint position biofeedback.[46] Patients were successfully trained using biofeedback to avoid genu recurvatum and to maintain slight knee flexion at midstance. The authors recognized the advantage of biofeedback in substituting for inadequate proprioception and facilitating greater accuracy in shaping patient responses.

Surgical Implications

A variety of surgical repairs and reconstructions have been advocated for both acute and chronic lateral ankle sprains. While these procedures address the mechanical component of instability, they do not consider proprioceptive restoration. The "anatomical" repair of the attenuated anterior talofibular and calcaneal-fibular ligaments was proposed initially by Brostrom.[8] Later modifications of the technique by Gould et al included mobilization of the lateral portion of the inferior retinaculum.[31] Hamilton has advocated a modified Brostrom procedure as superior to tendon graft reconstructive procedures since full motion is preserved and a near anatomic restoration of the soft tissues achieved.[35,35a] High-performance athletes have often reported greater confidence and stability on the operative ankle compared to the contralateral uninjured ankle.[35] The superior results with the modified Brostom procedure may be due to resetting the tension and therefore restoring the pattern of activity of the mechanoreceptors in the capsule and lateral ankle ligaments while also enhancing existing proprioceptors in the inferior extensor retinaculum.[35] Kennedy et al and Schutte et al have described

mechanoreceptors in the human anterior cruciate ligament consisting of both Ruffini and Pacinian corpuscles.[43,57] Current work on determining the neural histology and morphometry of the ankle joint capsule and lateral ligament complex is underway. Implications for surgical techniques based on neural histology may include modification of existing techniques using tendon grafts depleted of neural fibers for those utilizing neurally intact tissues.

Summary

The importance of proprioception in orthopedics has become increasingly evident in recent years. Implications for proprioceptive deficits in shoulder instability, cruciate injured knees, total knee replacement, and balance in the elderly population are some examples of areas that have been investigated. The capsule and ligamentous structures of the lateral ankle can no longer be viewed simply as a mechanical stabilizer. Equally important is the role for joint protection through a series of afferent inputs controlled on both conscious and subconscious levels with muscular reflexes to avoid placing the ankle joint in a position at risk for injury. Further research should be directed toward the development of practical clinical methods of assessing proprioception, clarifying factors involved in the athlete at risk, determining the underlying role of residual functional instability, and considering implications for lateral ankle ligament surgical repair and reconstruction.

Bibliography

1. Balduini FC et al: Management and rehabilitation of ligamentous injuries to the ankle, *Sports Med* 4:364, 1987.
2. Barrack RL, Skinner HB: The sensory function of knee ligaments. In Akeson W, O'Connor J, Daniel D, editors: *Knee ligaments, structure, function, injury and repair,* New York, 1990, Raven Press.
3. Beard DJ et al: Proprioception after rupture of the anterior cruciate ligament: an objective indication of the need for surgery? *J Bone Joint Surg* 75B:311, 1993.
4. Bilotta TW et al: Recurring distortions of tibiotarsal joint: evaluation using electrodynamography before and

after proprioceptive reeducation, Chir Organi Mov 73:65, 1988.

5. Bosien WR, Staples LS, Russell S: Residual disability following acute ankle sprains, *J Bone Joint Surg* 37A:1237, 1955.

6. Brand RL, Black HM, Cox JS: The natural history of inadequately treated ankle sprain, *Am J Sports Med* 5:248, 1977.

7. Brand RL, Collins MF, Templeton T: Surgical repair of ruptured lateral ankle ligaments, *Am J Sports Med* 9:40, 1981.

8. Brostrom L: Sprained ankles: Part I, anatomic lesions in recent sprains, *Acta Chir Scand* 128:483, 1964.

9. Brunt D et al: Postural responses to lateral perturbation in healthy subjects and ankle sprain patients, *Med Sci Sports Exerc* 24:171, 1992.

10. Bullard RH, Dawson J, Arenson DJ: Taping the "athletic ankle," *J Am Podiatr Assoc* 69:727, 1979.

11. Cooper PS et al: Proprioception in the cruciate deficient and reconstructed knee: a simple reproducible method of examination, poster presentation at the 61st AAOS meeting, New Orleans, LA, February 1994.

12. Deitz V, Berger W: Spinal coordination of bilateral leg muscle activity during balancing, *Exp Brain Res* 47:172, 1982.

13. Diener HC et al: Medium and long latency responses to displacements of the ankle joint in patients with spinal and central lesions, *Electroencephalogr Clin Neurophysiol* 60:407, 1985.

14. Diener HC et al: The significance of proprioception on postural stabilization as assessed by ischemia, *Brain Res* 296:103, 1984.

15. DiFabio RP et al: Influence of local sensory efference in the calibration of human balance responses, *Exp Brain Res* 80:591, 1990.

16. Feuerbach JW, Grabiner MD: Effect of the air cast on unilateral postural control: amplitude and frequency variables, *J Orthop Sports Phys Ther* 7:149, 1993.

17. Feuerbach JW, Grabiner MD: Comparison of an ankle orthosis and ankle taping on maximal, vertical and lateral jump performance, manuscript submitted for publication, 1993.

18. Feuerbach JW et al: Effect of an ankle orthosis and ankle ligament anesthesia on ankle joint proprioception, *AJSM* 22:223, 1994.

19. Fiore RD, Leard JS: A functional approach in the rehabilitation of the ankle and rear foot, *Athletic Training* 231, 1980.

20. Freeman NAR: Treatment of ruptures of the lateral ligament of the ankle, *J Bone Joint Surg* 47B:661, 1965.

21. Freeman NAR, Dean MRE, Hanham WF: The etiology and prevention of functional stability of the foot, *J Bone Joint Surg* 47B:678, 1965.

22. Freeman NAR, Wyke B: Articular reflexes of the ankle joint: electromyographic study of normal and abnormal influences of ankle joint mechanoreceptors upon reflex activity in the leg muscles, *Br J Surg* 54:990, 1967.

23. Freeman NAR, Wyke BD: The innervation of the cats knee joint, *J Anat* 98:299, 1964.

24. Fumich RM et al: The measured effect of taping on combined foot and ankle motion before and after exercise, *Am J Sports Med* 9:165, 1981.

25. Garn SN, Newton RA: Kinesthetic awareness in subjects with multiple ankle sprains, *Phys Ther* 68:1667, 1988.

26. Garrick JG: The frequency of injury, mechanism of injury, and epidemiology of ankle sprains, *Am J Sports Med* 5:241, 1977.

27. Garrick JG, Requa RK: Role of external support in the prevention of ankle sprains, *Med Sci Sports* 5:200, 1973.

28. Glencross D, Thornton E: Physician sense following joint injury, *J Sports Med* 21:23, 1981.

29. Glick JM, Gordon RB, Nishimoto D: The prevention and treatment of ankle injuries, *Am J Sports Med* 4:136, 1976.

30. Gordon DS: Pedal goniometer to assess ankle proprioception, *Arch Phys Med Rehabil* 69:461, 1988.

31. Gould N, Seligson D, Gassman J: Early and late repair of the lateral ligament of the ankle, *Foot Ankle* 1:84, 1980.

32. Greene TA, Hillman SK: Comparison of support provided by a semi-rigid orthosis and adhesive ankle taping before, during and after exercise, *Am J Sports Med* 18:498, 1990.

33. Gross MT: Effects of recurrent lateral ankle sprains on active and passive judgements of joint position, *Phys Ther* 67:1505, 1987.

34. Halata Z: The ultra structure of the sensory nerve endings in the articular capsule of the knee joint of the domestic cat (Ruffini corpuscles and Pacinian corpuscles), *J Anat* 124:717, 1977.

35. Hamilton WG: Personal communication, 1994.

35a. Hamilton WG, Thompson EM, Snow SW, The modified Brostrom procedure for lateral ankle instabilty, Foot & Ankle 14:1, 1993.

36. Harrington KD: Degenerative arthritis of the ankle secondary to long standing lateral ligament instability, *J Bone Joint Surg* 61A:354, 1979.

37. Isakov E et al: Response of peroneal muscles to sudden inversion of the ankle during standing, *Int J Sports Biomech* 2:100, 1986.

38. Jackson DW, Ashley RL, Powell JW: Ankle sprains in the young athlete, *Clin Orthop* 101:201, 1974.

39. Johnson MB, Johnson CL: Electromyographic response of peroneal muscles in surgical and non-surgical injured ankles during sudden inversion, *J Orthop Sports Phys Ther* 18:497, 1993.

40. Karlsson J, Andreasson GO: The effect of external ankle support and chronic lateral ankle joint instability, Am J Sports Med 20:257, 1992.

41. Kaumeyer G, Malone T: Ankle injuries: anatomical and biomechanical considerations necessary for the development of an injury prevention program, *J Orthop Sports Phys Ther* 1:171, 1980.

42. Kay DB: The sprained ankle: current therapy, *Foot Ankle* 6:22, 1985.

43. Kennedy JC, Alexander IJ, Hayes KC: Nerve supply of the human knee and its functional importance, *Am J Sports Med* 10:329, 1982.

44. Kimura IF et al: Effect of the air stirrup in controlling ankle inversion stress, *J Orthop Sports Phys Ther* 9:190, 1987.

45. Kisner C, Colby LA: Chapter 12. In *The ankle and foot in therapeutic exercise: foundations and techniques,* ed 2, Philadelphia, 1990, FA Davis.

46. Koheil R, Mandel AR: Joint position biofeedback facilitation of physical therapy and gait training, *Am J Phys Med* 59:288, 1980.

47. Lattanza L, Gray GW, Kantner RN: Closed versus open kinematic chain measurements of subtalar joint eversion: implications for clinical practice, *J Orthop Sports Phys Ther* 9:310, 1988.

48. Lephart SM et al: Proprioception following anterior cruciate ligament reconstruction, *J Sports Rehab* 1:188, 1992.

49. Lundin TM, Feuerbach JW, Grabiner MD: Effect of plantar and doriflexor fatigue on unilateral postural control, manuscript submitted for publication, 1983.

50. Mack RP: Ankle injuries in athletics, *Athletic Training* 10:94, 1975.

51. Moller-Larsen F et al: Comparison of three different treatments for ruptured lateral ankle ligaments, *Acta Orthop Scand* 59:564, 1988.

52. Myburgh H, Vaughn CL, Isaacs SK: The effects of ankle guards and taping on joint motion before, during and after a squash match, *Am J Sports Med* 12:441, 1984.

53. Nawoczenski DA et al: Objective evaluation of peroneal response to sudden inversion stress, *J Orthop Sports Phys Ther* 7:107, 1985.

54. Oatis CA: Biomechanics of the foot and ankle under static conditions, *Phys Ther* 68:1815, 1988.

55. Rarick L et al: The measurable support of ankle joint by conventional methods of taping, *J Bone Joint Surg* 44A:1183, 1962.

56. Sammarco GJ: Biomechanics of the foot and ankle injuries to the foot, *Athletic Training* 10:96, 1975.

57. Schutte MJ et al: Neural anatomy of the human anterior cruciate ligament, *J Bone Joint Surg* 69A:243, 1987.

58. Smith RW, Reischl S: The influence of dorsiflexion and the treatment of severe ankle sprains: an anatomical study, *Foot Ankle* 9:28, 1988.

59. Skinner HB, Barrack RL, Cook SD: Age related decline in proprioception, *Clin Orthop* 184:208, 1984.

60. Skinner HB et al: Effect of fatigue on joint position sense of the knee, *J Orthop Res* 4:112, 1986.

61. Sprigings EJ, Pelton JD, Brandell BR: An EMG analysis of the effectiveness of external ankle support during sudden ankle inversion, *Can J Appl Sport Sci* 6:72, 1981.

62. Staples LS: Result of study of ruptures of lateral ligaments of the ankle, *Clin Orthop* 85:50, 1972.

63. Stover CN: Air Stirrup management of ankle injuries in the athlete, *Am J Sports Med* 8:360, 1980.

64. Tropp H, Ekstrand J, Gillquist J: Stabilometry in functional instability of the ankle and its value in predicting injury, *Med Sci Sports Exerc* 16:64, 1984.

65. Zimmy ML, Schutte M, Dabezies F: Mechanoreceptors in the human anterior cruciate ligament, *Anat Rec* 214:204, 1986.

2

Rehabilitation Modalities, Trauma, Disease, and Pediatrics

7

Therapeutic Modalities for Foot and Ankle Rehabilitation

Jean Bloecher Cooper

Therapeutic modalities are widely used in both physical therapy clinics and athletic training facilities. There are many different types of modalities available to the clinician, ranging from the simplest, such as ice, to the more complex and expensive, such as interferential electrical stimulation. The clinician, therefore, has many choices when planning a treatment, and knowledge of the benefits and risks of each modality is essential in providing optimal care for each patient based on the diagnosis. Several factors must be taken into account before deciding on the appropriate modality, such as (1) whether the injury is acute (less than 3 weeks duration), subacute (3 to 6 weeks), or chronic (more than 6 weeks duration), (2) the goal of treatment, and (3) any medical condition of the patient that could put them at risk, such as the use of heat on the insensate foot of a diabetic. With careful planning and understanding of the rationale behind each modality, the greatest benefit can be achieved and healing time reduced significantly. Note that modalities are only one facet of a total treatment plan, used to enable the patient to progress with exercise and function-oriented activities toward the goals of independence and return to previous levels of activity.

Cryotherapy

Cold is delivered to the injured site by direct application. The energy transfer of this modality is through conduction. The amount of temperature change depends on the temperature gradient between the cold agent and the body part being treated, the length of time of treatment, and the type of agent used. There are several cold agents to choose from. A cold pack is generally a gel-filled pack that is kept in a freezer. It does not freeze to solid form and is therefore malleable and can be shaped to conform to an irregular body surface, such as the ankle. Gel packs do not cause as great a temperature drop as ice-filled packs.[6,74] They have, however, been reported to be very effective in the treatment of ankle inversion sprains for the reduction of edema.[95] Other techniques of cold application include slush or ice baths, contrast baths, and ice massage. An ice bath of 30° C has been shown to reduce edema more significantly than a bath of 20° C.[73] "Wet ice," or ice that is applied directly through a wet towel, produces a greater temperature reduction than ice that is contained in a plastic bag and applied with a wet towel.[6] Contrast baths combine the vasoconstrictive effects of cold with the vasodilative effects of heat to create a theoretical "pumping" mechanism within the vessels to decrease edema. Another method of delivery, ice massage, is discussed below.

At the time of injury, cold is the treatment of choice. The primary objectives are the reduction of inflammation, edema, hemorrhage, and pain. By adding elevation of the extremity, hydrostatic pressure is reduced, and combined with ice, edema is greatly diminished. Cold is also beneficial in reducing postexercise edema in the subacute patient. Physiologically, the application of cold agents results in arteriolar vasoconstriction (secondary to the effect of cold on smooth muscle), slowing of the local metabolism with a decrease in vasoactive agents, such as histamine, and elevation of the pain threshold. There is also a decrease in local hemorrhage and better lymphatic drainage from the site of injury because of the lower pressure on the extravascular fluid.[44] Stiffness may result from an increase in tissue viscosity.[77] Ice is believed to depress muscle spindle activity as well, which may bring about a decrease in muscle spasm and pain.[43] In the acute and subacute rheumatoid joint, cold may inhibit collegenase activity, thereby reducing cartilage destruction.[62,90]

Pain has been found to be inhibited by cold through a decrease in nerve conduction velocity. A decrease in skin temperature by 5° C is sufficient to cause a reduction in motor nerve activity.[38] As the temperature decreases, there is a corresponding decrease in sensory and motor nerve velocity, eventually causing synaptic transmission to be blocked. Small-diameter myelinated fibers are the first to be affected. In sensory nerves, the A fibers, which carry the sensation of sharp, pricking pain, are blocked before the C fibers, which produce a dull, burning sensation when activated. The effect on nerve conduction velocity depends on the amount of temperature decrease and the duration of treatment.[77]

Another theory about the mechanism of pain inhibition through the use of ice was postulated by Bansil and Maloney in 1984.[3] They studied the effects of ice packs on the production of prostaglandin E (PGE) postexercise and found that there was a significant change in pain and PGE levels in the control group that did not receive ice, versus essentially no fluctuation in PGE in the treatment group. They concluded that the possible mechanism for pain inhibition after acute trauma was suppression of PGE at the periphery.

Ice massage is one technique of delivering cold during the acute phase of injury or after exercise to decrease inflammation (Fig. 7-1). A paper cup is filled with water and frozen, then peeled down to expose about ½ inch of ice. Circular massage of the injured part is performed for approximately 5 minutes. The initial sensation is intense cold, followed by a burning sensation, then finally numbness. The area becomes hyperemic from reflex vasodilation.

In 1967, Waylonis studied the effects of ice massage on skin and subcutaneous temperature.[100] He found that after 5 minutes of ice massage to the calf, skin temperature dropped by 17.2° C. At a depth of 1 cm there was a 6.2° drop and at 2.0 cm a 1.1° drop in temperature. At the muscle layer (3 to 4 cm deep) there was little change. However, after approximately 20 minutes, there was a delayed drop in temperature at this level by 1.1 to 2.0° C. Waylonis was doubtful that this small change in temperature could cause anaesthetic effects at the muscle level. Surface anaesthesia was achieved after 4.5 minutes of ice massage. Skin temperature gradually returned to normal after 40 minutes, but anaesthesia was reported to last from 30 minutes to 3 hours. It was established that frostbite was not possible with ice massage, because skin temperature did not go below 14° C, even when ice massage was performed up to 10 minutes. Yackzan et al, in 1984, studied the effect of ice massage on muscle soreness resulting from exercise.[104] Contrary to the results of Bansil,[5] they

Rehabilitation Modalities, Trauma, Disease, and Pediatrics

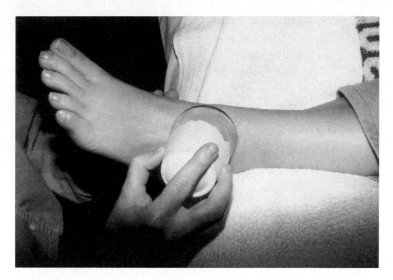

Fig. 7-1   Ice massage is used for cooling of a specific area. Analgesia occurs after approximately 4.5 minutes.

found no differences in muscle soreness or range of motion when applying ice massage immediately, 24 hours, and 48 hours after exercise. This may illustrate the difference between the effects of ice massage and ice packs on subcutaneous/muscle temperature. In a comparative study of ice massage and brief intense transcutaneous electrical nerve stimulation (see below), ice massage was found to be superior for providing immediate local analgesia.[102]

Waiting more than 36 hours after injury to apply ice can delay healing significantly. Hocutt et al found that patients with grade III ankle sprains who were treated with cryotherapy on day 0 or 1 were pain-free running and jumping after 6 days, whereas those who began using ice on day 2 went 11 days before they could run and jump without pain.[44] Contrasted with this, the use of heat on day 0 or 1 postinjury led to a recovery time of 14.8 days. Patients with grade IV ankle sprains who received ice on day 0 or 1 returned to running and jumping without pain 13.2 days postinjury, as opposed to those treated on day 2 with ice, who required a full 30.4 days to resume pain-free activity. Those who used heat on day 0 or 1 with grade IV sprains took 33.3 days to recover. Malone and Hardaker advocate immediate ice and daily taping for acute ankle

sprains in ballet dancers, to be discontinued once pain and swelling have resolved.[69]

Other research has compared cold and heat for treatment of acute injury. Cote et al studied the effects of cold, heat, and contrast baths on posttraumatic edema in grade I and II ankle sprains.[17] The treatments were given to three randomly assigned groups on the third, fourth, and fifth day after injury. The cold treatment group submerged the ankle in a cold bath of 50 to 60° F for 20 minutes. The heat treatment group submerged the ankle in a whirlpool at 102 to 106° F for 20 minutes. The group receiving contrast baths had the ankle fully submerged first in a whirlpool of 102 to 106° F for 3 minutes, then in cold water of 50 to 60° F for 1 minute for a total of 5 heat treatments and 4 cold treatments, ending with heat. Results for the third, fourth, and fifth days postinjury were evaluated. Edema reduction was achieved only by using cold on the first treatment day. By the third treatment day, contrast baths produced more edema than either cold or heat.

As shown above, cold is most beneficial in the acute phase of injury, primarily on the day of the injury or the next day. It should be noted, however, that there are situations where cold is contraindicated. Patients with hypersensitivity to cold may exhibit both local and systemic reactions, such as localized urticaria, sudden drop in blood pressure, dizziness, and tachycardia.[45] Cold should not be used in patients with peripheral vascular disease or Raynaud's syndrome, where vasoconstriction is undesirable. Cold has also been shown to have an adverse effect on wound healing, and it is therefore recommended to refrain from using ice over a wound for the first 2 to 3 weeks following injury.[77] In severe contusions, however, ice may be used daily without adverse effects until pain and edema have been completely resolved and the full range of motion has been restored.[49]

Thermal Agents

There are several methods available to the clinician with which to provide heat to an injured body part. The most commonly used include moist heat with hydrocollator packs, which heat through conduction, or whirlpool, which heats through conduction and convection. Other popular sources of thermal energy include therapeutic ultrasound and diathermy, which heat through conversion. Conduction is the transfer of heat between a surface and a moving fluid that are at different temperatures by the displacement of the fluid. Convection describes heat transfer through the movement of fluid from one place to another. It occurs more rapidly than conduction. One example is heat dissipation through vasodilation. Conversion occurs when nonthermal energy is converted to thermal energy. Moist heat is considered most effective for superficial heating, while ultrasound and diathermy are used when deep heating is desired.

Heat is indicated in the subacute and chronic phases of recovery for several reasons. It is beneficial for enhancing tissue healing, muscle relaxation, and tissue extensibility through increased tissue temperature, blood flow, and oxygenation.[76] In patients with soft tissue contractures, it is important that the patient perform stretching exercises during or immediately after receiving heat to achieve the greatest amount of elon-

gation. Heat has also been found to provide pain relief in patients with connective tissue disorders of the foot and ankle, such as rheumatoid arthritis. In these patients, whirlpool and contrast baths have been shown to offer the greatest relief of all the heat therapies.[4] Continuous heating for 20 minutes in a whirlpool at 45° C produces a significant increase in local blood flow, even at a tissue depth of 3.4 cm, resulting in a rise of skin, subcutaneous tissue, and muscle temperatures and local oxygen uptake. It has been found that continuous heating for longer than 20 or 30 minutes does not significantly alter these variables beyond the level achieved within the shorter time periods.[1] When heated in a whirlpool for 20 minutes, peak skin temperature is reached in 15 minutes,[1] whereas heating with a moist heat pack in which the heat is allowed to dissipate results in peak skin temperature at 8 to 10 minutes.[39]

Moist hot packs are generally kept in water that is heated between 71° and 79° C. The packs contain silica gel and are wrapped in thick terrycloth covers to prevent burns (Fig. 7-2). A treatment time of 20 minutes is used to achieve a temperature increase of 2° C at a depth of 1 cm in the muscle layer and 1° C at a depth of 2 cm. Deeper muscle tissue is insulated by the subcutaneous fat layer and also protected from significant temperature changes by vascular cooling responses.[39]

Whirlpool, or hydrotherapy, is beneficial for providing superficial heating along with the benefits of agitation (Fig. 7-3). The generally accepted temperature range for whirlpool treatments is 36.5° to 40.5° C. The mechanical stimulation of the skin receptors may play a role in the analgesia and relaxation associated with whirlpool treatments. By stimulating the large sensory afferents, pain input may be blocked.[99] Agitation alone has not been shown to increase local blood flow.[14] It is, however, beneficial in the mechanical debridement of open wounds and stimulation of the formation of granulation tissue. The thermal effect of the whirlpool aids in increasing local circulation, which brings in oxygen and nutrients to the area to promote wound healing.[99] It has been shown that 20 minutes of whirlpool is enough time to increase skin,

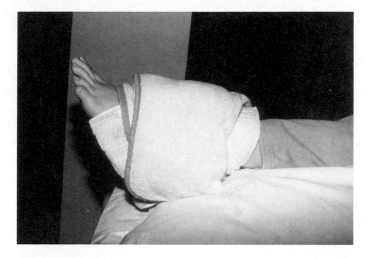

Fig. 7-2 Moist heat provides superficial heating. When used prior to stretching, soft tissue elongation is more easily attained.

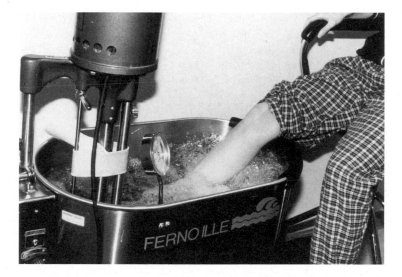

Fig. 7-3 Hydrotherapy allows the patient to exercise while heat is delivered through conduction and convection.

muscle, and joint capsule temperature in the foot.[9]

Along with increased blood flow comes enhanced capillary permeability, which leads to edema formation.[43] Whirlpool has been found to increase the level of edema in an extremity in both normal individuals and patients with pathological conditions and is therefore not indicated in acute injuries. The higher the temperature of the water, the greater the increase in edema.[67] In patients with cardiovascular or pulmonary disease, the temperature should be no greater than 38° C.[99] Whirlpool offers a medium for exercise in the presence of heat that, through the effects of increased tissue extensibility, can produce positive results in a chronic condition where

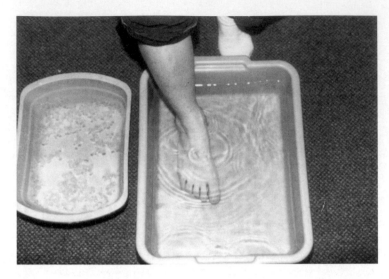

Fig. 7-4 Contrast baths are beneficial for metatarsalgia and heel pain, as well as subacute ankle sprains.

weakness and tissue shortening have occurred. Therefore, this is a modality that is not necessarily passive but rather allows the patient to participate in rehabilitation through active range of motion and stretching while it is being administered.

Contrast bath is another form of hydrotherapy (Fig. 7-4). This technique is used when the goals of treatment are edema and pain reduction. The theory is that through alternative vasoconstriction and vasodilation there is a pumping effect, but this has not been proven. The warm bath is kept at a temperature from 38° to 44° C, and the cold bath is from 10° to 18° C. There are different protocols for the duration of hot and cold immersion. Treatment time is generally 30 minutes, with the hot/cold ratio being 3:1 or 4:1 in terms of minutes. For decreasing edema and inflammation in the management of metatarsal and heel pain, beginning with cold and ending with cold has been found to be beneficial.[15,22] When started too soon, contrast baths tend to increase edema and are therefore not recommended for acute foot and ankle injuries.[17]

Therapeutic ultrasound is indicated for heating of deep tissues at 3 cm or more while allowing the superficial layers to remain at a safe temperature (Fig. 7-5). It has been advocated for the treatment of Achilles tendinosis and retrocalca-

neal bursitis.[59] Thermal effects are achieved with continuous mode ultrasound and include the following: increased local blood flow, increased tissue extensibility,[35] decreased joint stiffness and muscle pain/spasm, and increased nerve conduction velocity.[58] The higher the intensity, the greater the thermal effects. Continuous wave ultrasound produces a greater temperature increase than pulsed and is therefore used when inflammation is no longer acute. Therapeutic intensities range from 0.5 to 3.0 W/cm^2. However, continuous ultrasound with an intensity greater than 2.0 W/cm^2 may actually inhibit the repair process.[27] Frequency is inversely proportional to depth of penetration—the higher the frequency, the greater the attenuation and absorption in the superficial tissue. Therefore, for deeper penetration of heat, a unit that generates a lower frequency is desirable.

Ultrasound units generally come in 1.0- and 3.0-MHz frequencies. With a 1-MHz ultrasound beam, collagen has a high absorption capability. Therefore, tissue such as tendons, joint capsules, and bone, as well as scar tissue, absorbs a significantly higher amount of energy than does skin.[105] For this reason, to achieve tissue lengthening, it is most beneficial to combine ultrasound with stretching or to follow the treatment with prolonged stretching in order to achieve measur-

Rehabilitation Modalities, Trauma, Disease, and Pediatrics

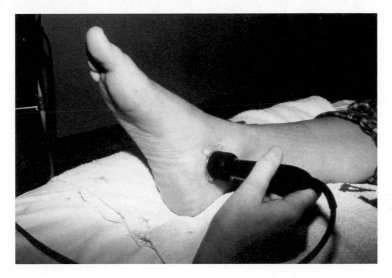

Fig. 7-5 Direct application of ultrasound over the posterior tibialis tendon using a small soundhead for better contact.

able muscle lengthening. It has been shown that the combination of static stretching and ultrasound to the triceps surae produces a greater increase in ankle dorsiflexion than static stretch alone.[101]

Ultrasound also produces nonthermal effects. Cavitation occurs as the gas bubbles in the tissues contract and expand from the condensation and rarefaction of molecules in the path of the ultrasound waves. This can alter diffusion across cell membranes and consequently affect cell function.[63] Unstable or transient cavitation may cause severe damage from the collapse of the gas bubbles. This occurs when too high an intensity is utilized during treatment.[32]

Acoustical streaming is another result of the mechanical pressure wave produced by the ultrasound.[105] This refers to circular fluid movement along cell membranes. Beneficial nonthermal effects include stimulation of tissue regeneration, soft tissue and bone repair, and an increase in blood flow and pain relief.[27,32] Nerve conduction velocity, however, is not affected by pulsed or nonthermal ultrasound.[58] Tendon repair has been shown to be influenced by treatment with this mode of ultrasound in variable ways. In a study on tenotomized and repaired rat Achilles tendons, pulsed low-intensity (0.5 W/cm^2) 1-MHz ultrasound was applied either on postoperative days 2 to 4 or on days 5 to 7. Tensile strength increased when ultrasound was applied earlier and actually decreased when applied in the later time period.[30] During the proliferative stage of repair, fibroblasts can be stimulated to produce more collagen when exposed to therapeutic levels of ultrasound, increasing tensile strength.[26] However, ultrasound applied later can inhibit collagen synthesis.[27]

Treatment of acute ankle sprains with ultrasound and ice has been found to be effective in decreasing pain and increasing the absorption of intracellular tissue fluid.[68] It is recommended that treatment with 0.5 W/cm^2 ultrasound at a pulsed duty cycle of 20% be used for 5 minutes, which may stimulate the release of histamine from the mast cells, accelerating the time of healing.[27] Pulsed ultrasound is also beneficial for the treatment of neuroma, within 3 months of development. Underwater application of 0.5 W/cm^2 at a frequency of 1 MHz is recommended and has shown good results.[85]

A coupling medium is required to transmit the ultrasonic waves. Gel has been proven to provide the best transmission.[24] Underwater ultrasound is also an excellent means of transmitting energy (Fig. 7-6). However, it has been shown

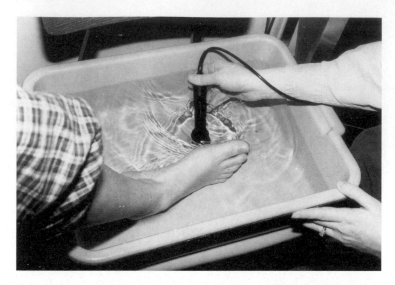

Fig. 7-6 Underwater ultrasound works well for deep heating of irregular surfaces.

to raise tissue temperature in human calf muscles by only 6% compared to a 13.9% increase with the use of a topical gel and direct application.[25] A metal whirlpool should not be used for this type of treatment, because some of the ultrasound energy is reflected by the metal and can cause an increase in intensity near the metal. When using ultrasound, the applicator head should be kept moving in slow, circular patterns. The conventional technique for application is a rate of 3 cm/sec, with each circle overlapping 50% of the previous circle.[58] The soundhead must be at an angle of less than 15 degrees to the skin surface or the energy will not be transmitted.[94] Precautions should be taken when using ultrasound over metal implants cemented with methyl methacrylate, which can become overheated. Only low dosages should be used.[64] Caution must also be exercised when applying ultrasound over insensate tissue, areas of reduced circulation,[4] and epiphyseal areas.[105] Care should be taken over bony prominences, such as a malleolus, because absorption is very high and excess heat may be generated causing pain and tissue damage. Ultrasound is contraindicated in the presence of malignant growth, infection, thrombophlebitis, and acute bone sepsis.[83]

The stationary technique of applying ultrasound is not recommended, because distribution of energy to the tissue is nonuniform and can result in "hot spots" and tissue damage. Stasis of blood flow, endothelial damage to veins, and platelet aggregation can occur, leading to clot formation.[26]

Phonophoresis is the introduction of antiinflammatory medication through ultrasound for reduction of pain and inflammation. A commonly used medication is hydrocortisone cream mixed with ultrasound gel. A recent study has shown that transmission of the ultrasound using this combination is virtually zero. Other preparations that contain corticosteroids but demonstrate 88% to 97% transmission include Lidex gel (fluocinonide 0.05%) and betamethasone 0.05% in ultrasound gel.[11] Another study, however, used phonophoresis with 10% hydrocortisone ointment and reported detectable amounts in the blood of four healthy subjects.[46] Unfortunately, this was not compared with topical application of the hydrocortisone without ultrasound. During phonophoresis, molecules are broken down into ionic compounds, which may create radicals to be used in chemical reactions. These molecules may be driven to tissue depths of up to 2 inches.[2] Pulsed ultrasound is recommended to avoid the thermal and therefore proinflammatory effects of continuous-mode ultrasound. Using the pulsed mode provides the same effect on ac-

Rehabilitation Modalities, Trauma, Disease, and Pediatrics

tive transport of ions through biological membranes, on cell membrane permeability, and on mechanisms for diffusion through the membranes as the continuous mode of ultrasound.[65] Ultrasound may also be used after injection of hydrocortisone to enhance its effects.[81]

Shortwave and microwave diathermies provide deep heat through conversion. Shortwave describes high frequency alternating currents at frequencies between 10 and 50 MHz, while microwave is in the range of ultra-high frequency on the electromagnetic spectrum. The depth of heating with diathermy is greater than with moist heat but not as great as with ultrasound.[56] Microwave diathermy is absorbed by tissues with higher water content, such as blood and muscle, than is shortwave diathermy, and produces deep heating at depths of 3 to 5 cm,[86] but significant heating of the subcutaneous fat layers does occur.[90] Indications for other thermal modalities are the same as for diathermy. However, shortwave and microwave diathermies are contraindicated in the presence of metal prostheses or implants. Patients with cardiac pacemakers should not be in the vicinity when this modality is in use.[56] Because ultrasound offers deep heating with less hazardous thermal and electromagnetic effects, it is used with much greater frequency in the clinical setting. For orthopedic diagnoses, shortwave and microwave diathermies are seldom considered the treatment of choice.[43]

Electrotherapy

The use of electrical stimulation as a therapeutic modality has become widespread for the treatment of pain, edema, inflammation, muscle weakness, and wound healing. There are many different electrical stimulators on the market. Some have been shown to be effective, others have not. Research exists supporting the use of electrical stimulation as a modality, but much more is needed to substantiate the claims of the manufacturers.

Transcutaneous electrical nerve stimulation (TENS) gained popularity in 1965 when Melzack and Wall published their "gate theory" of pain modulation.[75] The premise is that by electrically stimulating the large A-β fibers in the peripheral nerves, presynaptic inhibition of the T cells will occur, closing the "gate" on the slow-conducting, unmyelinated C fibers that transmit burning pain. It has also been postulated that endogenous opiates are released through the use of TENS, since the analgesic effect has been shown to reverse with the use of naloxone.[71] Electrode placement is important and may be based on acupuncture points or the location of the source of the pain. Dermatomal placement has also been suggested.[70] Foot and ankle conditions that have subjectively responded to TENS include sprains, fractures (operative and nonoperative), peripheral neuropathies, and postoperative soft tissue procedures.[71] TENS has also been shown to be very effective in the treatment of reflex sympathetic dystrophy or Sudeck's atrophy.[8,82] The neuroprobe is another electrical stimulator based on the gate theory of pain modulation, and it can pinpoint a very specific treatment area. Using standard therapy in conjunction with stimulation of auriculotherapy and acupuncture points with the Neuroprobe, second-degree ankle inversion sprains were treated and compared with those treated with standard therapy alone. Rehabilitation time was shown to decrease and ankle range of motion increase sooner with the use of this modality.[84]

Edema reduction has been studied using various types of electrical stimulation. Interferential current (5000 Hz) has been shown to reduce edema in ankle sprains (Fig. 7-7). It is also beneficial in the treatment of reflex sympathetic dystrophy. Because it uses medium-frequency biphasic pulses, capacitive skin resistance is much lower and the current is more comfortable than conventional electrical stimulation.[55] For reduction of edema, two phases of treatment are used: the first to stimulate sensory nerves to increase circulation, and the second to stimulate motor nerves to create a muscle "pump."[23] A study of rat hind limbs revealed that high voltage pulsed galvanic stimulation (HVPGS—greater than 100 V, frequency 2-100 Hz) did not affect trauma-induced edema.[78] Similar results were reported using monophasic pulsatile current with a pulse rate of 1000 Hz[61] and low voltage direct cur-

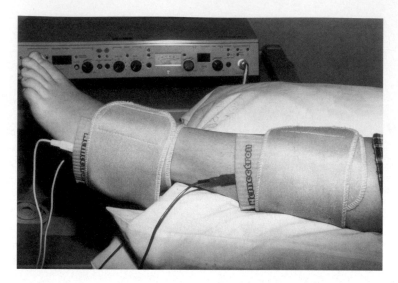

Fig. 7-7 Interferential current has been shown to be beneficial in the treatment of reflex sympathetic dystrophy and is more comfortable than conventional electrical stimulation because of the decreased capacitive skin resistance with this type of current.

rent.[50] In another study, when compared to ice for effect on pain, edema, and range of motion in acute lateral ankle sprains in human subjects, no difference was found using HVPGS.[92] Other authors, however, report good success in treating ankle and foot edema in the clinic with HVPGS.[10,72] A recent study supported these claims, examining the effect of 30 minutes of continuous, 120 Hz cathodal high voltage pulsed stimulation on trauma-induced edema in frog hind legs. Voltage was set at 10% below motor threshold. Results showed a significant reduction in edema in the treated limb for 4 to 7.5 hours following treatment when compared to the contralateral nontreated traumatized limb.[96] Similar results were reported in another study using similar treatment parameters.[7]

Blood flow has been studied using different modes of electrical stimulation. With the use of HVPGS, no change in blood flow at the popliteal artery was found when 10% and 30% of maximum voluntary contraction (MVC) of the plantarflexors was elicited, compared to a significant increase with active muscle contraction at the same intensity.[98] A study on rat hind limbs, however, showed a significant increase in blood flow at the femoral artery using HVPGS. Since muscle contraction was not elicited with each stimulation, a muscle pump effect could not explain the increase in blood flow in the noncontracting muscle. The authors attributed the mechanism to direct stimulation of the type III and IV afferent nerves.[79] Using a different type of stimulator that delivers a 2500 Hz sine wave modulated at 50 bursts/sec, Currier et al determined that blood flow at the popliteal artery could be increased by an average of 20% in humans at 10% and 30% of MVC of the gastrocnemius muscle.[20] This was supported by a study on rats that showed an increase in microvascular perfusion in the tibialis anterior and extensor digitorum muscles with the same type of stimulation. A significant change was found only when a muscle contraction was elicited.[13] A concombinant decrease in blood flow to the digital arteries in the fingers has been found in response to this type of stimulation to the lower extremities, as is found with active lower extremity exercise.[66]

Wound healing is accelerated with the use of low intensity direct current.[12,34,103] This has been attributed to the bactericidal effect of the cathode stimulation.[12,89] More recently, high voltage stimulation has also been found to be ef-

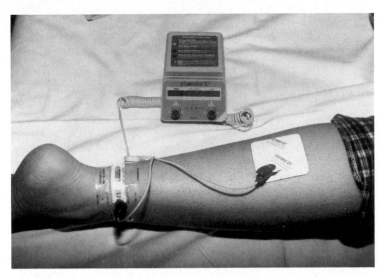

Fig. 7-8 Iontophoresis is used for delivery of an antiinflammatory agent in the treatment of Achilles tendinosis.

fective in augmenting tissue repair. An average healing rate of 44.8% per week was achieved with stage IV chronic ulcers, with all patients in the treatment group demonstrating complete healing by 7.3 weeks. This was compared to an increase in wound size of 11.6% per week in the control group. Three patients who were then switched over to the treatment group achieved 100% healing by 8.3 weeks. High voltage stimulation appears to show greater benefit than low intensity direct current or whirlpool in the treatment of chronic ulcers.[57] Another study showed that the proportion of patients healed with HVGS was 2.4 times higher than that of patients treated with a placebo.[97]

There are many studies of the effect of electrical stimulation on muscle strength and girth. Studies regarding increases in muscle girth in humans are inconclusive.[18] The use of electrical stimulation to produce training effects in normal muscle has not been shown to have an advantage over volitional exercise, but it does demonstrate an increase in strength when compared to nonexercise controls.[19,60,91] In a study of strength changes in ankle evertors following exercise or electrical stimulation at 35% MVC, Protas et al found no training effect.[87] The electrical parameters of the unit used were not stated,

but 60% MVC was necessary to achieve this effect, and few would tolerate the intensity of stimulation necessary to achieve this strong a contraction. Another study comparing HVPGS to isometric exercise found that exercise is more effective in increasing strength.[80] Electrical stimulation does, however, appear to have a role as an adjunct to exercise in the postoperative lower extremity. A group of patients who had undergone knee ligament surgery were divided into two groups: isometric exercise only and isometric exercise combined with electrical stimulation. Those receiving electrical stimulation achieved active contraction earlier and had less atrophy and more improved muscle function than those who performed exercise only.[31] This was supported in another study that demonstrated strength gains in the postsurgical knee in patients receiving electrical stimulation.[37] To summarize, electrical stimulation is most beneficial in helping to restore strength and function in the atrophied muscle following injury or surgery, when volitional contraction is inhibited by edema and pain.

Iontophoresis, or ion transfer, is the use of electrical stimulation to drive topical solutions of ions into tissue (Fig. 7-8). Galvanic, or direct, current must be utilized to create a negative and positive pole. Different substances may be used, depending on the desired effect. Analgesics, such as lidocaine, may be delivered to a depth of 3 cm of soft tissue under the active electrode.[16] Antiinflammatory agents are commonly prescribed for use in iontophoresis. In a study of patients with sprains of the anterior talofibular and calcaneofibular ligaments, seven out of eight had good to excellent results after one to three treatments of dexamethasone sodium phosphate (DSP) delivered by iontophoresis, with an increase in strength and reduction of pain.[40] The depth of penetration of DSP was studied in rhesus monkeys after a 20-minute treatment. Detectable amounts of the drug were found as deep as the joint capsule and cartilage of the ankle joint.[36] Clinically, iontophoresis with dexamethasone has been shown to improve muscle and joint function in the rheumatoid patient.[41,42] There is also radiographic evidence that calcium deposits resolve after treatment with acetic acid.[48]

The use of cold laser for the treatment of open foot lesions has been shown to enhance the healing process and provide analgesia in the acute phase.[29,47] It may also stimulate bone healing, with the best results seen using the helium-neon laser. The mechanism of tissue healing is believed to be through facilitation of adenosine triphosphate synthesis, mRNA production, collagen synthesis, fibroblast proliferation, and vascularization.[29] Tendon healing can be positively influenced by laser photostimulation through augmentation of tensile strength and energy absorption capacity of the injured tendon.[28] A case study of a patient with reflex sympathetic dystrophy of the foot of 4 months duration following a crush injury was described in which ten laser treatments were administered. Within 1 month the patient was pain-free and had full range of motion. Other orthopedic cases resistant to traditional treatment were reported to respond to this modality within a similarly short period of time.[54] Research supports the role of laser in the therapeutic treatment of posttraumatic joint disorders, myofascial pain, and rheumatoid arthritis.[5] Cold laser is still considered a new modality and requires more research before it is used routinely in the clinic.

External Compression

The use of mechanical intermittent external compression is an effective means of reducing foot and ankle edema. There are several different types of compression units on the market with varying parameters. Some units provide intermittent or sequential pressures that allow the lymphatic and venous vessels to fill during the deflation phase, then cause an acceleration of interstitial fluid movement during the compression phase (Fig. 7-9). A cycling period of 15 seconds was found to provide the best results for edema reduction in patients with ankle sprains.[93] The use of an external pressure device facilitates healing and allows the athlete to begin rehabilitation sooner.[88] A pneumatic impulse device was developed and described in 1990 by Gardner et al, based on the discovery of a venous pump present in the foot.[33] This pump is made up of the venous comitantes of the lateral plantar artery and is not activated by muscle contraction but by the passive flattening of the plantar arch. This longitudinal stretching of the veins occurs naturally during weight-bearing, effectively emptying the pump, after which the plantar muscles contract. The pump has been found to be fully operative in paraplegics during braced weight-bearing. Based on these findings, a device was created that rapidly inflates (in less than 0.4 seconds) a small pneumatic pad placed under the plantar arch within a slipper or under a cast. Upon inflation, the plantar arch is flattened and the venous pump empties. Not only has it been found to decrease edema following lower extremity trauma, but compartment pressures were altered in 4 out of 5 patients with tibial fractures whose pressures had exceeded 40 mmHg, thus avoiding the need for fasciotomies.

Manual Modalities

Various manual procedures are employed by the physical therapist that are extremely beneficial for reducing edema in the foot and ankle, breaking up scar tissue, decreasing pain and in

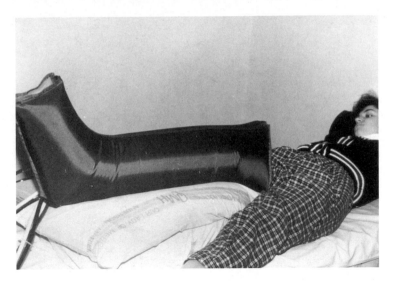

Fig. 7-9 Ankle and foot edema may be significantly reduced with the use of an external compression pump. Early reduction of extracellular fluid is important in the prevention of scar tissue formation.

flammation, elongating soft tissue, and increasing joint mobility. The use of manual techniques is also desirable in providing the patient with one-on-one treatment, and allows the therapist to constantly reassess and directly influence the course of the pathological process or sequelae of injury. The timing and degree of intervention are important so that acute inflammation is not aggravated and yet detrimental sequelae are prevented or reduced. Early mobilization following trauma or surgery has been shown to decrease pain and edema, prevent the development of scar adhesions, and increase synovial fluid lubrication within a joint. The use of ice after a manual technique allows gains to be made with less risk of reactive inflammation.

Lymphedema and postoperative swelling are common complaints that may be addressed manually and are found in both the active and inactive patient. Retrograde massage of the foot and ankle with the lower extremity elevated is effective in reducing edema by providing external pressure through distal to proximal massage, essentially "milking" the fluid away from the foot while hydrostatic pressure is minimized by the position of the extremity (Fig. 7-10).[21] The procedure should be pain-free. The ankle pump can also be stimulated by passive stretching of the

longitudinal arch. Another technique that is popular in Europe and becoming recognized in the United States is manual lymph drainage. This is a skilled technique that specifically utilizes the lymph system to achieve edema reduction through gentle manual intervention. It has been found to be effective in reducing limb volume and discomfort.[51]

Friction massage is performed over an area of soft tissue adhesions perpendicular to the direction of the fibers. Deep transverse friction massage was advocated by Cyriax to promote increased mobility and extensibility of a structure.[21] This technique is believed to encourage longitudinal orientation of the scar tissue as it is produced instead of allowing the disorganized array of collagen fibers that occurs with healing.[52] In cases of tendinitis, where the inflammation has become chronic and reticent to treatment, friction massage may be effective in creating an acute inflammatory response, thereby stimulating soft tissue healing and resolution of the inflammation, especially at the tendon-bone interface.

Manual stretching is indicated for treatment of soft tissue shortening. The use of heat prior to or during stretching creates greater elasticity of the tissue, permitting more significant length in-

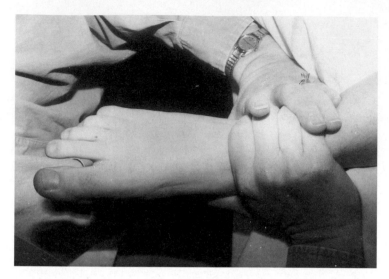

Fig. 7-10 Retrograde massage is beneficial for edema reduction and can be incorporated with other soft tissue techniques, such as stimulation of the venous pump and friction massage.

creases to be achieved. A low load, prolonged stretch has been found to be the most effective technique for achieving elongation of soft tissue. Ballistic stretching should be avoided since it may trigger the stretch reflex and cause muscle contraction. A technique using reciprocal inhibition is often employed by having the patient contract the antagonist muscle, resulting in relaxation of the tight muscle and allowing greater stretch. In the case of tight plantar flexors, the patient contracts the dorsiflexors against resistance, and the ankle is passively dorsiflexed. Another stretching technique called contract-relax, in which the patient isometrically contracts the tight muscle, or gastrocnemius in this case, then relaxes as the ankle is passively moved into more dorsiflexion, works through autogenic inhibition. Contraction of the tight muscle causes firing of the Golgi tendon organ, resulting in relaxation of that muscle.[53]

Joint mobilization is a manual technique used to increase the mobility of a joint and decrease pain. The technique addresses the accessory motions of a joint, referred to as roll and glide, which must accompany physiological, or voluntary, motion. These are often restricted when range of motion is decreased. Graded oscillations from I to IV are applied while the joint is dis-

tracted, varying from small to large amplitude at different parts of the range. Small amplitude oscillations are effective in decreasing joint pain and may allow relaxation of the muscles crossing that joint. Larger amplitude oscillations are indicated for joint restrictions caused by a tight joint capsule, ligaments, or scar tissue. In a patient with an equinus deformity resulting from intraarticular restriction, joint mobilization is an effective tool for gaining motion at the ankle joint. Similarly, decreased mobility in the foot resulting from pathology, trauma, or prolonged immobilization in a cast is an indication for mobilization. Pain reduction and increased shock absorption capabilities will result as the joints of the foot and ankle regain accessory movements.

Summary

Therapeutic modalities are used for the purpose of increasing circulation, promoting healing, and decreasing inflammation, pain, and edema. Early mobilization, in conjunction with specific modalities, has been shown to prevent the detrimental sequelae of inflammation, edema, and disuse and to shorten rehabilitation time. Complete rehabilitation of the foot and ankle must address the underlying biomechanics and include a comprehensive strengthening and stretching program as determined by the evaluation. Modalities allow the progression of the patient to the point where exercise can be tolerated and are therefore an important part of the rehabilitation process.

Bibliography

1. Abramson D et al: Changes in blood flow, oxygen uptake and tissue temperatures produced by a topical application of wet heat, *Arch Phys Med Rehabil* 42:305, 1961.
2. Antich TJ: Phonophoresis: the principles of the ultrasound driving force and efficacy in treatment of common orthopaedic diagnoses, *J Orthop Sports Phys Ther* 4:99, 1982.
3. Bansil CK, Maloney MA: Mechanism of pain inhibition by ice in acute trauma (abstract), *Phys Ther* 64:745, 1984.
4. Bardwick PA: Physical modalities for treating the foot affected by connective tissue diseases, *Foot Ankle* 3:41, 1982.
5. Beckerman H et al: The efficacy of laser therapy for musculoskeletal and skin disorders: a criteria-based meta-analysis of randomized clinical trials, *Phys Ther* 72:483, 1992.
6. Belitsky RB, Odam SJ, Hubley-Kozey C: Evaluation of the effectiveness of wet ice, dry ice, and cryogen packs in reducing skin temperature, *Phys Ther* 67:1080, 1987.
7. Bettany JA, Fish DR, Mendel FC: Influence of high voltage pulsed direct current on edema formation following impact injury, *Phys Ther* 70:219, 1990.
8. Bodenheim R, Bennett JH: Reversal of a Sudeck's atrophy by the adjunctive use of transcutaneous electrical nerve stimulation, *Phys Ther* 63:1287, 1983.
9. Borrell R et al: Comparison of in vivo temperatures produced by hydrotherapy, paraffin wax treatment, and Fluidotherapy, *Phys Ther* 60:1273, 1980.
10. Brown PS: Ankle edema and galvanic muscle stimulation, *Physician Sports Med* 9:137, 1981.
11. Cameron MH, Monroe LG: Relative transmission of ultrasound by media customarily used for phonophoresis, *Phys Ther* 72:142, 1992.
12. Carley P, Wainapel S: Electrotherapy for acceleration of wound healing: low intensity direct current, *Arch Phys Med Rehabil* 66:443, 1985.
13. Clemente FR, Barron KW: The influence of muscle contraction in the degree of microvascular perfusion in rat skeletal muscle following transcutaneous neuromuscular electrical stimulation, *J Orthop Sports Phys Ther* 18:488, 1993.
14. Cohen A, Martin G, Wakim K: The effect of whirl-pool bath with and without agitation on the circulation in normal and diseased extremities, *Arch Phys Med Rehabil* 30:212, 1949.
15. Cooper DL, Fair J: Contrast baths and pressure treatment for ankle sprains, *Physician Sports Med* 7:143, 1979.
16. Costello C, Emran A, Sabbahi M: Penetration of lidocaine into the deep tissues with iontophoresis (abstract) *Phys Ther* 72:S105, 1992.
17. Cote DJ et al: Comparison of three treatment procedures for minimizing ankle sprain swelling, *Phys Ther* 68:1072, 1988.
18. Currier DP: Electrical stimulation for improving muscular strength and blood flow. In Nelson RM and Currier DP, editors: *Clinical electrotherapy,* East Norwalk, Conn, 1987, Appleton & Lange.
19. Currier DP, Mann R: Muscular strength development by electrical stimulation in healthy individuals, *Phys Ther* 63:915, 1983.
20. Currier DP, Petrilli CR, Threlkeld AJ: Effect of graded electrical stimulation on blood flow to healthy muscle, *Phys Ther* 66:937, 1986.
21. Cyriax J: *Textbook of orthopaedic medicine,* ed 10, vol 2, London, 1980, Bailliere & Tindall.
22. D'Ambrosia RD: Conservative management of metatarsal and heel pain in the adult foot, *Orthopedics* 10:137, 1987.
23. De Domenico G: *Interferential stimulation: a monograph,* 1988, Chattanooga Group, Chattanooga, TN.
24. Docker M, Foulkes DJ, Patrick MK: Ultrasound couplants for physiotherapy, *Physiotherapy* 68:124, 1987.
25. Draper DO, Sunderland S, Kirkendall DT, Ricard M: A comparison of temperature rise in human calf muscles following applications of underwater and topical gel ultrasound, *J Orthop Sports Phys Ther* 17:247, 1993.
26. Dyson M: Mechanisms involved in therapeutic ultrasound, *Physiotherapy* 73:116, 1987.
27. Dyson M: Therapeutic applications of ultrasound. In Nyberg WL, Ziskin MC, editors: *Biological effects of ultrasound (clinics in diagnostic ultrasound),* New York, 1985, Churchill Livingstone.
28. Enwemeka CS et al: The biomechanical effects of Ga-As laser photostimulation on tendon healing (abstract), *Phys Ther* 72:S67, 1992.
29. Enwemeka CS: Laser photostimulation, *Clin Manage Phys Ther* 10, 24, 1990.
30. Enwemeka CS: Inflammation, cellularity, and fibrillogenesis in regenerating tendon: implications for tendon rehabilitation, *Phys Ther* 69:816, 1989.
31. Eriksson E, Haggmark T: Comparison of isometric muscle training and electrical stimulation supplementing isometric muscle training in the recovery after major knee ligament surgery, *Am J Sports Med* 7:169, 1979.
32. Gann N: Ultrasound: current concepts, *Clin Manage Phys Ther* 11:64, 1991.
33. Gardner AM et al: Reduction of post-traumatic swelling and compartment pressure by impulse compression of the foot, *J Bone Joint Surg* [Br] 15:229, 1990.

34. Gault WR, Gatens PF Jr: Use of low intensity direct current in management of ischemic skin ulcers, *Phys Ther* 56:265, 1976.

35. Gersten JW: Effect of ultrasound on tendon extensibility, *Am J Sports Med* 34:662, 1955.

36. Glass JM, Stephen RL, Jacobson SC: The quantity and distribution of radiolabeled dexamethasone delivered to tissue by iontophoresis, *Int J Dermatol* 19:519, 1980.

37. Godfrey CM et al: Comparison of electrostimulation and isometric exercise in strengthening the quadriceps muscle, *Physiotherapy Can* 31:265, 1979.

38. Griffen JE, Karselis TC: *Physical agents for physical therapists,* Springfield, Ill, 1982, Charles C Thomas.

39. Halvorson GA: Therapeutic heat and cold for athletic injuries, *Physician Sports Med* 18:87, 1990.

40. Harris PR: Iontophoresis: clinical research in musculoskeletal inflammatory conditions, *J Orthop Sports Phys Ther* 4:109, 1982.

41. Hasson SM et al: Effect of iontophoretically delivered dexamethasone on muscle performance in a rheumatoid arthritic joint, *Arthritis Care Res* 1:177, 1988.

42. Hasson SM et al: Exercise training and dexamethasone iontophoresis in rheumatoid arthritis, *Physiotherapy Can* 43:11, 1991.

43. Hillman SK, Delforge G: The use of physical agents in rehabilitation of athletic injuries, *Clin Sports Med* 4:431, 1985.

44. Hocutt JE, Jaffe R, Rylander CR, Beebe JK: Cryotherapy in ankle sprains, *Am J Sports Med* 10:316, 1982.

45. Horton BT, Brown GE, Roth GM: Hypersensitiveness to cold with local and systemic manifestations of a histamine-like character: its amenability to treatment, *JAMA* 107:1263, 1936.

46. Howes BR, Olsen J: Absorption of 10% topical hydrocortisone during phonophoresis, *Phys Ther* 71(suppl):S113, 1991.

47. Kahn J: Electrotherapy with podiatric conditions, *Clin Manage Phys Ther* 8:6, 1988.

48. Kahn J: Acetic acid iontophoresis, *Phys Ther Forum* :9, 1991.

49. Kalenak A: Athletic injuries: heat vs. cold, *Am Fam Physician* 12:131, 1975.

50. Karnes JL, Mendel FC, Fish DR: Effects of low voltage pulsed direct current on edema formation following impact injury (abstract), *Phys Ther* 71:S116, 1991.

51. Kepics JM, Newton RA: Edema reduction by manual lymph drainage in patients with upper limb lymphedema after breast cancer surgery (abstract), *Phys Ther* 72:S115, 1992.

52. Kessler RM: Friction massage. In Kessler RM, Hertling D, editors: *Management of common musculoskeletal disorders,* Philadelphia, 1983, Harper & Row.

53. Kisner C, Colby LA: *Therapeutic exercise: foundations and techniques,* ed 2, Philadelphia, 1990, FA Davis.

54. Kleinkort JA, Foley RA: Laser acupuncture: its use in physical therapy, *Am J Acupuncture* 12:51, 1984.

55. Kloth L: Interference current. In Nelson RM, Currier DP, editors: *Clinical electrotherapy,* East Norwalk, Conn, 1987, Appleton & Lange.

56. Kloth L: Shortwave and microwave diathermy. In Michlovitz S, editor: *Thermal agents in rehabilitation,* Philadelphia, 1986, FA Davis.

57. Kloth LC, Feedar JA: Acceleration of wound healing with high voltage, monophasic, pulsed current, *Phys Ther* 68:503, 1988.

58. Kramer JF: Ultrasound: evaluation of its mechanical and thermal effects, *Arch Phys Med Rehabil* 65:223, 1984.

59. Labropoulos PA: Indications for surgery. In Hurwitz SR et al, editors: *Foot and ankle pain,* Charlottesville, Va, 1988, Mitchie.

60. Laughman RK et al: Strength changes in the normal quadriceps femoris muscle as a result of electrical stimulation, *Phys Ther* 63:494, 1983.

61. Lea JA et al: The effect of electrical stimulation on edematous rat hind paws (abstract), *Phys Ther* 72:S116, 1992.

62. Lehmann JF, deLateur BJ: *Therapeutic heat and cold,* ed 3, Baltimore, 1982, Williams & Wilkens.

63. Lehmann JF, Herrick JF: Biologic reactions to cavitation, a consideration for ultrasound therapy, *Arch Phys Med Rehabil* 34:86, 1953.

64. Lehmann JF et al: Ultrasound: considerations for use in the presence of prosthetic joints, *Arch Phys Med Rehabil* 61:502, 1980.

65. Licht S, editor: *Therapeutic heat and cold,* New Haven, Conn, 1965, Elizabeth Licht.

66. Liu H, Currier DP, Threlkeld AJ: Circulatory response of digital arteries associated with electrical stimulation of calf muscle in healthy subjects, *Phys Ther* 67:340, 1987.

67. Magness J, Garrett T, Erickson D: Swelling of the upper extremity during whirlpool baths, *Arch Phys Med Rehabil* 51:297, 1970.

68. Makuloluwe RT, Mouzas GL: Ultrasound in the treatment of sprained ankles, *Practioner* 218:586, 1977.

69. Malone TR, Hardaker WT Jr: Rehabilitation of foot and ankle injuries in ballet dancers, *J Orthop Sports Phys Ther* 11:355, 1990.

70. Mannheimer JS: Electrode placements for transcutaneous electrical nerve stimulation, *Phys Ther* 58:1455, 1978.

71. Mannheimer JS, Lampe GN: Electrode placement techniques. In Mannheimer JS, Lampe GN, editors: *Clinical transcutaneous electrical nerve stimulation,* Philadelphia, 1984, FA Davis.

72. McCluskey GM, Blackburn TA Jr, Lewis T: A treatment for ankle sprains, *Am J Sports Med* 4:158, 1976.

73. McMaster WC, Liddle S: Cryotherapy influence on posttraumatic limb edema, *CORR* 150:283, 1980.

74. McMaster WC, Liddle S, Waugh TR: Laboratory evaluation of various cold therapy modalities, *Am J Sports Med* 6:291, 1978.

75. Melzack R, Wall PD: Pain mechanisms: a new theory, *Science* 150:971, 1965.

76. Michlovitz S: Biophysical principles of heating and superficial heat agents. In Michlovitz S, editor: *Thermal agents in rehabilitation,* Philadelphia, 1986, FA Davis.

77. Michlovitz S: Cryotherapy: the use of cold as a therapeutic agent. In Michlovitz S, editor: *Thermal agents in rehabilitation,* Philadelphia, 1986, FA Davis.

78. Mohr T, Akers TK, Landry RG: Effect of high voltage stimulation on edema reduction in the rat hind limb, *Phys Ther* 67:1703, 1987.

79. Mohr T, Akers TK, Wessman HC: Effect of high voltage stimulation on blood flow in the rat hind limb, *Phys Ther* 67:526, 1987.

80. Mohr T, Carlson B, Sulentic C, Landry R: Comparison of isometric exercise and high volt galvanic stimulation on quadriceps femoris muscle strength, *Phys Ther* 65:606, 1985.

81. Neumann MM: Nonsurgical management of pain secondary to peripheral nerve injuries, *Orthop Clin North Am* 19:165, 1988.

82. Newman MK, Kill M, Frampton G: The effects of ultrasound alone and combined with hydrocortisone injections by needle or hydrospray, *Am J Phys Med* 37:206, 1958.

83. Oakley EM: Dangers and contraindications of therapeutic ultrasound, *Physiotherapy* 64:173, 1978.

84. Paris DL, Baynes F, Gucker B: Effects of the Neuroprobe in the treatment of second-degree ankle inversion sprains, *Phys Ther* 63:35, 1983.

85. Patrick MK: Applications of therapeutic pulsed ultrasound, *Physiotherapy* 64:103, 1978.

86. Policoff LD: Effective use of physical modalities, *Orthop Clin North Am* 13:579, 1982.

87. Protas EJ, Dupuy T, Gardea R: Electrical stimulation for strength training (abstract), *Phys Ther* 64:751, 1984.

88. Quillen WS, Rouillier LH: Initial management of acute ankle sprains with rapid pulsed pneumatic compression and cold, *J Orthop Sports Phys Ther* 4:39, 1982.

89. Rowley B et al: The influence of electrical current on an infecting microorganism in wounds, *Ann NY Acad Sci* 238:543, 1974.

90. Schroeder MA: Physical modalities for foot pain, *Clin Phys Ther* 15:231, 1988.

91. Selkowitz DM: Improvement in isometric strength of the quadriceps femoris muscle after training with electrical stimulation, *Phys Ther* 65:186, 1985.

92. Smith W, Michlovitz SL, Watkins MP: A comparative study of ice and high voltage stimulation for ankle sprain (abstract), *Phys Ther* 65:684, 1985.

93. Starkey JA: Treatment of ankle sprains by simultaneous use of intermittent compression and ice packs, *Am J Sports Med* 4:142, 1976.

94. Summer W, Patrick MK. *Ultrasonic therapy,* New York, 1964, Elsevier.

95. Taber CM et al: The effect of cold gel pack application on local limb volume following inversion sprain of the ankle (abstract), *Phys Ther* 72:S105, 1992.

96. Taylor K et al: Effects of a single 30-minute treatment of high voltage pulsed current on edema formation in frog hind limbs, *Phys Ther* 72:73, 1992.

97. Unger P, Eddy J, Raimastry S: A controlled study of the effect of high voltage pulsed current (HVPC) on wound healing (abstract), *Phys Ther* 71:S119, 1991.

98. Walker DC, Currier DP, Threkeld AJ: Effects of high voltage pulsed electrical stimulation on blood flow, *Phys Ther* 68:481, 1988.

99. Walsh M: Hydrotherapy: the use of water as a therapeutic agent. In Michlovitz S, editor: *Thermal agents in rehabilitation,* Philadelphia, 1986, FA Davis.

100. Waylonis GW: The physiologic effect of ice massage, *Arch Phys Med Rehabil* 48:37, 1967.

101. Wessling KC, DeVane DA: Effects of static stretch versus static stretch and ultrasound combined on triceps surae muscle extensibility in healthy women, *Phys Ther* 67:674, 1987.

102. Whipple-Ellsworth A et al: A comparison of the analgesic effects of ice massage and brief intense transcutaneous electrical nerve stimulation (abstract), *Phys Ther* 72:S69, 1992.

103. Wolcott LE et al: Accelerated healing of skin ulcers by electrotherapy: preliminary clinical results, *South Med J* 62:795, 1969.

104. Yackzan L, Adams C, Francis KT: The effects of ice massage on delayed muscle soreness, *Am J Sports Med* 12:159, 1984.

105. Ziskin M, Michlovitz S: Therapeutic ultrasound. In Michlovitz S, editor: *Thermal agents in rehabilitation,* Philadelphia, 1986, FA Davis.

8

Rehabilitation of Fractures and Sprains of the Ankle

Stephen F. Conti

David A. Stone

Ankle ligament sprains are among the most common orthopedic injuries. It is estimated that ankle injuries constitute between 10% and 15.5% of all injuries in sport, with 85% of these involving a sprain of the lateral ligament complex. Orthopedic surgeons, emergency room physicians, physical therapists, coaches, and trainers are often called upon to evaluate and treat this condition. However, the clinical presentations and differential diagnosis may be confusing due to diffuse swelling and ecchymosis. During athletic contests a "golden period" exists immediately following these injuries when there is minimal swelling and an accurate physical examination can be performed. Professionals involved in the care of athletes should be familiar with the initial assessment and treatment of ankle injuries. A proper diagnosis is imperative if effective treatment is to be instituted in a timely fashion. Evaluation of the patient several days after injury must be done efficiently with a logical treatment algorithm in mind. Issues of patient comfort, immobilization

for ligament healing, and physical therapy for range of motion, peroneal strengthening, and proprioceptive training must be coordinated in such a manner as to maximize the restoration of function following injury. Unfortunately, this is one of the most controversial areas in orthopedic surgery. Disagreement over the criteria used to diagnose the extent of ligament damage and a lack of prospective, randomized studies have made it difficult to uniformly group together patients with similar injuries to compare various treatment protocols.

Ankle fractures are less common than sprains. The ankle can tolerate large loads in compression, but the forces necessary to produce rotational injuries are small. This explains how severe ankle fractures can result from apparently minor twisting injuries. Bony disruptions may be obvious on radiographic examination, but most indirect ankle fractures also have associated ligamentous injury of some degree. Therefore, the complicated patterns of ankle injury seen with fractures can only be properly understood if they are analyzed in terms of both bone and ligament injuries.

Direct or indirect violence may cause ankle injury. Indirect trauma is the result of abnormal talar movement either exceeding physiologic motion in a normal plane or due to pathological talar movements within the mortise. Traditionally, this motion is described as movements of the foot relative to the leg. In practice, these injuries occur most commonly with the foot fixed and the leg rotating around the talus. Athletes involved in contact sports may sustain direct trauma resulting in fracture. They are especially prone to indirect fracture patterns as well as injury such as stress fracture. In this chapter, a rational approach to treating and rehabilitating ankle ligament sprains and ankle fractures is presented with emphasis on the rehabilitative aspects of care.

Anatomy of the Ankle Joint and Lateral ligament Complex

The ankle joint is formed by the articulation of the distal tibia and fibula with the talus. The joint approximates a uniaxial hinge with motion occurring around a line drawn through the tips of the medial and lateral malleoli. The tibiofibular mortise is externally rotated 15 to 20 degrees relative to the knee joint axis. Normal ranges of passive ankle dorsiflexion are 15 to 20 degrees with 40 to 50 degrees of plantarflexion. Approximately 5 to 6 degrees of talar rotation is possible within the mortise in the horizontal plane.

The lateral ankle ligament complex consists of the anterior talofibular (ATF), calcaneofibular (CF), and posterior talofibular (PTF) ligaments. Since subtalar instability has been associated with lateral ankle ligament injury, the lateral talocalcaneal (LTC) ligament should be included in this group.

The ATF courses distally from the anterior lateral malleolus to insert on the talus. It is a thickening of the anterior ankle joint capsule. When the ankle is in neutral position, the ATF is parallel to the long axis of the talus and is relaxed. As the ankle is plantarflexed, the ATF becomes

progressively more taut.[3] It is the main stabilizer to ankle inversion stress when the ankle is plantarflexed. During an inversion plantarflexion injury, the ATF ruptures after the ankle joint capsule.[10] It has the weakest tensile strength of the three lateral ankle ligaments.[1] Rupture of the ligament produces a tear in the ankle joint capsule, with hemarthrosis and ecchymosis from the subcutaneous extravasation of hemorrhage. Dorsiflexion of the ankle results in maximum apposition of the ATF.[12]

The CF runs obliquely plantarward and slightly posteriorly from the tip of the lateral malleolus to the calcaneus. It is extraarticular in relationship to the ankle joint but is intimately associated with the peroneal sheath. The fibers of the CF tighten as the ankle moves from plantarflexion to dorsiflexion, and it is in a position of dorsiflexion that the CF acts as a primary stabilizer of the ankle to inversion stress. Tearing of the ligament may be associated with a rent in the peroneal sheath or a split of the peroneal tendon. The PTF connects the posterolateral tubercle of the talus to the lateral malleolus. The ligament plays a role in providing stability against external rotation of the ankle, particularly in the plantarflexed position. The LTC is the most variable of the ligaments previously discussed. In anatomic dissections, the appearance of the LTC varies from that of a discrete ligament to having no identifiable structure with anterior fibers of the CF attaching to the talus rather than the calcaneus. It tends to parallel the much larger CF ligament.

The deltoid ligament is classically described as consisting of two parts. The superficial deltoid fibers originate from the anterior colliculus of the medial malleolus and insert on the navicular, talus, and calcaneus in a fan-shaped pattern. The deep deltoid runs from the posterior colliculus of the medial malleolus to the talus. It is a short, taut structure, which provides the majority of the ligamentous support on the medial side of the ankle. The deltoid ligament also has the highest load to failure of all the ligaments about the ankle.[1] The deltoid does not significantly contribute to anterior stability of the ankle. Following division of both the deep and superficial fibers, there is no increased anterior instability of the ankle. Lateral translation of the talus is primarily inhibited by the fibula. An intact deltoid will allow up to 3 mm lateral talar translation if the fibula is resected. Valgus talar tilting is prevented by the deep deltoid ligament. Following a valgus stress the superficial deltoid will tear before the deep fibers. Rupture of both deltoid fibers is necessary for valgus tilting of the talus in the mortise to occur. Following an inversion injury with the foot in plantarflexion, the lateral ankle ligaments will tear followed by the deltoid ligament.[10]

Ankle stability is a complex issue, with a number of separate but interrelated factors contributing to the overall stability of the talus in the mortise. Both bony and ligamentous support must be considered in the assessment of stability. Range of motion must constantly be balanced against the need for stability. Both must be present and complement each other for the ankle to function properly. When viewed from above, the talus is wider anteriorly than posteriorly, an average of 4 millimeters. This originally led to the view that the talus was unstable in plantarflexion. Subsequently it has been shown that the malleoli remain apposed to the talus in all positions of the ankle. With progressive dorsiflexion, the malleoli separate 1.5 mm and the lateral malleolus externally rotates 5 to 6 degrees. Inman noted that the trochlea has a larger radius laterally than medially. He suggested that the trochlea is a segment of a cone, which allows for stable ankle motion to occur with minimal separation of the malleoli. Early studies examining the contribution of individual ligaments to ankle stability were performed in unloaded cadaver specimens. More recent investigations have described loading as an important contributor to ankle stability. The deltoid ligament is the primary stabilizer to eversion in the unloaded specimen. Inversion restraint occurs primarily by the CF and secondarily by the ATF in all unloaded positions of the ankle. In both eversion and inversion in the loaded state, stability is provided by the articular surface/bony configuration of the mortise. In unloaded external rotation the CF is the primary restraint, while in internal rotation the ATF and deltoid ligaments are primary restraints. Under load the articular

surface again provides nearly as much stability.

Normally the talus moves within physiological limits within the ankle mortise in the sagittal plane with little motion occurring in coronal (tilting) or horizontal (rotational) planes. Studies have shown that in unloaded specimens the ATF and CF provide restraint against inversion and rotation stress, while in specimens that were physiologically loaded the articular surface provides primary stability in all planes.[7,11,12,13] In fact one study[13] concluded that with physiological weight-bearing the articular surface provided 30% stability in rotation and 100% stability in inversion. This suggests that most lateral ankle sprains are not caused by loaded inversion stress. Many occur in relatively unloaded conditions such as following a fall while landing on the lateral side of the heel or may be due to rotational stress. In most cases the anterior ankle joint capsule tears along with the ATF first followed by the CF. An isolated injury of the CF may occur if the foot is in dorsiflexion at the time an inversion stress is applied.

Medial ankle sprains are much less common than their lateral ligamentous counterparts. Both superficial and deep deltoid ligaments must tear before significant valgus tilting of the talus can be demonstrated radiographically. Isolated rupture of the deltoid ligament is rare. Most deltoid injuries are associated with lateral ligament tears, syndesmotic injuries, or fibula fractures.

The ankle syndesmosis is formed by the articulation of the distal tibia and fibula and their ligamentous supporting structures. The interosseus membrane connects the tibia and fibula in the leg. Bony anatomy of the distal tibia and fibula provides some stability to the syndesmosis. The distal fibula is held in the concave peroneal recess and bound by anterior and posterior tubercles of various size. Four identifiable ligaments that provide most of the stability of the syndesmosis can be defined between the tibia and fibula at the ankle. These include the anteroinferior tibiofibular ligament (AITF), posteroinferior tibiofibular ligament (PITF), transverse tibiofibular ligament (TTF), and the interosseus ligament (IO). The AITF runs from the anterolateral tubercle of the tibia to the anterolateral malleolus. The most distal fascicle has been described as a separate entity and may be responsible for some cases of anterolateral talar impingement following a sprain. The PITF originates on the posterolateral tubercle of the tibia and inserts on the posterior aspect of the lateral malleolus. Deep and inferior to the PITF is the TTF, which covers the posterior aspect of the tibiotalar joint and deepens the joint. The IO ligament connects the distal tibia and fibula just above the plafond for a distal of 1 to 2 cm.

Experimental sectioning of the AITF ligament results in a separation of the distal tibia and fibula of 4 to 12 mm according to various authors. In each study, including the IO ligament in the sectioning results in additional widening. Isolated AITF rupture results in 1 to 2 degrees of additional external rotation of the fibula, and including the IO ligament increases this approximately 1 degree. Sectioning of the PITF alone results in an approximately 1-mm increase in internal rotation of the fibula.

Mechanism of Injury

Most lateral ankle sprains are the result of plantarflexion and inversion stress to the ankle. The body may be relatively stationary while the foot is moved into forced inversion, as in a basketball player coming down from a rebound, or the foot may be fixed while the rest of the body rolls over the ankle, as in a runner who makes a sudden cut. Pure inversion with the foot in a neutral position is uncommon. Rotational moments with the foot in various positions may cause a series of ligamentous and bony injuries as well. This is described in the Lauge-Hansen classification of ankle fractures. In this scheme, the position of the foot is described first followed by the direction of the injuring force. For example, in a supination–internal rotation type of injury, the foot is supinated and an internal rotation force is applied through the tibia causing injury to both the ATF and CF ligaments. Axial loading across the ankle may cause injury alone or in combination with the above. This may result in intraarticular fractures of the distal tibia (so-called pilon fractures) or talus. Complex patterns of injury may occur if rotational moments are combined with axial loading forces.

Medial ankle sprains are most often caused by excessive eversion of the heel, although forced plantarflexion and dorsiflexion can cause deep deltoid rupture. Isolated injuries are rare, and associated lateral ligamentous injuries, syndesmosis injuries, or fibula fracture can occur in conjunction with a deltoid tear.

Syndesmosis sprains are believed to be most commonly caused by external rotation stress applied through the foot. The AITF ligament tears first, followed by the IO ligament and membrane. Continued external rotation results in a proximal fibula fracture (Maisonneuve fracture). Usually the PITF ligament is preserved, resulting in an incomplete diastasis between the distal tibia and fibula. Another mechanism is a pure abduction force of the talus against the lateral malleolus. In this instance a tear of the deep deltoid or fracture of the medial malleolus would have to occur concurrently. Lastly, forced hyperdorsiflexion of the ankle has been implicated as a mechanism of syndesmotic disruption in some cases.

Stress fractures are the clinical expression of an imbalance between microtraumatic and reparative processes in the body. Ordinarily bone undergoes both degradation and appositional growth in response to applied stress. When the rate of repetitive microtrauma exceeds the rate of repair, a stress fracture is produced. Typically this is seen in athletes who suddenly increase or change their training routine. Long-distance runners and those involved in repetitive activity are especially susceptible to this injury. Additionally it has been suggested that runners with significantly pronated feet may be susceptible to lateral malleolar stress fractures due to increased stress on the malleolus at heel strike.

Physical Examination

Physical examination of the acutely injured ankle may provide valuable information to the clinician. Violation of the skin producing an open injury should be obvious and signal an emergent need for prompt orthopedic evaluation. Proper assessment necessitates removal of all apparel below the knee. Any gross deformity should be noted. Range of motion of the ankle, subtalar, and midfoot regions should be tested actively and passively. Systematic palpation of the ankle should begin over the medial malleolus and deltoid ligament and progress to the lateral malleolus and lateral collateral ligaments individually. It is important to palpate anteriorly over the distal tibiofibular syndesmosis as well as over the proximal fibula for areas of tenderness. Tendons around the ankle should be palpated for tenderness and determined to be intact. Dorsalis pedis and posterior tibial artery pulses should be assessed using a standard notation, such as 0 = not palpable, 1+ = diminished, 2+ = normal. A comparison to the contralateral foot is helpful if the pulse is not normal. Doppler evaluation is useful if swelling limits the examiner's ability to palpate a pulse. As discussed later, there is a significant incidence of peroneal and posterior tibial nerve neuropraxias following grade II and grade III sprains. Therefore, light touch and pinprick sensation should be evaluated and documented. In the ankle seen several hours after injury, areas of swelling and ecchymosis should be noted. The circumference of the injured ankle should be compared to that of the uninjured one. It has been shown that if it is increased by 4 cm, there is a 70% incidence of ligament rupture. Isolated tenderness over the ATF is associated with a 52% incidence of rupture, while tenderness over the CF represents a 72% probability of rupture. If both the ATF and CF are tender and the circumferential swelling is greater than 4 cm, the incidence of major ligament damage increases to 92%.

Sagittal and coronal instability should be tested clinically with the anterior drawer and talar tilt tests. Some confusion exists regarding performance of the anterior drawer test. It does not test pure anterior translation of the talus under the tibial plafond unless ATF and deltoid ligaments are torn but rather assesses anterolateral rotatory instability of the ankle. In most ankle sprains the medial side of the ankle remains intact. Attempts at anterior translation of the talus produce a rotational motion in the horizontal plane, the deltoid ligament functioning as the axis around which anterior displacement of the lateral side of the talus occurs. The test should be performed in slight plantarflexion with one hand cupped around the heel and the other hand over the anterior aspect of the distal tibia. With the foot fixed, a posteriorly directed force is applied to the anterior aspect of the distal tibia. Assessment is aided by comparison of the injured and uninjured ankles. Visual inspection of the anterolateral corner of the ankle will reveal the presence of a sulcus sign, with significant anterior displacement of the talus on the mortise. The talar tilt test should be performed to evaluate the competency of the CF ligament and is defined by the angle formed by the tibial plafond and the dome of the talus. Controversy exists regarding patient positioning for the test. Neutral to slight plantarflexion of the ankle with the knee bent is acceptable. Care must be exercised in interpreting the test clinically since force is exerted through the ankle and subtalar joints in producing this deformation. Subtalar instability may manifest as an apparent exaggeration of talar tilt, so the examiner must visualize and palpate the anterolateral corner of the ankle to determine where the coronal plane motion is being produced. Radiographic confirmation is advised in all cases of suspected clinically significant ligament laxity.

Valgus stress may be applied to the ankle to assess deep deltoid ligament competency, usually under X-ray control. Syndesmosis injury is suspected when there is point tenderness over the AITF ligament. In subtle cases, the diagnosis may be aided by the use of provocative tests that reproduce the patient's pain. These include external rotation stress on the ankle with the foot in neutral position and compression of the tibia and fibula together about 10 cm above the tip of the lateral malleolus.

Radiographic Evaluation

The ankle radiographic series is one of the most commonly ordered musculoskeletal radiographic examinations in emergency rooms. The yield of radiographs demonstrating a fracture, however, is less than 15%. Attempts to define discriminating guidelines for the use of radiography in ankle injuries have met with some early success. A 100% sensitivity was obtained in a recent prospective study if any one of the following three criteria were met: bone tenderness at the posterior edge or tip of the medial or lateral malleolus or inability to bear weight both immediately and in the emergency department. A similar sensitivity for a foot X-ray series occurred if there was bone tenderness at the navicular or the base of the fifth metatarsal or an inability to bear weight both immediately and in the emergency department.

The initial radiographic evaluation of an acute ankle injury must include anteroposterior (AP), mortise, and lateral views of the ankle and an AP view of the foot. Any proximal fibular tenderness must be examined with an AP and lateral view of the entire leg. Ankle arthrography and peroneal tenography have limited use in evaluating ankle injuries due to their invasiveness and their high incidence of false-negative results. Stress radiography is used to estimate the extent of functional ligament damage. Anterior drawer testing is useful in evaluating the ATF and anterior ankle capsule. The talar tilt test will determine the competency of the CF. Since the CF is almost always associated with concomitant ATF tearing, some authors may bypass the anterior drawer test and only perform the talar tilt test to document that significant ankle ligament injury has occurred. External rotation stress X-rays are used to determine competency of the deep deltoid ligament. This is especially important in supination–external rotation injuries when there is a typical lateral malleolus fracture with questionable deltoid ligament tenderness. Inversion stress views may be helpful in determining isolated subtalar instability in patients with symptoms of instability but no talar tilt. Special techniques to perform these views are well described in the literature.

Bone scans are useful as screening tests for osteochondral lesions of the talus, occult (stress) fractures around the ankle, and syndesmosis injuries. Computed tomography (CT) scanning is often helpful in assessing subtle syndesmotic widening. Magnetic resonance imaging (MRI) is a useful tool, which can assess the extent of osteochondral lesions and also most accurately visualize soft tissue damage. This may include tendon pathology and ligament injury. Even the superior peroneal retinaculum can be evaluated in suspected cases of peroneal tendon subluxation.

Subtalar arthrography has been proposed as a method of objectively documenting the presence of sinus tarsi syndrome. A posterior injection of dye into the subtalar joint is performed, with loss of the normal microrecesses and cutoff of dye at the interosseus ligament in this condition.

Classification of Ankle Sprains and Fractures

The classification of ankle sprains varies, but they are generally divided into three grades of injury:

- Grade 1 sprain is defined as injury to the ATF ligament. Most schemes view the injury as having some fibers within the ligament that are stretched, but the ligament itself remains competent, with no evidence of laxity. There is swelling, but since the ligament is mostly intact, little ecchymosis is present.
- Grade 2 sprain involves complete tearing of the ATF ligament with a partial tear of the CF ligament. Swelling and ecchymosis occur around the lateral malleolus. Signs of mild anterior instability can be elicited on stress testing.
- Grade 3 sprain is a dislocation of the ankle with the ATF and CF ligaments ruptured and variable damage to the PTF ligament. Extensive swelling and ecchymosis are present, with gross instability of the ankle noted on stress testing.

Various schemes have been used to classify ankle fractures. The two most widely accepted are the Lauge-Hansen and Weber classifications.

Lauge-Hansen System

This system classifies ankle fractures based on position of the foot at the time of injury and the direction of the applied force. Four categories of injury are described:

- Supination-adduction fracture

Two stages are noted:

Stage 1: transverse fracture of the lateral malleolus below the syndesmosis or a tear of the lateral collateral ligaments (unusual)

Stage 2: stage 1 plus a fracture of the medial malleolus

- Supination-eversion fracture (eversion means external rotation of the foot relative to the leg)

Four stages are noted:

Stage 1: rupture of the AITF and IO ligaments

Stage 2: stage 1 plus a spiral oblique fracture of the lateral malleolus above the syndesmosis

Stage 3: stage 2 plus injury to the PITF ligament or fracture of the posterior lip of the tibia.

Stage 4: stage 3 plus a fracture of the medial malleolus or rupture of the deltoid ligament.

- Pronation-abduction fracture

Three stages are noted:

Stage 1: fracture of the medial malleolus or tear of the deltoid ligament

Stage 2: stage 1 plus rupture of the AITF and PITF ligaments alone or in combination with a fracture of the posterior lip of the tibia

Stage 3: stage 2 plus an oblique fracture of the fibula at the level of the syndesmosis

- Pronation-eversion fracture

Four stages are noted:

Stage 1: Fracture of the medial malleolus or tear of the deltoid ligament

Stage 2: stage 1 plus injury to the ATF and PTF ligaments

Stage 3: stage 2 plus a fracture of the fibula several centimeters above the syndesmosis

Stage 4: stage 3 plus a fracture of the posterior lip of the tibia secondary to avulsion of the PITF and TTF ligaments.

Weber Classification

The Lauge-Hansen scheme was based on cadaver specimens and describes both ligamentous and bony injury in controlled experimental situations. It is often cumbersome and difficult to apply clinically. Of interest are the unique fibular fractures produced by each type of injury. An easier system to apply, and one that can be used to determine the appropriate treatment for ankle fractures, was developed by Weber. It includes three groups based on the type of fibular fracture produced.

- Type A: the fibula is fractured at or below the level of the tibial plafond, thus leaving the syndesmotic ligaments intact. A vertical fracture of the medial malleolus may accompany the fibula fracture. There may be a small area of articular compression at the medial corner of the ankle as well. This roughly corresponds to the Lauge-Hansen supination-adduction fracture.

- Type B: the fibula fracture begins at the level of the tibial plafond and is usually spiral in configuration. Injury of the deltoid-medial malleolus complex can also occur in this type of fracture. The type B fracture correlates with the Lauge-Hansen supination-external rotation fracture.

- Type C: the fibula fracture occurs above the level of the tibial plafond with rupture of the syndesmosis. Medially there is an injury of the medial malleolus-deltoid complex with an avulsion fracture of the malleolus or tear of the ligament. These fractures may be subdivided based upon the exact location of the fibula fracture. Two eponyms are commonly used. Duyputren fractures occur 4 to 5 cm above the syndesmosis, while Maisonneuve fractures occur in the proximal one third of the fibula.

Isolated injury to the ankle may occur that does not readily fit into one of the above categories. Superficial deltoid ligament sprains may occur and can present as tenderness over the ligament without evidence of talar instability. Occasionally these occur as avulsions of the anterior colliculus of the medial malleolus. Ruptures of the superficial and deep deltoid ligaments occur as a result of plantar hyperflexion. These may be accompanied by fracture of the lateral malleolus. Widening of the medial mortise, and a radiographic medial clear space greater than 3 mm, indicates rupture of the deep deltoid ligament. Chip fractures of the anterior or posterior colliculus are variations of these injuries. They represent avulsions of the superficial or deep deltoid ligaments, respectively.

Pure ankle dislocations are a separate category of ankle injury. Extensive soft tissue trauma is manifested by gross instability of the ankle to manual stress testing. Careful neurovascular examination is mandatory before and after closed reduction is performed. These tend to be high energy injuries, although they have been reported in sports such as basketball when simply coming down from a lay-up.

Nerve injury has been shown to occur in association with inversion injuries to the ankles.[8] Grade I sprains showed no abnormalities on clinical or electrodiagnostic testing. Grade II sprains had a 17% incidence of peroneal nerve injury, with 10% demonstrating abnormalities in the posterior tibial nerve by electromyography (EMG). Sensory abnormalities were exhibited in only 10% of patients; each in the peroneal nerve distribution. Resolution had occurred by 1 month after injury. Marked differences were demonstrated in the clinical findings for patients with grade III sprains when compared to those who sustained grade II ankle injuries. Grade III sprains showed an 86% incidence of peroneal nerve abnormalities on EMG and an 83% incidence of posterior tibial nerve injury. Abnormal sensation in the peroneal nerve distribution was noted in 54% of patients. More than one half of the deficits developed over a period of 3 to 5 days after injury, with normal sensation noted immediately after injury. Return to normal sensation required 5.8 weeks. The postulated etiology in these cases was traction injury sustained at the time of injury. In terms of rehabilitation, the time required to return to full activity was 1.3 weeks for grade II sprains and 5.3 weeks for grade III sprains. Nerve injury may account for the persistent inability to push off forcefully during ambulation and the visible gastrocnemius muscle atrophy seen in grade III ankle sprains. This may account in part for the longer period of morbidity and prolonged rehabilitation required in the more serious injuries. Osteochondral or transchondral fractures of the talar dome may also occur. A high index of suspicion must exist to diagnosis these lesions.

Berndt and Harty[2] performed an extensive study and classified osteochondral lesions into four different stages of severity:

Stage 1: A small area of compression of subchondral bone

Stage 2: A partially detached osteochondral fragment

Stage 3: A completely detached osteochondral fragment remaining in the crater. Two instances have been reported in which the osteochondral fragment had inverted upon itself[6]

Stage 4: A displaced osteochondral fragment

These lesions are classically described as being located anterolaterally or posteromedially on the talar dome. Lateral lesions are consistently wafer-shaped and associated with a history of trauma. Medial lesions are deeper and more cup-shaped The majority can be associated with trauma, but many are thought to result from an avascular process. Symptoms of ankle discomfort after apparent healing of an ankle sprain should clue the clinician to search for osteochondral lesions. Displaced fragments may cause grating or locking sensations. Plain X-rays of the ankle may reveal the lesion. AP and mortise views in 20 degrees of plantarflexion are often helpful in visualizing more posteriorly located lesions. Bone scan may be positive but is nonspecific. CT and MRI are able to visualize the extent of the defects more accurately than plain films or bone scan.

Talar neck fractures are an uncommon form of ankle injury in the athlete. These are usually associated with high energy trauma. The mechanism of injury most commonly is a forced dorsiflexion moment about the ankle. Hawkins[5] classified these fractures into three types:

Type I: Nondisplaced fracture through the talar neck

Type II: Displaced fracture with subtalar subluxation or dislocation

Type III: Displaced fracture with both subtalar and ankle subluxation or dislocation

Type IV: Displaced fracture with subluxation or dislocation of the subtalar and talonavicular joints (as described by Canale et al)

Two major problems are classically described in association with talar neck fractures. One is an increasing incidence of avascular necrosis (AVN) of the talar body with successive types of neck fractures. Type I fractures have a less than 10% incidence of AVN, while type II and type III fractures are associated with an approximately 50% and 85% incidence of AVN, respectively. Type IV fractures can be expected to have AVN in a high percentage of cases due to extensive disruption of primary sources of blood supply. A second problem encountered in talar neck fractures is degenerative arthritis of the ankle and subtalar joints. Both AVN and arthritis are more common with increasing displacement of the talar body; however, it is not possible to predict whether a given individual will develop these complications.

Various other fractures may occur around the ankle and should be sought after in patients with a history of ankle trauma but no obvious fracture on routine radiographic examination. Fracture of the posterior process of the talus must be differentiated from an os trigonum. Often a CT scan is helpful in this regard. Fracture of the lateral talar process or anterior superior process of the calcaneus are uncommon fractures that must be looked for carefully. Fractures of the base of the fifth metatarsal as well as cuboid fractures may occur and cause lateral ankle pain and swelling that must be differentiated from lateral ligament sprains. We have seen patients with inversion injuries who are tender over the sinus tarsi with small bone fragments seen just lateral to the anterior process of the calcaneus, which we believe represents avulsion of the origin of the extensor digitorum brevis muscle.

Stress fractures can also develop in the distal tibia and fibula. These occur when repeated microfractures occur at a rate that exceeds the body's ability to repair them. A history of a recent increase in activity may often be elicited. Runners are prone to this injury, especially if they have undergone a change in training pattern. Initially the pain may be generalized to the medial or lateral ankle, but it gradually becomes localized to one point on the bone. Palpation may reveal the sensitive spot. Weight-bearing is painful, and symptoms are reproduced with forced internal or external rotation of the ankle. X-rays may not become positive for 4 to 6 weeks. A bone scan or MRI will permit early diagnosis. Fibula stress fractures are often associated with pronation of the foot and increased force on the fibula. For recurrent stress fractures in the same leg, a leg length discrepancy should be sought. Talar neck stress fractures may occur in the athlete with symptoms as described above.

Finally, tendon injuries may occur and simulate ankle sprains. Peroneal tendon subluxation/dislocation results from resisted ankle dorsiflexion and eversion. Acutely, the patient may complain of pain and swelling around the lateral malleolus, and pain may be reproduced with resisted ankle dorsiflexion and eversion. Palpation of the subluxation or dislocation may be difficult. Chronic injuries present with tenderness isolated to the superior peroneal retinaculum, and palpation detects the dislocation. Peroneal tendon tears are associated with severe inversion injuries to the ankle and may be a source of chronic lateral ankle pain following such injuries. Tenderness may be isolated to the peroneus brevis tendon, and discomfort may be reproduced with resisted eversion. Most commonly the tear occurs as the tendon courses around the lateral malleolus. Posterior tibial tendon tears may rarely occur in association with twisting injuries of the ankle. These may be avulsions or intrasubstance tears. Pain is described along the medial ankle as well as extending into the arch. Swelling and tenderness are noted over the course of the tendon. Inversion weakness can be demonstrated. The patient initially will be unable to rise on the toes of the affected foot and later will notice flattening of the arch and progressive valgus of the hindfoot.

Initial Treatment of Ankle Injury

Open ankle fractures and dislocations require urgent medical treatment. Open ankle fractures require irrigation and debridement in the operating room followed by open reduction and internal fixation. Ankle dislocations should be reduced immediately. The patient's neurovascular status, both prereduction and postreduction, should be documented carefully to determine the extent of initial nerve injury and any changes that may have occurred with reduction. If the reduction is stable, then either plaster immobilization or early surgical repair of the ankle ligaments is undertaken. Controversy exists over which form of treatment is best for this injury. Those who favor cast immobilization cite the fact that most patients with Grade III sprains do well without surgery and those with long-term instability obtain excellent results with subsequent lateral ankle ligament reconstruction. Proponents of early surgical repair feel the incidence of late instability is less and function is better than with either cast immobilization or later reconstruction. If the reduction is unstable, then the ankle joint can be held with percutaneous pins or the ankle ligaments may be immediately repaired.

Nondisplaced ankle fractures may be treated in a nonweight-bearing short leg cast until radiographic evidence of healing has taken place. Following cast removal the patient is begun on progressive weight-bearing ambulation training. Active and passive range of motion exercises of the ankle and subtalar joints should begin immediately. Once 80% of the range of motion is restored, strengthening can begin. Displaced ankle fractures should be treated with anatomic open reduction and internal fixation. Techniques proposed by the AO/ASIF are the most widely accepted methods of repair and are beyond the scope of this chapter. The goal of rigid, stable internal fixation is to allow range of motion exercises to begin soon after surgery. Nonweight-bearing must continue until bony healing is demonstrated on X-ray. Ideally, patients should begin active range of motion of the ankle and subtalar joints once uncomplicated soft tissue healing is assured. This usually corresponds to postoperative day 10. In cases where fixation of the fracture fragments is less than ideal or when patient compliance is a concern, a short leg cast with the ankle in neutral position should be applied.

The treatment of the large majority of lateral ankle sprains in the young healthy patient is by functional rehabilitation. Jackson et al treated mild and moderate sprains (using a classification based on function) within an average of 8 and 15 days respectively, using a regimen consisting of rest, ice, compression, and elevation. This was followed by taping with progressive weight-bearing, active range of motion exercises, strengthening and endurance exercises, and proprioceptive training. Their results were uniformly excellent, and several authors[2-4] have effectively employed this form of treatment with more severe sprains. Moreover, Staples and Jackson et al discussed the problems of treatment by cast immobilization without rehabilitation for severe sprains. In Staples' study, almost 40% of young patients treated by immobilization for 3 to 8 weeks had residual symptoms; mostly pain, weakness, or functional instability. Whereas immobilization is appropriate for older or disabled patients, it remains a symptomatic treatment and is ineffective in the young. In addition, the effects of immobilization on articular cartilage[6] and muscle strength and endurance[7] may create more problems for the young patient whose goal is to return to sports. In Staples' study, muscle weakness persisted in almost half of the patients who remained symptomatic following casting. Stress radiographs demonstrated anatomic instability in almost half the patients, whether or not they were symptomatic. Freeman also compared early mobilization of ankle sprains with cast immobilization and surgery and found function best in the early mobilization group. Some combination of immobilization followed by rehabilitation may be appropriate for severe sprains, as detailed by Smith, who employed casts for 3 to 6 weeks in grade III sprains before initiating rehabilitation, and Hamilton, who advocated casting grade II sprains for 3 weeks before rehabilitation, but simple immobilization alone would appear to be ineffective.

The specific treatment program for ankle sprains remains the same in principle from sport to sport, but some subtle sport-specific differences exist. The goal of early treatment should be to minimize pain and swelling. When the natural pumping action of the calf muscles is lost due to pain, and the patient is unable to exercise the leg, edema and tissue fibrosis can result. This can lead to adhesions in joint capsules and ligaments and stiffness.[9] Prevention is traditionally accomplished with the use of rest, ice, a compression wrap, and elevation (RICE). Ice or cold packs are usually prescribed for 20-minute applications,[1] but frequency of application is usually not discussed. Rewarming studies have shown that the ankle requires more than 2½ hours to return to normal skin temperature,[10] and complications from the use of ice are rare. Intermittent pneumatic compression devices have proven more effective than simple Ace bandages,[11] but the effects of these at the tissue level are poorly understood, and potential injury caused by their use cannot be estimated. Some authors[9] recommend semirigid taping with a horseshoe-shaped pad around the lateral malleolus to apply specific localized pressure. If tape is used to control swelling, it can also be used to add stability to the ankle during therapeutic exercises. No consensus exists on this practice. Our experience is that this form of treatment is often poorly tolerated by patients because pressure is applied directly over an area of tenderness with resultant discomfort. Recently the use of commercial units to deliver cold and compression (Aircast Cryocuff, Jobst) has become popular (Fig. 8-1). These units are portable, convenient, easy to use, and routinely available in most clinics. We do not routinely aspirate the effusion or inject local anesthetics to initiate early rehabilitation. If possible, some type of protection to the injured ligament should be provided. A variety of ankle braces that allow protected early motion are available, and the treating physician should be familiar with them. None has been proven superior to the others in testing, and we believe that comfort and shoe fit should determine this decision.

Usually, active range of motion exercises can be started within the first 2 to 4 days after injury. These exercises are a prelude to the more aggressive therapy prescribed later in the rehabilitation process. They traditionally consist of "alphabet exercises" or simple dorsiflexion/plantarflexion movements that allow the calf muscles to function as pumps and reduce swelling. They

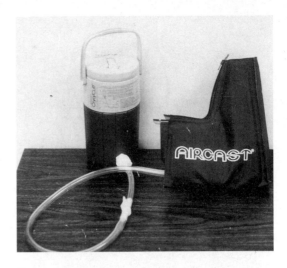

Fig. 8-1   These units can provide cold and compression simultaneously to acutely injured ankles.

are guided by pain, never done with resistance, and usually prescribed in high repetitions (20 to 40) once or twice a day.[10] The use of manual distraction and passive stretching of the anterior capsule, commonly referred to as A-P glides, has been advocated by some authors (Fig. 8-2). The athlete should be allowed to progress with these at a comfortable pace; and as motion improves, gentle Achilles tendon and ankle dorsiflexor tendon stretching can be started (Fig. 8-3 A and B). Passive warming has been shown to increase the extensibility of the musculotendinous unit and may decrease the risk of "overstretch." If possible, the athlete should warm up for 5 minutes before stretching. When this is not possible, heat should be applied to muscles at risk before stretching. In an animal model to evaluate the biomechanical effects of stretching it has been found that stretching is most effective in the first 18 seconds and the first 4 repetitions. We recommend that patients hold all stretches for 20 seconds and repeat them 4 to 5 times. Restoration of full range of motion is important, especially for ballet dancers for whom subtle loss of plantarflexor flexibility may produce problems going *en pointe* after a sprain. We do not routinely incorporate galvanic stimulation, ultrasound, or other modalities into our rehabilitation scheme unless pain or swelling persists.

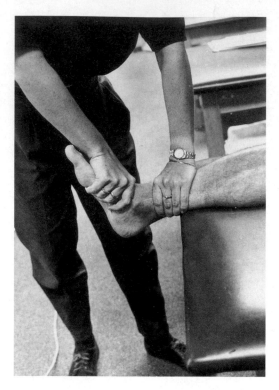

Fig. 8-2 Technique for performance of the A-P glide.

As soon as pain permits, strengthening exercises can be initiated. Isometrics can usually be started fairly quickly, especially in dorsiflexion/plantarflexion, and progression to isotonic exercises with elastic tubing or some other resistance device for eversion/inversion should follow (Fig. 8-4). Hamilton noted that plantarflexion exercises, such as toe raises, do not restore peroneal strength. He also believed that dancers should perform peroneal strengthening exercises in plantarflexion. Staples thought that peroneal weakness in particular was a cause of persistent symptoms after ankle sprains and "should be a part of any of the therapy regimens under consideration." Peroneal weakness has been found in 22% of all ankle sprains and in 66% of ankles with residual symptoms. Strengthening exercises progressing from elastic tubing to weights or isokinetic exercises can be prescribed at the physician or therapist's discretion. Machines that utilize free weights are often more difficult to use than rubber tubing or isokinetics and should be

the final progression in the rehabilitation process (Fig. 8-5). However, all strengthening programs should be sport-specific in that the type of contraction (isometric, eccentric, concentric), speed of contraction (fast vs. slow), and position of ankle (dancers and fencers, for example, have different requirements) should all be taken into account. In the early phases of strength development, exercises should start with high repetitions and low weights. This program is maintained for at least 3 to 4 weeks before becoming more specific. This phase of rehabilitation should also include cardiovascular conditioning, as well as the conditioning of the rest of the leg for return to play.

Proprioception training is also important in the rehabilitation of the sprained ankle. The role of proprioceptive deficits in the development of the chronically unstable ankle has been debated by a variety of authors. Freeman believed that ankle injury leads to proprioceptive deficits and functional instability. In contrast, Staples noted them as a cause of persistent symptoms but did not consider them important to his study. More recently, Tropp was able to reduce the rate of ankle sprain by using stabilometric training on a balance board, and Rebman noted a reduction in chronic sprains after incorporating proprioception training into a rehabilitation program. In his protocol, patients performed exercises for only 2 minutes twice per day and were encouraged to make their own balance board for home use. Proprioception exercises usually begin as simple standing and balancing on one leg (Fig. 8-6). This is followed by a progression of exercises using some type of balance board, initially seated and then standing. The biomechanical ankle platform system (BAPS) is popular (Fig. 8-7), although other systems (e.g., KAT) are available (Fig. 8-8).

In the final phase of rehabilitation, a series of functional progressions is instituted to restore agility, confidence, and ultimately, performance. This phase usually does not begin until the athlete has painless full range of motion, strength that is within 15% to 20% that of the unaffected ankle, and walks without a limp. However, if a pool is available, barre exercises or running in a pool can be started earlier, usually when the ath-

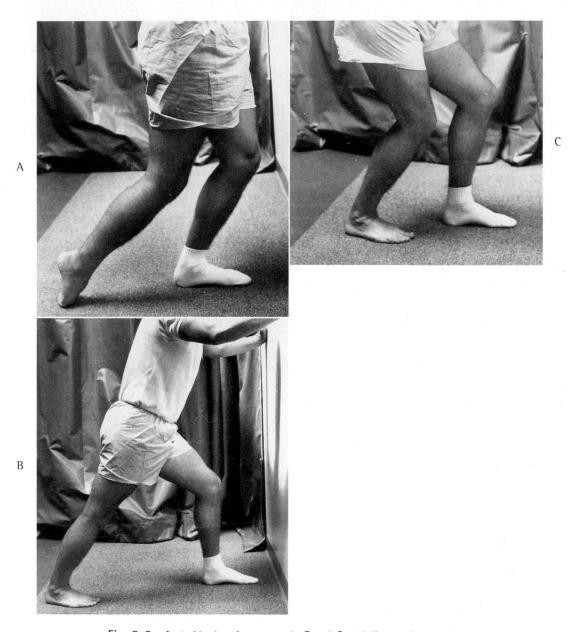

Fig. 8-3 **A,** Ankle dorsiflexor stretch. **B** and **C,** Achilles tendon stretch.

lete can walk without a limp or toe raise without pain. The basic functional progression is walk-jog-run-cut-drill-practice-play. Cuts are generally divided into side step and crossover maneuvers and must be accomplished with both speed and precision. Commonly athletic trainers or therapists will ask the athlete to cut on their command, not at the athlete's whim. As the progression is completed, the athlete resumes practice, initially for easy drills and later for scrimmaging. When practice is well tolerated, the athlete is cleared to play. The goal of the rehabilitation process is to produce a functionally stable ankle with full range of motion and normal strength that requires no further treatment.

The prognosis for mild to moderate sprains is

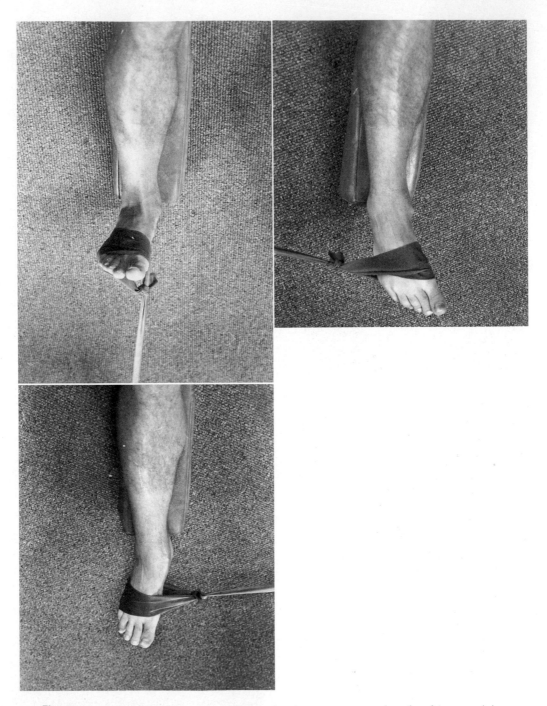

Fig. 8-4 Rubber tubing exercises can be used to incorporate strength and endurance training.

Rehabilitation Modalities, Trauma, Disease, and Pediatrics

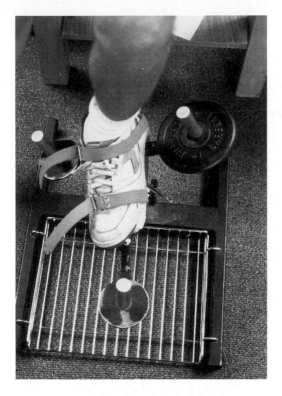

Fig. 8-5 These machines incorporate free weights into ankle rehabilitation.

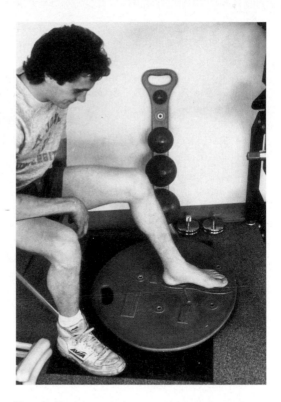

Fig. 8-7 Biomechanical ankle platform system (BAPS).

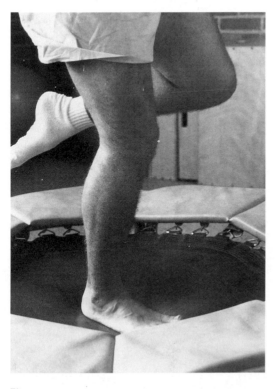

Fig. 8-6 Balancing on one leg on a trampoline can help restore proprioception.

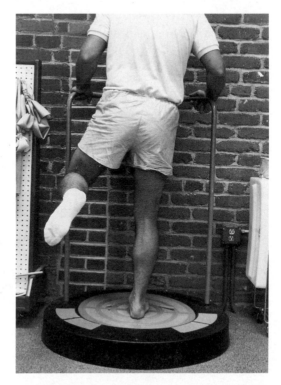

Fig. 8-8 KAT system for proprioception training.

generally regarded as good. Jackson observed that mild sprains required about 8 days of treatment and moderate sprains about 15 days. McConkey noted that few patients treated with functional rehabilitation requested further treatment. The ultimate prognosis of any individual sprain, however, is not the problem. Patients who have recurrent sprains ultimately require some type of reconstruction if they develop mechanical instability or recurrent symptoms, and these patients may be relatively common. Smith,[2] for example, in his survey of high school basketball players discovered that 70% had a previous sprain, 80% of those with a sprain had multiple sprains, and 50% had residual symptoms. In Tropp's study of soccer players, the control group represented untreated players: 25% of athletes who had a previous sprain were reinjured, compared to 11% of those who had never had a sprain. These results agree poorly with those of Konradsen, who compared early mobilization with casting in grade III ankle sprains and demonstrated 95% mechanical stability at 1 year, with residual symptoms in 13% of functionally treated ankles and 9% of casted ankles. He noted that the best prognostic factor after an ankle sprain may not be extent of injury "but rather functional demand put on the ankle by the patient."

If persistent ankle symptoms result from a severe sprain in a young athlete, some type of prophylactic brace to maintain athletic performance and reduce symptoms is indicated. Ideally this brace should permit full range of motion and allow normal ankle kinematics. The best studied and oldest form of protection has been taping, initially espoused by Quigley. Perguson was able to demonstrate that tape improved reaction time of the peroneal muscles to almost normal levels, attributing the improvement to a proprioceptive function. The concern over the use of tape is often that it loosens usually in less than 1 hour and that it is expensive, averaging about $1.75 per day. Rovere demonstrated the benefit of a laced stabilizer in a retrospective study done with college football players. While the study's design was not perfect, over a 6-year period the combination of a lace-up ankle support and a low-top shoe proved superior to tape and a low-top or high-top shoe. A variety of lace-up and semi-

rigid ankle supports are now available commercially. They do not appear to affect athletic performance, but more testing needs to be done to determine their effectiveness.

Syndesmosis injuries are rare but important causes of ankle pain. Hopkinson found only 15 syndesmosis sprains in a review of 1344 ankle sprains over a 41-month period at West Point. Average time of recovery was almost twice that of patients with severe ankle sprains (55 vs. 28 days). Taylor noted an average recovery time of 31 days in football players with syndesmosis injuries. Diagnosis can be made by an external rotation stress or "squeeze test." Staples noted partial injury to the distal ATF ligament at surgery in 7 of 27 patients and felt the ligament healed predictably. Heterotopic ossification develops fairly frequently but in and of itself does not require treatment. The development of a symptomatic tibiofibular synostosis often does require resection.

Nitz demonstrated that 86% of grade III ankle sprains had peroneal nerve injury on EMG. Bosein noted a 22% incidence of peroneal nerve symptoms in his review of the complications of ankle sprains. Persistent paresthesias in a peroneal nerve distribution should be followed but rarely need exploration since most spontaneously resolve.

Persistent pain following an ankle sprain is unusual and usually requires investigation. The most common etiology is an osteochondral fracture of the talar dome, which occurs in about 7% of sprains. Impactive loading appears to be the mechanism, resulting in a laceration of the articular cartilage and fracture of the underlying microtrabeculae. The usual presentation is persistent pain, with swelling and occasional locking. Standard radiographs are often negative. MRI remains the imaging modality of choice. Lesions are usually either posteromedial or anterolateral. The posteromedial injury usually occurs by inversion and internal rotation, while the anterolateral occurs by eversion and dorsiflexion. Medial lesions are considered more stable and can often be treated by immobilization. Lateral lesions often require surgical fixation with absorbable pins for larger fragments and excision of smaller pieces.

Anterior ankle synovitis following recurrent sprains is also a cause of persistent pain. Typically it presents as morning stiffness and pain, with increased swelling following athletic activity. Conservative care is often unsuccessful, but arthroscopic partial synovectomy is usually effective. Anterior impingement syndrome, secondary to spurs on the talar neck, is a common cause of synovitis in dancers and football linemen. Scranton has classified distal tibiotalar spurs into four groups: types 1, 2, and 3 can be successfully treated with arthroscopic resection, while the larger type 4 spurs do best with ankle arthrotomy and open excision.

Peroneal tendon subluxation and dislocation can often be confused with an ankle sprain. Traumatic subluxation, as described by McConkey, occurs by a plantarflexion/inversion mechanism. It presents as refractory clicking and instability of the lateral ankle, and the clicking can be reproduced by vigorously everting and dorsiflexing the foot against resistance. Frank dislocation is most often seen in skiers and may be difficult to diagnose acutely if swelling and ecchymosis are present. The mechanism of injury is usually forced dorsiflexion inside the ski boot during a fall. Pain is usually more proximal and behind the malleolus than with an inversion sprain, and manual muscle testing of the peroneals is more painful than with an ankle sprain. An attempt at conservative care is recommended by some authors acutely, but surgery is recommended in all chronic cases. If the tendon can be reduced closed, a short leg cast can be applied with careful molding over the lateral malleolus in the acute situation. Reconstructions of chronic subluxations/dislocations involve combinations of deepening the groove behind the lateral malleolus and repair of the superior peroneal retinaculum.

Rehabilitation of the ankle after a fracture is similar to that for sprains. Ankle fractures that are treated nonoperatively require immobilization with the inevitable accompanying stiffness and muscle atrophy. The goal of operative treatment is early range of motion to reduce these sequelae.

In summary, acute ankle sprains are not innocuous lesions that can be treated passively, especially in the athlete. While the treatment of severe sprains remains controversial, a substantial body of information now exists indicating that simple immobilization is not adequate treatment. Controversies also exist regarding prophylaxis of ankle sprains, and most of the ankle braces on the market have yet to be tested. Finally, ankle sprains that do not respond to rehabilitation often have a secondary injury, which should be looked for carefully.

Bibliography

1. Attarian DE et al: Biomechanical characteristics of human ankle ligaments, *Foot Ankle* 6:54, 1985.
2. Berndt AL, Harty M: Transchondral fractures (osteochondritis dissecans) of the talus, *J Bone Joint Surg* 41A:988, 1959.
3. Dias LS: The lateral ankle sprain: an experimental study, *J Trauma* 19:266, 1979.
4. Garrick JG: The frequency of injury, mechanism of injury and epidemiology of ankle sprains, *Am J Sports Med* 5:241, 1977.
5. Hawkins LG: Fractures of the neck of the talus, *J Bone Joint Surg* 52A:991, 1970.
5a. Inman VT: *The joints of the ankle,* ed 1. Baltimore, Williams & Wilkins, 1976.
6. Kenny CH: Inverted osteochondral fracture of the talus diagnosed by tomography, *J Bone Joint Surg* 63A:1020, 1981.
7. McCullough CJ: Rotatory stability of the load-bearing ankle, *J Bone Joint Surg* 62B:460, 1980.
8. Nitz AJ, Dobner JJ, Kersey D: Nerve injury in Grades II and III ankle sprains, *Am J Sports Med* 19:177, 1985.
9. Renstrom P et al: Strain in the lateral ligaments of the ankle, *Foot Ankle* 9:59, 1988.
10. St. Pierre R et al: A review of lateral ankle ligament reconstructions, *Foot Ankle* 3:114, 1982.
11. Smith RW, Reischl S: Treatment of ankle sprains in young athletes, *Am J Sports Med* 14:465, 1986.
12. Smith RW, Reischl S: The influence of dorsiflexion in the treatment of severe ankle sprains: an anatomical study, *Foot Ankle* 9:28, 1988.
13. Stormont DM et al: Stability of the loaded ankle, *Am J Sports Med* 13:295, 1985.

9

Reflex Sympathetic Dystrophy

G. James Sammarco

Mitchell first reported reflex sympathetic dystrophy (RSD) in the mid-19th century.[7] He described an unrelenting, burning pain reported to him by soldiers who had sustained penetrating wounds to a major nerve trunk in the American Civil War.[20] Many reports of neurovascular dysfunction related to the sympathetic nervous system have since appeared in medical literature. Symptoms and signs of this syndrome are similar to Mitchell's original description, with some exceptions. Patients' with RSD seem to display differing causes, onset of symptoms, and response to treatment.[31] The term *reflex sympathetic dystrophy syndrome* has been used to characterize this group of disorders because of the wide variety of causes, presentation, and course of the condition.[30]

Anatomy and Physiology

The sympathetic nervous system is the thoracolumbar division of the autonomic nervous system. The parasympathetic nervous system is the craniosacral division of the autonomic system (Fig. 9–1). The autonomic nervous system, along with the endocrine system, helps to regulate internal human function and cannot be controlled voluntarily.[1]

Afferent sympathetic neuron cell bodies are locate in the lateral horn of the spinal cord from the first throacic to the third lumbar level. The axons pass up or down several vertebral levels before entering the paravertebral ganglia chain through the white ramus communicans (Fig. 9–2). The axons then travel up or down several additional levels before synapsing with the postganglionic neuron. They may synapse with other postganglionic neurons also. The postganglionic neuron receives input from other preganglionic neurons. Some preganglionic axons pass through the paravertebral chain of ganglia to synapse in the prevertebral ganglia. The lower three lumbar and first sacral ganglia supply only the legs, with no visceral connections.

The afferent sympathetic fibers carry information into the spinal cord and synapse in the spinal cord gray matter (Fig. 9–2). The preganglionic axon then travels out the spinal nerve to the paravertebral ganglia where it synapses. The post ganglionic axon then returns back to the spinal nerve through the gray ramus communicans and out the spinal nerve to the skin, providing vaso-

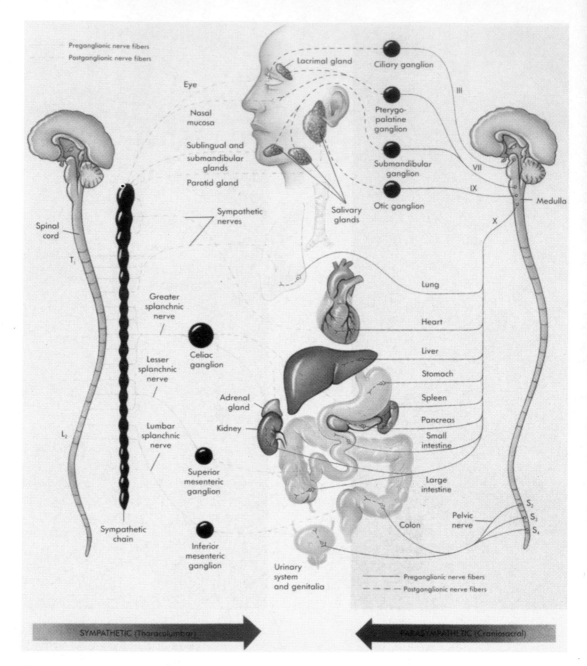

Fig. 9-1 In the sympathetic division of the autonomic nervous system, preganglionic fibers begin in the spinal cord (intermediolate: nucleus) and pass to peripheral autonomic ganglia. The postganglionic fibers pass from the peripheral ganglia to effector organs. In the parasympathetic division of the autonomic nervous system, preganglionic fibers begin in the brainstem and presacral segments and pass to peripheral ganglia. Post ganglionic fibers pass from the ganglia to the effector organs. The hypothalamus helps regulate the system as does the supranuclear regulatory apparatus of the CNS. Preganglionic fibers are indicated by *solid lines,* and postganglionic fibers are indicated by *broken lines*. (From Seeley RR, Stephens TD, Tate R. *Anatomy and physiology,* St Louis, 1989 Times Mirror/Mosby college Publishing. Used by permission.)

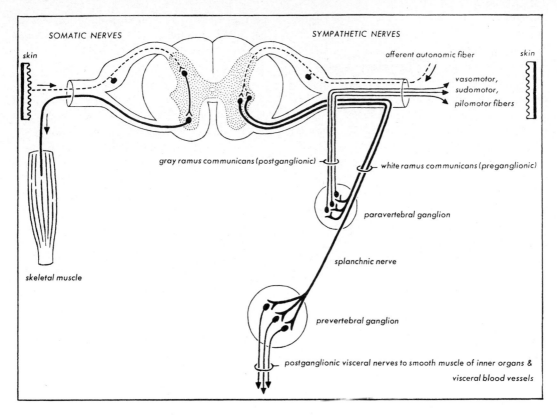

Γig. 9-2 Sympathetic outflow form the spinal cord and the course of sympathetic fibers. *Heavy lines* are preganglionic fibers. *Thin lines* are postganglionic fibers. (Adapted from Pick S: *The autonomic nervous system,* Philadelphia, 1970, JB Lippincott.)

motor, sudomotor, and pilomotor innervation.

In the lower extremities, the sympathetic regulatory system functions as a vasomotor control including the control of constriction and dilation of the blood vessels; sudomotor function with regulation of sweating; and piloerection, hair movement. The neurotransmitter for most of the sympathetic system is norepinephrine. The blood vessels, piloerector muscles, and sweat glands receive only sympathetic innervation, but the sweat glands respond only to acetylcholine.

The sympathetic nervous system functions in both the excitatory and inhibitory modes. Alpha receptors are generally excitatory. Beta receptors are inhibitory. These fibers are found in bronchial muscles and the sinoatrial node of the heart.

Diagnostic tests and therapeutic regimens for RSD often include drugs that block nerve function. Local anesthetic agents block the lumbar

paravertebral sympathetic chain for diagnosis of lower extremity disease. With a successful sympathetic block, both sensation and motor function remain intact. With an incomplete block, sympathetic symptoms also remain. A complete blockade of all somatic and sympathetic systems is then necessary. Local anesthetics such as lidocaine or bupivacaine (Marcaine) are used. An epidural block in the lower extremity has been found to be effective. Intravenous regional anesthesia is used only for the upper extremity.

Several theories have been published concerning the development of hyperactivity of the sympathetic nervous system following an injury and occasionally even without injury. Livingston[24] suggested that a "vicious cycle of reflexes" caused chronic irritation of a peripheral nerve following trauma leading to increased afferent input to the central nervous system (CNS). This caused pain and stimulated the internuncial pool of neurons in the lateral and anterior horn of the spinal cord. This stimulation, in turn, increased sympathetic and efferent motor activity.

Melzak[20] felt that the substantia gelatinosa in the spinal cord modulated afferent impulses before they reached the effector neurons. He theorized that afferent impulses are then transmitted by the small (C) and large (A) neural fibers to the substantia gelatinosa. Preferential stimulation of small (C) fibers would suppress the substantia gelatinosa and facilitate more afferent impulses to flow into the spinal cord. If the large (A) fibers were preferentially stimulated, the substantia gelatinosa would have an enhanced inhibitory tone, and block afferent impulses. Selective continuous stimulation of small (C) fibers could possibly allow unrestrained afferent impulses to the spinal cord and to other interconnecting routes.

Schott[28,29] concluded that the CNS plays an important role in RSD. He gave several reasons for this. Causalgia occurs in diseases confined to the CNS and it occurs in phantom limb pain. An unusual distribution of pain can occur such as a stocking-like distribution in the leg or even in the contralateral leg. Also, a paradoxic widespread pain distribution may occur following sympathetic nervous system injury. Moreover, peripheral sympathetic blockage is effective even when the CNS and the central interactions can cause motor, sensory, and psychological changes.

Janig[36] believed that central lesions, peripheral nerve lesions, and "chronic excitation of visceral and deep somatic afferents" could precipitate RSD. These lesions caused changes in processing information in the spinal cord and brain and in coupling between sympathetic post ganglionic axons and afferent axons in the periphery. This coupling causes orthodromic impulse activity to the spinal cord and antidromic afferent activity to the periphery, with the possible development of an "axon response" in peripheral tissues. With changes of innervation in the sympathetic system, supersensitivity to circulating catecholamines, other blood-borne substances, and other autonomic effector organs develops. In addition, stimulation of visceral afferents such as angina pectoris could also produce symptoms of RSD.

Roberts, Stanton-Hicks and collegues[25,36] re-ported a theory based on the assumption that spinal sensory neurons receive excitatory input from low-threshold mechanoreceptors. These mechanoreceptors are influenced by injury. The neurons are sensitized by stimulation and become hyperexcitable. Subsequent sympathetic activation of the low-threshold mechanoreceptors produces excessive discharging of the hyperexcitable neurons, resulting in spontaneous pain. Further discharging by the low-threshold mechanoreceptors leads to excessive firing of the sensory neurons and characteristic sensitivity to touch (allodynia).

The many different variations of RSD have one characteristic in common—sympathetically maintained pain. In 1864 the term "causalgia" was first used.[29] Pain usually started within a week of injury. The sciatic nerve was the most commonly affected nerve in the lower extremity. Pain spread beyond the area of the specific damaged nerve to include the entire extremity of contralateral extremity.[29]

Sudeck's atrophy,[28] reported in 190, described radiograph changes including bony resorption in the involved extremity. Swelling and redness of the extremity were also reported.

In 1940 Homans used the term *minor causalgia* for patients having RSD but without nerve injury and *major causalgia* for those with nerve injury.[20]

Other terms used include[11]: postraumatic pain syndrome, postraumatic osteoporosis, postraumatic dystrophy of the extremities, RSD, sympathetic dystrophy, mimocausalgia, algoneurodystrophy, shoulder-hand syndrome, algodystrophy, reflex sympathetic imbalance, and RDS syndrome.

Disease Stages

There are three distinct stages of RSD.[34,36] Determining which stage the patient is in at the time of diagnosis helps in planning treatment and in determining prognosis. The first stage, called acute, begins from the time of onset and lasts 3 months. It is believed to be the result of denervation of the sympathetic nervous system. Symptoms include burning pain, prolonged painful sensation to touch (hyperpathia) increased blood flow to the extremity, elevated skin temperature, dependent redness of the leg, localized edema, accelerated hair and nail growth, and joint stiffness with decreased active and passive range of motion.

The second stage is called the dystrophic phase. Symptoms in this stage are related to increased activity in the sympathetic nervous system. They include: persistent hyperpathia and burning pain, decreased blood flow the leg, decreased skin temperature, decreased hair growth and brittle nails, spreading brawny edema, pale cyanotic color, muscle stiffness, atrophy, and localized osteoporosis. Psychological changes and severe physical disability of the leg are present. This phase may be present for as long as 3 months.

The third stage is that of severe atrophy. There is less hyperpathia and burning pain; normal blood flow; a return to normal local skin temperature; coarse hair and rigid nails; smooth, glossy skin with subcutaneous atrophy; atrophic muscles; arthrofibrosis of joints with tendon and muscle contractures; localized osteoporosis; and a chronic pain syndrome personality.

Clinical Symptoms

Diagnosis begins with a good history. Certain symptoms are common.[26,36] The patient has pain and tenderness in the leg, foot, or a part of the foot. Hyperpathia and allodynia may be present. Pain is characteristically out of proportion to the injury and is often described as "burning", that is, hyperalgesia. The leg may be swollen and may have an increased or decreased vasomotor reaction with sweating or dryness of the skin. Diseases known to precipitate RSD include: myocardial infarction, angina pectoris, arthritis, and herpes zoster. Brain tumors, head injury, cervical fractures, and subarachnoid hemorrhage can also produce it. Orthopedic causes include, fractures, sprains, amputations, and surgical procedures during which nerves are manipulated or otherwise traumatized. Onset may occur quite early in the postoperative period and has been reported as beginning even in the recovery room following surgery. Intramuscular injections near the sciatic nerve or lateral femoral cutaneous nerve[15] have been reported to trigger it and it has been reported to occur with diabetic neuropathy.[27]

Onset of complaint begins with postoperative or posttraumatic pain that gradually increases and becomes continuous. The physician or the therapist may think that the pain is due to the patient's hypersensitivity or a mechanical problem such as a tight cast or brace, but symptoms rapidly increase beyond physical findings. Pain at rest, pain with active and passive motion, and pain at night are characteristic. Burning pain often involves the leg from just above the injury site or surgical wound distally in a stocking-like distribution. Pain may also be localized without the distribution of a peripheral nerve or spinal dermatome. The patient may be unable to tolerate even the weight of a sheet on the foot at night. Symptoms may advance to include the entire lower extremity as well as the bowel and bladder and may prevent any voluntary motion of the leg without triggering muscle spasm. Crutches are necessary. Chronic spasm may lead to joint contracture including ankle equinus and toe felxion. In the severest stages, the patient is unable to tolerate pain and may demand amputation. The patient often is unable to work, leading to social problems that complicate the treatment and the prognosis.[36]

RSD occurs in males and females equally at all ages. It is most common in adolescent girls.[13] Adolescents and children may have a spontaneous onset of symptoms without a history of injury. The clinical course in children is shorter than in adults. Simple noninvasive modalities are usually effective and the outcome is good.[10,35]

Radiographs

After a history and physical examination, radiographs are obtained. Localized osteoporosis is seen as early as 3 to 4 weeks after onset of symptoms. Soft tissue swelling and subperiosteal bone resorption are often present. These findings are not specific for RSD and may also be seen in other conditions such as hyperparathyroidism, thyrotoxicosis, and conditions with high bone turnover.

Special Studies

A three-phase tehnetium bone scan is helpful in making an RSD diagnosis.[36] Increased blood flow into the affected leg causes increased bone metabolism. Early perfusion and blood-pool studies may show increased flow to the ankle and foot. Delayed images may show increased periarticular activity in bone if symptoms have been present for more than 6 weeks.[6,16] Children may have decreased uptake in all three phases.[11]

Lumbar sympathetic block with 5 ml of 0.25% bupivacaine injected with a spinal needle directed into the paravertebral sympathetic plexus is an important test. An image intensifier may be used to guide the needle tip to the correct anatomic site. This technique greatly increases the accuracy of the needle position and the validity of the test. After injection, a warm flush is felt by the patient in the leg distally. The burning pain may be relieved for more than 2 hours. Even though the test may not relieve the pain, RSD cannot be ruled out.[36]

Schwartzman and McLellan[31] described a diagnostic epidural spinal block performed at 10-minute intervals with the following solutions in order of sequence: (1) 5 ml normal saline (placebo) followed by (2) 5 ml 0.25% procaine hydrochloride (critical sympathetic concentration), and (3) 5 ml 0.5% procaine hydrochloride (critical motor concentration). The lowest level of procaine that relieves pain indicates whether the pain is sympathetically maintained, peripheral somatic, or centrally produced.

Treatment

Treatment of RSD is directed toward relieving the symptoms while eliminating their cause. This may be difficult because the cause of the syndrome is not understood. The nickname "the orphan disease" has been applied to this condition because the symptoms are often overwhelming and the treatment response may be limited. The initial treating physician often refers the patient to a specialist and the treatment process is repeated. Treatment is directed at interrupting the abnormal sympathetic input and the mechanisms that support it. It also is directed at the targets of the disease including the bones, joints, and muscles.[36]

Level I

After diagnosis is established, antiinflammatory medication and physical therapy are prescribed. Physical therapy is given daily and includes active range of motion and flexibility exercises, a tilt board, and progressive ambulation. Ultrasound, contrast baths, and hydrotherapy are also prescribed. The therapist should concentrate on those modalities that are the most successful in reducing pain and increasing function. The patient or athlete should not be forced beyond his or her tolerance. Supervised therapy is recommended throughout the course of the disease, sometimes for as long as a year. Painful physical therapy sessions may cause increased pain and prolong the symptoms. Progress in a therapy program at the patient's own rate allows him or her some control over the symptoms.

In addition to antiinflammatory medication, that is, nonsteroidal anti-inflammatory drugs, a tricyclic antidepressant such as Amitriptyline, 25 mg for sleep, is prescribed. The dose may be increased to 50 mg if the patient is able to tolerate it. Desipramine has also been used. Tricyclic medication reduces hypersensitivity in the affected foot and may secondarily treat the accompanying depression. Phenoxybenzamine has been prescribed as a chemical sympathectomy with some success.[31] Medications including propranolol, calcium channel blockers, prazosin nifedipine (Procardia), phenytoin, and calcitonin have been used, but their true effectiveness is unknown.[31,34,36]

Transcutaneous nerve stimulation (TENS) also has been used as a treatment.[36] Its mechanism of action is unknown, but Melzak reported that it produced stimulation of both large (A) and small (C) fibers blocking pain transmission. The TENS unit may be used early in the disease to enhance physical therapy.

Corticosteroids have been used but they do not treat the sympathetic system itself. Instead they seem to act on the peripheral tissue effects of RSD by stabilizing basement membranes, decreasing capillary permeability, and reducing perivascular inflammation.

Narcotic medication is not used in the treatment of RSD in Level I. Such medication does not relieve sympathetic pain and may lead to dependency with no relief of pain.[2]

Level II

When treatment modalities have been tried and been found to be ineffective for 4 to 8 weeks after the diagnosis of acute RSD, additional treatment is indicated.

Lumbar sympathetic blocks used in diagnosis are often an effective treatment modality and occasionally result in dramatic pain relief. Sympathetic blocks may be repeated, with the patient receiving up to ten blocks over a several-week period. The blocks are repeated when symptomatic improvement begins to deteriorate, initially within a few days and later at weekly intervals. As long as the blocks give enough pain relief to allow physical therapy, they may be continued. If pain relief is incomplete with the sympathetic block, an epidural spinal anesthetic may be effective.[4] If an indwelling catheter is inserted, intermittent injections may be performed for up to 1 week.[5,19]

For chronic cases of RSD, unresponsive to sympathetic blocks, dorsal column stimulators can be implanted in the spinal cord. Pain relief may be expected in 50% of patients. If all treatment fails, a morphine pump can be implanted. A daily dose of 30 mg of intrathecal morphine is recommended.

Surgical Treatment

If sympathetic blocks provide good but short-lived relief of pain, the patient may benefit from a lumbar sympathectomy. Long-term results are good in carefully selected patients.[17,23,36]

An important consideration in the treatment is related to precipitating trauma because unresolved treatment issues for the injury may be part of the cause of RSD. They include: nerve scarring or entrapment, retained internal fixation devices, malunion, and nonunion.[30] There is controversy with respect to surgical intervention in order to remove the offending condition. Broken or misplaced plates and screws and malunion or nonunion with obvious deformity should be corrected early in the course of the disease.[2] This may be difficult because the patient may not be able to tolerate cast immobilization. Alternatively, surgical intervention for RSD has been known to worsen symptoms. The need for surgical intervention must therefore be based on all factors and the patient advised of the potential benefits and risks of surgery.

Ankylosis, deformity, and muscle contracture are all results of chronic disease. It is important to recognize that surgery for these conditions will have a limited objective. Although the deformity may be corrected, symptoms of RSD may not be completely relieved.

There is a psychological component to any chronically painful condition. Although there is no evidence that RSD is caused by psychological factors as the dystrophy progresses the patient often develops dependency, depression, insomnia, and personality changes.[36] Successful treatment not only of the painful disorder but of the patient as a whole will require appropriate attention to this aspect of the disease.[20] This often involves psychiatric therapy as well as a social service consultation and rehabilitation counseling.

The best results of treatment occur if the diagnosis is made early and therapy is instituted before chronic atrophic changes develop.[5,36] When the disease reaches its chronic stage, even if pain relief is achieved, permanent changes such as arthrofibrosis and weakness preclude a return to normal function.

References

1. Adams RD, Victor M: *Principles of neurology,* New York, 1977, McGraw-Hill.

2. Amadio PC: Pain dysfunction syndromes, *J Bone Joint Surg [Am]* 70:944-949, 1988.

3. Beresford HR: Iatrogenic causalgia: legal implications, *Arch Neurol* 41:819-820, 1984.

4. Cicala RS, Jones JW, Westbrook LL: Causalgic pain responding to epidural but not to sympathetic nerve blockade, *Anesthet Analg* 70:218-219, 1990.

5. Cooper DE, DeLee JC, Ramamurthy S: Reflex sympathetic dystrophy of the knee, *J Bone Joint Surg [Am]* 71:365-369, 1989.

6. Davidoff G, Morey K, Amann M, et al: Pain measurement in reflex sympathetic dystrophy syndrome, *Pain* 32:27-34, 1988.

7. Davidoff G, Werner R, Cremer S, et al: Predictive value of the three-phase technetium bone scan in diagnosis of reflex sympathetic dystrophy syndrome, *Arch Phys Med Rehabil* 70;135-137, 1989.

8. Davies JAH,s Beswick T, Dickson G: Ketanserin and guanethidine in the treatment of causalgia, *Anesth Analg* 66:575-576, 1987.

9. Demangeat J, Constantinesco A, Brunot B, et al: Three-phase bone scanning in reflex sympathetic dystrophy of the hand, *J Nucl Med* 29:26-32, 1988.

10. Dietz F, Mathews KD, Montgomery WJ: Reflex sympathetic dystrophy in children, *Clin Orthop* 285:225-231, 1990.

11. Doury P: Algodystrophy: reflex sympathetic dystrophy syndrome, *Clin Rheumatol* 7:173-180, 1988.

12. Escobar PL: Reflex sympathetic dystrophy, *Orthop Rev* 15:646-651, 1986.

13. Goldsmith DP, Vivino FB, Eichenfield AH, et al: Nuclear imaging and clinical features of childhood reflex neurovascular dystrophy: comparison with adults, *Arthritis Rheum* 32:480-485, 1989.

14. Holland JT: The causalgia syndrome treated with regional intravenous guanethidine, *Clin Exp Neurol* 15:166-173, 1978.

15. Horowitz SH: Iatrogenic causalgia, *Arch Neurol* 41:821-824, 1984.

16. Intenzo C, Jim S, Millin J, et al: Scintigraphic patterns of the reflex sympathetic dystorphy syndrome of the lower extremities, *Clin Nucl Med* 14:657-661, 1989.

17. Jebara VA, Saade B: Causalgia: a wartime experience—report of twenty treated cases, *J Trauma* 27:519-524, 1987.

18. Kesler RW, Saulsbury FT, Miller LT, et al: Reflex sympathetic dystrophy in children: treatment with transcutaneous nerve stimulation, *Pediatrics* 82:728-732, 1988.

19. Ladd AL, DeHaven KE, Thanik J, et al: Reflex sympathetic imbalance. Response to epidural blockade, *Am J Sports Med* 17:660-668, 1989.

20. Malkin LH: Reflex sympathetic dystrophy syndrome following trauma to the foot, *Orthopaedics* 13:851-858, 1990.

21. Mandel S, Rothrock RW: Sympathetic dystrophies, *Postgrad Med* 87:213-218, 1990.

22. McKain CW, Urban BJ, Goldner JL: The effects of intravenous regional guanethidine and reserpine, *J Bone Joint Surg [Am]* 65:808-811, 1983.

23. Mockus MB, Rutherford RB, Rosales C, et al: Sympathectomy for causalgia, *Arch Surg* 122:668-672, 1987.

24. Procacci P, Maresca M: Reflex sympathetic dystrophies and algodystrophies: historical and pathogenic considerations, *Pain* 31:137-146, 1987.

25. Roberts WJ: A hypothesis on the physiological basis for causalgia and related pains, *Pain* 24:297-311, 1986.

26. Rowlingson JC: The sympathetic dystrophies, *Int Anesthesiol Clin* 24:117-129, 1983.

27. Schapira D, Barron SA, Nahir M, et al: Reflex sympathetic dystrophy syndrome coincident with acute diabetic neuropathy, *J Rheumatol* 15:120-122, 1988.

28. Schott G: Clinical features of algodystrophy: is the sympathetic nervous system involved? *Funct Neurol* 4:131-134, 1989.

29. Schott G: Mechanisms of causalgia and related clinical conditions, *Brain* 109:717-738, 1986.

30. Schutzer SF, Gossling HR: The treatment of reflex sympathetic dystrophy syndrome, *J Bone Joint Surg [Am]* 66:625-629, 1984.

31. Schwartzman JR, McLellan TL: Reflex sympathetic dystrophy, *Arch Neurol* 44:555-561, 1987.

32. Schwartzman RJ, Kerrigan J: The movement disorder of reflex sympathetic dystrophy, *Neurology* 40:57-61, 1990.

33. Seale KS: Reflex sympathetic dystrophy of the lower extremity, *Clin Orthop* 243:80-85, 1989.

34. Shelton RM, Lewis CW: Reflex sympathetic dystrophy: a review, *Dermatology* 22:513-520, 1990.

35. Silber TJ, Majd M: Reflex sympathetic dystrophy syndrome in children and adolescents, *Am J Dis Child* 142:1325-1330, 1988.

36. Stanton-Hicks M, Janig W, Boas RA: *Reflex sympathetic dystrophy,* Workshop held in Kelkheim, West Germany, Oct 15–17, 1988, Boston, 1990, Kluwer.

37. Tahmoush AJ, Malley J, Jennings JR: Skin conductance, temperature and blood flow in causalgia, *Neurology* 33:1483-1486, 1983.

10

Rehabilitation of the Diabetic Foot and Ankle

Stephen F. Conti

Arleen Norkitis

Diabetes mellitus is a systemic disease that affects an estimated 14 million people in the United States. It affects all ages, with manifestations ranging from asymptomatic borderline hyperglycemia to severe multisystem organ failure. The activity levels of diabetic people vary as well. Children, adolescents, and young adults may remain as active as their nondiabetic counterparts. Middle-aged and older diabetics are enjoying a healthier life-style and a longer life expectancy due to advances in medical care. Each of these group's desire to remain active places them at increased risk to suffer an insult or injury to their feet.

Disorders of the foot and ankle in diabetic patients can be as diverse as the disease's manifestations. Metabolic abnormalities can affect the foot and ankle causing changes that directly increase the diabetic's susceptibility to injury. Concomitant neuropathy and vascular insufficiency states may delay the recognition of injury by the patient or decrease its perceived seriousness. Rehabilitation of the diabetic foot requires an understanding of the changes in structure and function that occur in diabetes as well as the pathophysiology of injury in these patients. Early recognition and prompt treatment of injuries is imperative. Professionals that have the most contact with the diabetic patient must assume increasing responsibility for recognizing the potential seriousness of what would be a minor injury in a nondiabetic. This includes orthopedic surgeons, primary care physicians, physical therapists, coaches, and athletic trainers. The goal of rehabilitation is often different in diabetics than in nondiabetics with similar injuries. Vigilance and an awareness of the unusual presentations of early injury are the keys to preventing and treating foot and ankle problems in these patients. Finally, attention must always be given to the general medical status of the diabetic patient since ophthalmological, cardiovascular, renal, and neurological conditions may decrease their ability to follow a standard exercise or physical therapy regimen. Consultation with a physician is important in providing a safe environment for the diabetic to maximally recover.

Diabetes Mellitus—The Disease

Diabetes mellitus is a disease characterized by abnormal carbohydrate metabolism. Both genetic and environmental factors contribute to its development. However, the importance of each may not be readily discernible in a given individual. The cause of diabetes is debated, and current theories focus on attributing different etiologies to the different types of disease states seen in the diabetic population. Genetic factors play a role in all types of diabetes, as shown by the observation that the condition tends to aggregate in families. Viral infection may be the environmental agent responsible for some cases of insulin-dependent diabetes mellitus, while obesity clearly plays a role in many cases of noninsulin-dependent disease. A multifactorial etiology probably best categorizes most cases of diabetes mellitus, with genetic and environmental factors playing a role in its development. Current research focuses on attempting to clearly define the subgroups of disease so that more specific treatments can be offered in the future.

Three main categories of diabetes mellitus have been described. Type I, or insulin-dependent diabetes, usually affects people under the age of 40 years, who require daily insulin injections to control their hyperglycemia. They lack sufficient endogenous insulin for proper cellular metabolism of carbohydrates. This leads to a wide range of metabolic abnormalities. A lack of exogenous insulin can result in life-threatening complications in these patients. The onset of symptoms is usually abrupt, with thirst, excessive urination, increased appetite, and weight loss developing over a several day period. Occasionally the disease is heralded by ketoacidosis during illness, a period of stress, or following surgery. Characteristically, the plasma glucose level is elevated while the endogenous insulin level is low. Treatment of the ketoacidotic state is complicated and requires skilled medical care. Long-term control of plasma glucose levels is accomplished through careful monitoring and administration of insulin through injection. Type II, or noninsulin-dependent diabetes, insidiously affects older, usually obese patients. Symptoms begin more gradually than in the younger insulin-dependent diabetic. Plasma insulin levels are often elevated but less than expected for the patient's degree of hyperglycemia, resulting in a relatively insulin-deficient state. More importantly, especially in obese patients, there exists an insulin resistance that involves both a decreased number of insulin receptors and a postreceptor defect. Therefore, the insulin that the patient produces is less likely to effect a change in the plasma glucose levels. Weight reduction in the obesity-hyperglycemic syndrome often causes a return to euglycemia and return of insulin responsiveness. Type II diabetes is often adequately controlled by a combination of diet, exercise, weight-loss, and oral hypoglycemics, although insulin is sometimes used to more accurately regulate blood sugar levels. Hemoglobin A1C levels are used as a measure of the degree of long-term serum glucose control. Gestational diabetes mellitus is a hyperglycemic state that occurs in women during pregnancy. Foot involvement is minimal since the condition usually resolves following delivery.

Complications from Diabetes Mellitus

The complications of diabetes may be divided into acute and chronic types. Acutely, patients may experience problems with suddenly elevated or depressed serum glucose levels. Insulin-dependent diabetics are prone to ketoacidosis, which involves hyperglycemia, metabolic acidosis, and ketonemia. This is usually the result of insulin deficiency combined with emotional or physical stress. It begins clinically with anorexia, nausea, and vomiting, coupled with increased urine formation. Abdominal pain may occur. Altered consciousness or coma then results, with alterations in respirations. Early in its course, serum electrolyte abnormalities (hyponatremia) can develop if the patient vomits repeatedly and replenishes by drinking pure water. Coaches and athletic trainers must be cognizant of this presentation so that immediate medical evaluation and care may be sought. Noninsulin-dependent diabetics may develop nonketotic hyperosmolar coma, which is similar to ketoacidosis except that it occurs insidiously, usually in elderly, debilitated patients. The onset occurs over several days, with altered mental status being an early warning sign. Again, early recognition and treatment is important to lessen the morbidity of this condition.

Both groups are also subject to hypoglycemic states, with warning signs of sweating, hunger, and palpitations, which may progress to coma or death. Much more disconcerting is the fact that some patients may have no warning at all. Since exercise lowers the need for insulin, extreme care must be taken with diabetics who wish to begin a generalized exercise regimen for cardiovascular fitness. Suddenly starting an aerobic program while maintaining the same diet and insulin dosage without proper glucose monitoring could precipitate a hypoglycemic state. Immediate treatment involves oral intake of glucose in the form of fruit juice or a candy bar. Diabetics should be encouraged to bring these with them during periods of exercise. Ideally, methods of monitoring plasma glucose levels during periods of increased physical activity should be available to the diabetic patient. Again, physicians, coaches, and athletic trainers must demonstrate continued vigilance in caring for these patients. Diabetics must also receive education on recognizing the early warning signs of hypoglycemia and how to adjust their medication during periods of increased physical activity.

Chronic complications include ophthalmological, cardiovascular, and renal problems, which are beyond the scope of this chapter. Both cardiovascular and renal abnormalities can lead to fluctuating chronic pedal edema, making proper shoe fit difficult. Two long-term complications that affect the foot and ankle are neuropathy and vascular disease. Diabetic neuropathy is the most common and often the most troublesome complication. Frequently the diagnosis is difficult to make because the manifestations are nonspecific and the disorder may be manifested either clinically or subclinically, with abnormalities detectable only by careful testing. The prevalence of neuropathy in diabetic populations ranges from zero to 93%.[1] The wide range oc-

curs because of the differing criteria used by various authors to define neuropathy. The Diabetes Control and Complications Trial demonstrated that tight regulation of serum glucose levels reduced the incidence and severity of neuropathy.[4] However, despite extremely poor control of their diabetes, up to fifty percent of all diabetic subjects never develop symptoms of neuropathy, even after more than 20 years duration of disease.

Sensory, motor, and autonomic neuropathy combine to cause dysfunction in the foot. Sensory neuropathy affects small nerve fibers followed by large fibers. The longest nerves are affected first, so that the initial symptoms appear in the feet in most cases. This is manifested first with the loss of thermal sensitivity, reduced light touch, and pinprick, followed by reduced vibratory sensation and depressed tendon reflexes. Electrodiagnostic testing demonstrates slowing of nerve conduction velocities as one of the earliest abnormalities. However, nerve conduction velocity does not appear to be related to the severity of symptoms. Motor neuropathy usually follows sensory loss and results in denervation of intrinsic foot musculature. An imbalance between the intrinsic and extrinsic control of the toes causes hyperextension of the metatarsophalangeal joints, with flexion deformities of the proximal interphalangeal joints. With time these clawtoe deformities become increasingly pronounced and fixed. Areas of irritation from shoe wear may then occur on the dorsum of the proximal interphalangeal joints or over the tips of the toes (Fig. 10-1). Additionally, hyperextension of the metatarsophalangeal joint results in increased plantar pressure beneath the metatarsal heads. This leads to painful metatarsalgia or plantar ulceration beneath the metatarsal heads. Autonomic neuropathy affects both sympathetic and parasympathetic nerve fibers, with parasympathetic dysfunction preceding sympathetic dysfunction.[4,7] Cardiovascular abnormalities are manifested first and include an increase in resting heart rate, abnormalities to Valsalva's maneuver, and loss of the immediate heart-rate response to standing.[7,10] Sympathetic failure may be clinically related to postural hypotension, sweating disturbances, and hypoglycemic un-

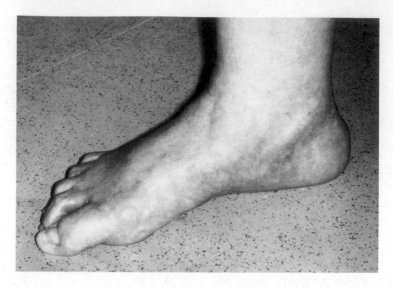

Fig. 10-1 Typical diabetic foot demonstrating fixed hammertoes.

awareness. Lack of sweating results in skin that is dry and prone to fissuring. This compromises the plantar skin, making it more susceptible to shear stress injury as well as bacterial superinfection. Callus formation and neuroarthropathy may be related to autonomic dysfunction as well.[6,7,13] Direct injury to the small myelinated and unmyelinated sympathetic nerve fibers responsible for pain and temperature may be responsible for painful peripheral neuropathy. This is often the earliest symptom and heralds the onset of neuropathy. The discomfort produced may be intense at first but usually diminishes over the course of several years. Decreased pain is an indication that the nerves are functioning less well and the neuropathy is becoming more severe.

Vascular complications are common in diabetics. Patients with diabetes are 15 times more likely than nondiabetics to have peripheral vascular disease, and it ranks second only to heart disease as the most costly of diabetic complications requiring hospitalization. The incidence of peripheral vascular disease increases with age and duration of disease. It has been estimated that the cumulative incidence of vascular disease in diabetics is 15% at 10 years and 45% at 20 years after initial diagnosis of the disease. Diabetes appears to augment atherosclerosis, especially in populations with other risk factors such as smoking, hyperlipidemia, and hypertension. The atherogenic effect of diabetes causes accelerated changes in the larger proximal vessels above the knee. Bilateral iliac and femoral stenosis is common. Unique to diabetes is a symmetrical narrowing of all three vessels just below the trifurcation (Fig. 10-2). The importance of this becomes apparent during planned revascularization procedures. Standard bypass techniques such as femoral-popliteal anastomoses are usually not advisable in diabetics. Instead, complicated bypass procedures such as reverse vein grafts, which course from the proximal femoral vessels to arteries in the foot, are often necessary. Foot pain as a result of intermittent claudication is possible and must be differentiated from neuropathic pain. History and physical examination supplemented by noninvasive Doppler studies are necessary to distinguish these two conditions. Arteriograms are useful as a preoperative anatomic guide to determine a candidate's suitability for vascular reconstruction. If the patient does not reconstitute a named vessel below the blockage, then bypass is not possible.

Rehabilitation, Modalities, Trauma, Disease, and Pediatrics

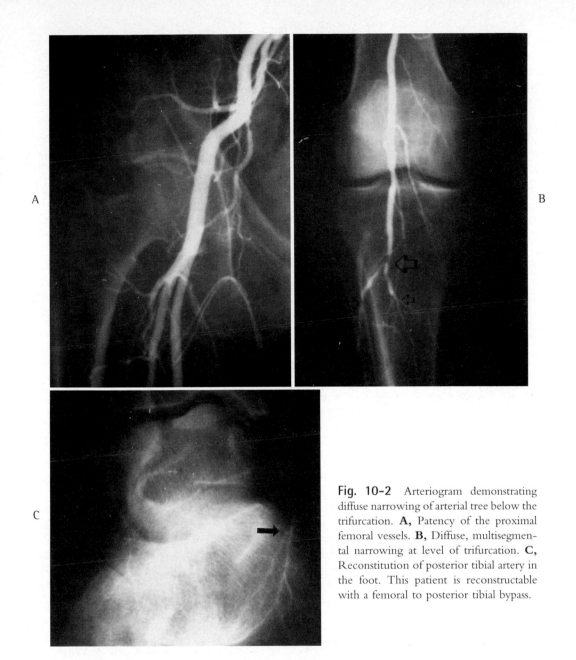

Fig. 10-2 Arteriogram demonstrating diffuse narrowing of arterial tree below the trifurcation. **A,** Patency of the proximal femoral vessels. **B,** Diffuse, multisegmental narrowing at level of trifurcation. **C,** Reconstitution of posterior tibial artery in the foot. This patient is reconstructable with a femoral to posterior tibial bypass.

Structure and Function of the Diabetic Foot

The foot has several functions, which include acting as a rigid base of support for the body while maintaining suppleness to accommodate to uneven ground, dissipating shock during gait, and absorbing transverse leg rotation. Compromising any one of these will predispose a person to injury. The diabetic foot is often stiff and weak, making injury from minor trauma an ever present possibility.

The human foot is composed of 26 bones and

over 50 joints that allow it to be quite flexible at times and rigid when necessary. The bones are connected by capsules and ligaments, which allow for joint motion to occur within defined physiological limits. These structures are composed of collagen fibers meshed within a ground substance. The collagen provides significant tensile strength, while the ground substance allows for some degree of flexibility. Each material is found in a well-controlled local molecular environment that maintains its unique properties. All human tissue undergoes a process known as nonenzymatic glycosylation of collagen, whereby sugar moieties are attached to collagen molecules causing a slight alteration of their ionic charge. In nondiabetics this reaction occurs continually at a very low level with no adverse consequences. In hyperglycemic states this same process occurs at a substantially accelerated rate, which leads to increased cross-linking of collagenase-resistant collagen fibers. The collagen no longer maintains its special properties, making tissues less resilient. Since this includes capsules and ligaments, joints become gradually stiffer and less mobile, making the foot more rigid. This in turn causes excessive stress to be transmitted to certain joints, predisposing the cartilage and bone on either side of the joint to fracture and fragmentation. In addition, a stiff foot is less able to accommodate to uneven terrain, predisposing it to injury. Excessive production of bone has been shown to occur in diabetics at ligamentous attachment sites, contributing to the problem of stiffness. Tendons can be similarly affected due to their collagen content.

Diminished muscle strength further contributes to the risk of injury. Muscles are weakened due to the nonenzymatic glycosylation of collagen that occurs in the connective tissue within the muscle belly. Also, impairment of the neurological reflexes that muscles participate in to protect adjacent joints results in joints that are less able to resist nonphysiological loads. Clinically, ankle dorsiflexors, inverters and everters, and intrinsics have been demonstrated to be weak in diabetic patients.[5,11,12,14] Rehabilitation of these muscle groups may require

specific strengthening exercises to prevent significant gait abnormalities.

Articular cartilage and the supporting subchondral bone are abnormal in the diabetic foot. Insulin is required for glucose uptake into cartilage as well as for the oxidation of carbon dioxide and for collagen synthesis. A lack of insulin results in cartilage that does not tolerate repetitive physiological trauma or compression well. In addition, insulin-dependent diabetics are more likely to develop osteopenia than are age-matched nondiabetics. The suspected causes include microangiopathy, sympathetic neuropathy, hyperemia, infection, and various metabolic abnormalities.[2,4,9] The generalized osteopenia of diabetes predisposes to fracture and subchondral bone collapse, making the joint more vulnerable to injury.

Neuropathy is the most significant factor responsible for injuries and the serious complications seen in the diabetic foot. Sensory abnormalities result in decreased plantar sensation and make recognition of injury by the patient unreliable. Patients with neuropathy may not notice an area of irritation or a blister on their feet. With continued unprotected activity, even seemingly minor skin lesions may be allowed to progress, ultimately leading to ulceration. This includes seemingly minor blisters that can rapidly form large ulcers. Direct trauma such as stepping on a pin may not be felt by the patient, leading to superficial or deep infection (Fig. 10-3). Equally important, sprains and strains may go unrecognized by the patient and untreated. Torn capsules and ligaments are not reflexely immobilized by the neuropathic patient in the same way they would be in someone with normal sensation. This results in unprotected weight-bearing with subluxation of joints and instability. These abnormalities may then continue, resulting in osteoarthropathy, collapse of the normal weight-bearing architecture of the foot, increased plantar pressures, and plantar skin breakdown (Fig. 10-4). Motor neuropathy causes severe fixed clawtoe deformities due to intrinsic muscle weakness. This increases pressure beneath the metatarsal heads, contributing to focal increases in plantar pressure. More proximal lesions cause subtle or overt muscle im-

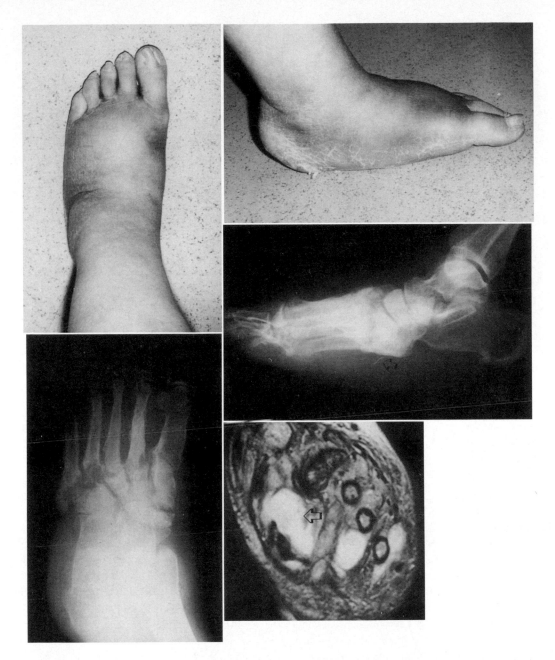

Fig. 10-3 A 53-year-old female presented with sepsis and a swollen left foot. Initial radiographs reveal Charcot midfoot changes and a pin in plantar aspect of the foot. Magnetic resonance imaging of the foot demonstrates the surrounding abscess.

balances in the foot, leading to gait abnormalities with the potential for injury. As a general rule, midfoot Charcot changes result in plantar pressure abnormalities, while hindfoot neuroarthropathy results in significant instability of the involved joints (Fig. 10-5). Autonomic neuropathy, as noted previously, is responsible for the characteristic lack of sweating noted in diabetic feet. The skin becomes less supple and more vulnerable to shear stress injury.

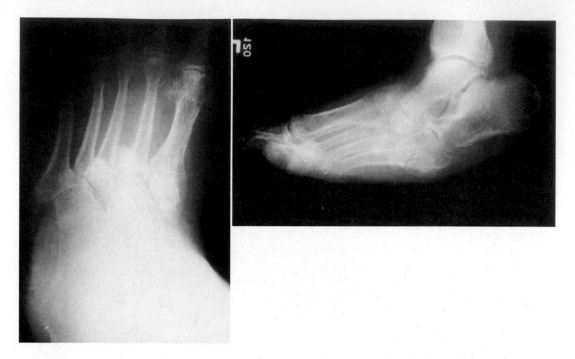

Fig. 10-4   Typical Charcot midfoot with fragmentation of the tarsometatarsal and intertarsal joints and collapse of arch.

General Care of the Diabetic Foot

With a knowledge of the pathophysiologic processes that commonly occur in the diabetic, it is possible to formulate a simple, rational plan to care for the diabetic foot. The single most important principle to be remembered is that continual education is the key to preventing foot problems in the diabetic. Those responsible for the care of these patients must reinforce the principles of good foot care at every opportunity and at the same time provide support as patients learn to cope with their disease and the life-style changes that accompany it. Surprisingly, it has been our experience that even diabetics with long-standing disease may have never had formal instruction on proper foot care. Both verbal and written material should be supplied to patients on their initial physician visit. Preventing plantar ulceration and other serious foot disorders must receive as much attention and effort as treating these conditions once they occur.

Regardless of age or severity of clinical symptoms and signs, all diabetics should adhere to the following guidelines in caring for their feet:

1. Feet should be washed and dried daily with a mild soap and water solution. Harsh, perfumed soaps can cause excessive drying of the skin. Autonomic neuropathy decreases the sweating response, making the skin dry. This results in an increased likelihood of forming skin fissures and subsequent bacterial infection. Additionally, plantar skin that is dry is less supple and resilient, making it more likely to be damaged by shear forces leading to ulceration. Caution must be exercised even in preparation for the bath. The temperature of the water should be checked with the elbow or a thermometer prior to immersing the feet to prevent accidental scalding.

2. A moisturizer should be applied to the skin after bathing to prevent drying. The exception is in the intertriginous spaces between the toes, which should be kept dry with powder to prevent fungal infection.

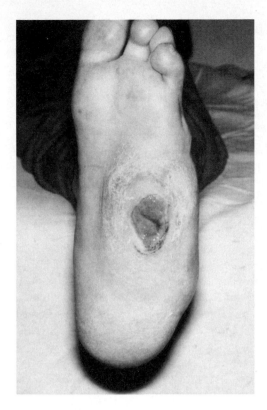

Fig. 10-5   Diabetic neuropathic midfoot ulcer.

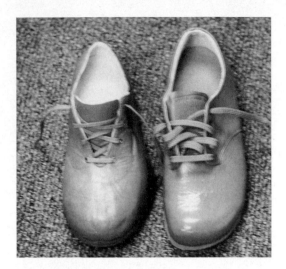

Fig. 10-6   Trilaminate Plastazote orthotics and extradepth shoes.

3. Nail care is very important and should be performed regularly by the patient, a family member, or physician. The nails should be trimmed straight across to prevent them from becoming ingrown. The corners should not be cut short. Fungal infections of the toenails are common and are probably the result of increased tissue glucose levels as well as an increased susceptibility to infection. Hyperkeratotic nails should be burred down with a high-speed tool such as the Dremel Mototool (Emerson Electric) to prevent dorsal/plantar pressure on the toe from contact with the shoe toebox. Nailplate removal should be performed with extreme caution since the distal circulation may be inadequate to allow successful healing.

4. Barefoot walking, even for short periods of time, should be discouraged. Penetration of the sole by foreign bodies such as pins is common and may lead to infection and abscess formation. Shoes must be properly made and fit well. Anyone with foot deformity must obtain shoes to accommodate their feet. High, wide-toebox shoes made of soft leather uppers with a single seam are appropriate. Over-the-counter athletic sneakers are adequate for many people to pursue recreational activities in. Evidence exists that custom-molded orthotics made of viscoelastic material, such as Plastazote, help to more evenly redistribute plantar pressure, and these are recommended for anyone at risk for plantar ulceration (Fig. 10-6). Recent studies suggest that pressure distribution over the soles of diabetic feet changes over a relatively short time (3 years). Therefore, orthotics and shoes need to be reevaluated at 6-month intervals, with remanufacturing necessary following any evidence of a change in the structure of the foot. Also, since the viscoelastic material used to make orthotics may permanently deform with time, it is important that these be evaluated by a pedorthotist at 6-month intervals.

5. Wearing two pairs of thin athletic socks is advisable for recreation. Orthotics and shoes can decrease peak plantar pressures,

but they do not reduce the shear stress that may play a role in the development of ulcers. In theory it is postulated that by wearing two pairs of socks a portion of the shear will occur between the socks, diminishing that which occurs between the skin and the sock.

6. New shoes should be broken in gradually. A typical wearing-in schedule might include wearing the shoes for 1 hour per day for 1 week and increasing this by 1 hour per day each week thereafter. Visual inspection of the foot every hour is mandatory during this time. Even custom shoes should not be taken out of the box and worn all day immediately, since they require a period of break-in as well.

7. Daily inspection of the feet must be performed by the patient or by someone caring for the patient. This should include the dorsal and plantar aspects as well as the areas between the toes. A mirror is useful to allow inspection of the sole. Trauma to the toes and nails, breaks in the skin, areas of erythema, new onset swelling, or change in the shape of the foot should be evaluated by a physician.

Recognition and Management of Acute Injury

It has already been noted that diabetics are at increased risk for sustaining injury. Injured nondiabetics protect their extremities because pain prevents them from weight-bearing. Neuropathy may not allow diabetics to recognize and protect their feet or ankles following an injury. They continue to walk painlessly, causing increasing damage to their feet. One theory regarding the etiology of neuroarthropathy begins with injury to capsules and ligaments surrounding joints. If appropriate immobilization allows complete healing, then no further complications will ensue. However, if the injury goes unprotected, then subluxation of the joint will occur followed by dislocation. Abnormal joint forces then occur across cartilage

and bone that are weakened by the factors previously discussed. The result is neuroarthropathic changes, collapse of the normal architecture of the foot, elevated areas of plantar pressure, and subsequent ulceration or instability of the foot.

A variety of schemes have been used to describe the neuropathic arthropathies. Neuropathic joints can be classified as acute or chronic. The acute phase is often precipitated by minor trauma and is characterized by swelling, erythema, increased temperature, joint effusion, and bone resorption. Chronic changes include cartilage fibrillation, loose body formation, subchondral sclerosis, and marginal osteophytes. The gradual absorption of fine debri and hematoma with callus formation is noted as well. Proliferative changes occur, with new bone formation resulting in decreased joint mobility and increased stabilization of the foot. Eichenholtz[2] divided the disease process into three radiographically distinct stages. The stage of development represents the acute, atrophic phase. The stage of coalescence is noted by a lessening of edema, absorption of fine debri, and healing of fractures. The final phase, or stage of reconstruction, is accompanied by further repair and remodeling of bone in an attempt to restore stability.

The initial care of the diabetic foot following injury is critical to successful rehabilitation of the patient. A high index of suspicion must exist to recognize that injury has occurred since symptoms may be minimal. Any diabetic with swelling in the foot or ankle must be considered to have sustained an injury until proven otherwise. Immediate cessation of activity and medical evaluation is absolutely mandatory.

The acute onset of swelling in the diabetic foot requires a careful physical examination to assess the presence of clinically significant neuropathy and radiographic evaluation to search for evidence of bone or joint abnormalities. If patients demonstrate no acute changes on radiograph, they should be placed into a total contact cast and given crutches or a walker to decrease weight on the extremity. Elevation above the level of the heart must be strictly enforced. The patient is seen at weekly intervals for a cast change and inspection of the foot. When swelling has abated, the patient may begin weight-bearing as tolerated in a brace or without protection and is started on a physical therapy regimen. Typically, resolution of the acute injury is heralded by decreased swelling and temperature of the skin. Newer, more quantifiable and reproducible techniques to assess healing are being investigated. One promising technique involves determining skin temperature differences between the injured and uninjured foot.[3] The acute inflammatory process is felt to be resolved when the temperature difference between feet is less than 3° C.

If the radiographs demonstrate an acute change in the appearance of a joint (i.e., subluxation or dislocation), consideration is given to early surgical reduction and stabilization using internal fixation and fusion. This has been shown to provide long-term stability to the structure of the foot and prevent the late sequelae of Charcot change and collapse. Minor degrees of subluxation may be successfully managed in a nonweight-bearing cast until radiographic evidence of bony consolidation has occurred or complete ligament healing has taken place. This requires a minimum period of immobilization of 3 months. Acute swelling in the presence of chronic radiographic joint changes and midfoot arch collapse requires total contact casting until the acute process has resolved, followed by consideration for orthotic management vs. surgical reconstruction of the foot. The advantages of orthotic and brace management of deformed feet are that it is often effective in stabilizing the deformity and preventing recurrent ulceration. It is also non-invasive, the complication rate is low, and it does not require hospitalization. The advantages of surgical reconstruction are that it can provide a foot that is more normally shaped, functions better, and can fit into over-the-counter footwear with a very low rate of ulcer recurrence. Preliminary data on surgical reconstruction have shown this to be a way of reestablishing the normal weight-bearing structure of the foot to prevent ulceration and improve gait. After healing in a cast or surgery, the patient can then begin a planned program of general and specific foot-oriented physical therapy.

Physical Therapy for the Diabetic Foot

General Exercise Guidelines in Diabetes

The presence of diabetes requires special considerations before beginning an exercise program. These relate to the type, control, and complications of the disease. In general, healthy and well-controlled individuals do not need a medical examination prior to the onset of an exercise program. Those with Type I diabetes for longer than 10 years and Type II obese patients should undergo physical examination to detect any coronary artery disease, retinopathy, nephropathy, or neuropathy (autonomic or sensory) that could put them at risk.

The role of exercise in the treatment of Type II diabetes is well established. Physical training will improve insulin sensitivity, encourage weight loss, reduce cardiovascular risk factors, and improve control of blood sugar levels. In fact some patients with Type II diabetes can be well controlled on a regimen of exercise and diet only. Conversely, the Type I diabetic will not experience the same type of metabolic control through physical training but can reduce the quantity of insulin needed per day.

The acute consequences of exercise (hypoglycemia) has caused controversy regarding the general recommendations for exercise in the Type I diabetic. Similar complications can be experienced by the Type II diabetic when treatment involves the use of insulin or sulfonylureas. An exercise program for these individuals should only be undertaken when the patient clearly understands the actions of these chemicals and has discussed the need for modifications of dosage/diet when exercising with a physician. When beginning an exercise program, more frequent monitoring of blood glucose level will help the individual and physician determine appropriate changes in medication dosing.

Normal response to exercise maintains blood glucose level. In diabetes this normal homeostatic mechanism is impaired, and close attention must be paid to blood sugar level, timing of exercise in relation to meals, and insulin dosage to avoid hypoglycemia and ketoacidosis. The risk of hypoglycemia during exercise is related to lowered blood glucose levels when the liver is unable to supply glucose at a pace sufficient for skeletal muscle use. In fact skeletal muscle continues to have a higher level of glucose uptake for up to 12 hours after exercise, which poses the possibility of postexercise hypoglycemia. These episodes are not uncommon 4 to 6 hours after exercise. Ketoacidosis may occur in individuals who exercise when in a poor state of metabolic control (hypoinsulinemia). Hypoinsulinemia prevents transfer of glucose into the liver and muscles and contributes to reduced stores of glycogen in these tissues. This impaired aerobic endurance requires utilization of free fatty acids for fuel production and the possibility of ketoacidosis.

Timing of exercise is important in diabetics. It is best to exercise when blood sugar is between 100 and 250 mg/dl. If blood sugar is less than 100 mg/dl, a preexercise snack is necessary and is probably a good habit for all patients. If blood glucose is greater than 250 mg/dl and urine ketones are negative, then exercise is allowed. Additional snacks (15 to 30 g of carbohydrate) should be eaten at 30-minute intervals if exercise is to continue for more than 30 minutes. After exercising, extra food may be required for up to 24 hours because of the increased metabolism brought on by exercise. However, late night snacks should be avoided, especially in the Type I diabetic, because of the possibility of rebound hypoglycemia while sleeping.

Following are some general guidelines to use in regulating the timing and dosage of insulin when exercising. Only a physician must make these decisions. Ideally a reduced dose of insulin should be taken 1 hour before exercise. The dosage of intermediate-acting insulin should be decreased by 30% to 35%. If supplemental insulin is needed following exercise, then the additional insulin should be taken with the evening meal. A regimen of intermediate and short-acting insulin might omit or reduce the need for short-acting insulin by 50%. If the insulin regimen includes several doses of short-acting insulin, the dose prior to exercise should be reduced by 30% to 50%, with postexercise doses adjusted based on glucose monitoring. Individuals on continuous subcutaneous infusion should eliminate or decrease the mealtime bolus and decrease the basal infusion rate during exercise. If the normal amount of insulin has already been taken, additional food must be eaten before exercising.

There is no indication to restrict the physical activity of healthy, well-controlled children, adolescents, and young adults except to avoid the acute complications of hypoglycemia and ketoacidosis. In the older diabetic the presence of associated conditions (such as coronary artery disease) will restrict the type of exercise that may be performed. The presence of retinopathy or nephropathy precludes exercise that sustains a systolic blood pressure greater than 180 to 200 mmHg. The type and amount of aerobic exercise that will lead to this rise in blood pressure vary with the individual and need to be determined by testing. Problems can develop with activities such as weight lifting, exercise associated with Valsalva's maneuvers, or positions in which the head is lower than the waist. Autonomic neuropathy reduces maximum heart-rate response and impairs sweating response. These factors significantly reduce aerobic capacity and predispose to hyperthermia. Exercising in heat and high humidity is contraindicated. In addition, autonomic neuropathy predisposes the individual to silent or painless myocardial infarction, which further complicates an exercise prescription. Sensory neuropathy predisposes diabetics to foot injury, suggesting that swimming and biking may be more appropriate exercise than walking or running.

Glucose requirements are relatively unchanged when the exercise intensity is less than 30% to 50% of maximum (Vo_2). Metabolic demands increase with intensity and duration of exercise. Type I diabetics with cardiovascular disease or older patients should limit physical activity to 30 to 40 minutes at 50% to 70% of Vo_2 max. Since Vo_2 max is not easily measured in the physical therapy clinic or on the athletic field, one can use 50% to 70% of the maximum heart rate as a guide.

Physical Therapy Examination of the Foot

A thorough evaluation must be completed before beginning an ankle or foot rehabilitation program. Ideally this evaluation should include measurement of active and passive range of motion (ROM), strength, and swelling; observation of gait, posture, balance, and coordination; and compilation of complete medical history including current injury. When evaluating the diabetic foot, additional considerations are needed because of the potential sequelae of any neuropathic and vascular complications. These additional considerations are evaluation of sensory level, vascular status, skin temperature, foot deformities, callus formation, and footwear.

The results of quantitative evaluation of sensation will influence many of the rehabilitative decisions in the care of the diabetic foot. Semmes-Weinstein monofilaments and the Biothesiometer are tools commonly used for assessing sensation. Semmes-Weinstein monofilaments are a series of inexpensive plastic or nylon monofilaments of different thicknesses (Fig. 10-7). Each monofilament is numbered according to the logarithm of the pressure it exerts. When applied perpendicular to the skin, each monofilament bends when a specific amount of pressure is applied, allowing for quantitative measure of touch/pressure sensation. Inability to feel the 5.07 Semmes-Weinstein monofilament has been defined as loss of protective sensation and indicates that significant sensory neuropathy is present. Loss of protective sensation means that an individual is unable to feel sufficient pain to reflexly splint the limb and prevent skin injury from occurring. This damage can be severe, such that a nail may penetrate through the sole of the shoe into the foot with the person only becoming aware of this when they are unable to remove the shoe or a trail of blood is noticed. The Biothesiometer measures vibration perception threshold. An inability to feel 35 V on the machine is probably suggestive of sensory neuropathy. Biothesiometers are not easily standardized between models and are expensive, suggesting that this modality is more appropriate in specialized clinics treating and investigating diabetic foot problems.

Typical physical therapy evaluation of vascular status includes palpating pulses and observing for signs of peripheral vascular disease. While this may be adequate, especially in the younger athlete, a more accurate assessment of circulation can be obtained by Doppler. This can provide the ankle brachial index (ABI), which is a ratio of the brachial systolic blood pressure to the

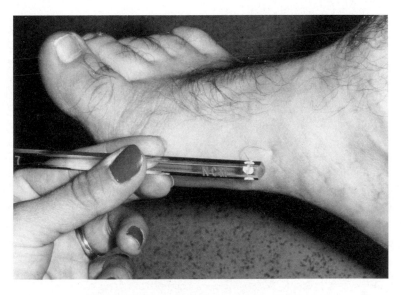

Fig. 10-7 Semmes-Weinstein monofilaments.

ankle systolic blood pressure. Hallux systolic pressures can also be obtained by Doppler, but a more accurate assessment can be obtained by using a plesmograph. An ABI of less than 0.45 or a hallux pressure of less than 40 mmHg raises concern that circulation is inadequate to promote healing of an ulceration. An ankle systolic pressure of over 200 mmHg or an ABI over 1.5 suggests calcified arteries. Calcified arteries artificially raise the ankle systolic blood pressure, making the ABI less reliable. This is because the sphygmomanometer must exert increased pressure to collapse the stiffened walls of calcified vessel.

Skin temperature will be elevated with increased blood flow as a result of inflammation of any cause. Increased skin temperature of one midfoot or ankle compared to the same site on the contralateral foot may be a warning sign of an early Charcot process or an indication of continuing neuroarthropathic fragmentation. Skin temperature should be assessed throughout the rehabilitation process by using thermography, infrared skin thermometers, or the dorsum of the hand. Thermography is an accurate method of measuring temperature but is expensive and inconvenient for frequent screening. A hand-held infrared skin thermometer can be easily used in the clinic to assess skin temperature. The feet should be placed in a device to prevent drafts across the feet, such as a cardboard box, for 10 minutes before using the infrared skin thermometer. Use of the dorsum of the examiner's hand can be adequate to assess temperature differences between feet for routine screening purposes.

Evaluation of footwear, deformities, and callus formation are important in the prevention of ulceration. Improperly fitting footwear and formation of plantar callus contribute to the development of ulcers. Deformities can make proper shoe fit difficult and can cause callus formation. Shoe fit should be assessed while the patient is standing. The typical diabetic shoe is made of a soft leather upper with a single seam. It is custom made to accommodate all deformities. The sole should be lightweight and flared to provide a stable base for support. A properly fitting shoe should be approximately ¼ to ½ inch longer than the longest toe and should bend at the first metatarsal head when the heel is lifted off the ground. The width of a shoe is appropriate when one can pinch a small piece of the shoe material while running the fingers across the toebox. Recurrent ulceration in the same place may indicate improperly fitting footwear or inadequately modified footwear. Long-term studies of plantar pressure in diabetics have shown that over a 3-year period the pressure distribution over the sole changes significantly in many patients.[3] Additionally a large percentage of recurrent ulcers occur at sites different from those of previous ulcers, suggesting a change in the plantar pressure distribution pattern with time. The most obvious explanation is that the static or dynamic structure of the foot is altered with time. This may be due to the biochemical changes that occur in the ligaments and muscles, as discussed previously, or to progressive neuroarthropathy and collapse of the arch or increased instability of the hindfoot. Vigilance and constant reassessment of the need for new footwear are keys to the successful prevention of plantar ulceration.

Goals of Rehabilitation

When protective sensation is preserved, there is a relatively low risk of developing diabetes-related foot problems. Therefore, treatment goals for rehabilitating injuries in the nonneuropathic foot should be no different than in nondiabetic patients. Some additional guidelines, however, are related to education regarding diabetic foot problems, general care, and proper shoe fit. When circulation is compromised, proper shoe fit is crucial in order to avoid ulceration.

Treatment of the Neuropathic Foot

Loss of protective sensation prevents a person from sensing pain before permanent injury occurs. The lack of pain sensation allows patients with neuropathy to walk with little pain, even on large ulcerations, foot fractures, and dislocations. Treatment must substitute for the protective pain mechanism in order to be successful in rehabilitating the neuropathic foot.

Ulceration is a common occurrence in the diabetic foot. As long as the vascular status is adequate and no deep infection is present, ulcers will heal with appropriate pressure relief.

When the ulcer is on the plantar surface of the foot, pressure relief must be either nonweight-bearing with crutches or the use of a total contact cast. Unloading nonplantar ulcers can be as simple as removing the offending footwear and replacing it with a healing sandal. A healing sandal can be made by placing a soft cushioned insole inside a cast boot. In the event of infection or vascular insufficiency, appropriate consultation should be sought. These must be dealt with first before ulcer healing can take place.

Sprains, strains, and contusions are common foot and ankle injuries. In a neuropathic individual these injuries may be painless even in the presence of swelling, increased skin temperature, and hematoma. Typically an individual's level of pain is what guides treatment of these injuries. However, in the neuropathic individual, one cannot rely on pain level as an assessment of the degree of recovery. When considering this and the fact that neuropathy often begins with a soft tissue injury, it becomes evident that treatment protocols must be drastically changed. All sprains, strains, and contusions resulting in a hot, swollen foot require either nonweight-bearing or immobilization, preferably in a total contact cast. The cast is often the more desirable choice because one does not have to rely on patient compliance to protect the foot. This protective phase should continue until the inflammatory stage has resolved. Traditional signs, including reduction in skin temperature and resolution of swelling, redness, and/or hematoma, should be used as guidelines. A skin temperature differential of less than 3°C between feet shows some promise of being an objective indicator that the inflammatory process is finished. Because of the risk of neurarthropathy, a radiograph should rule out any early bony changes before completing the protective phase of treatment.

Management of fractures and dislocations of the neuropathic foot and ankle is controversial. As previously discussed, any subluxation or dislocation should be treated with early open reduction and primary fusion. Fracture care should follow the principles established for nondiabetics. Nonoperative treatment should be employed whenever possible. The decision to proceed with operative intervention must take into account the patient's overall medical condition, integrity of the skin, and adequacy of the distal circulation. Evaluation of the dorsalis pedis and posterior tibial artery pulses, midfoot TcPo$_2$, and digital arterial Doppler waveforms and pressures are useful in this assessment. The presence of neuropathy requires some special considerations, however. First, these injuries can take much longer to heal than similar injuries in nondiabetics. Therefore, patients need to be immobilized for a much longer period of time. A minimum of 3 months of cast immobilization is recommended. Very importantly, an individual cast should not be left on for more than 2 weeks at a time and must be changed if it is loose, damaged, or painful. Second, one should monitor skin temperature as a means of assessing the resolution of the inflammatory component of the injury. Persistently elevated temperatures may place the patient at risk of developing Charcot arthropathy, and continued cast immobilization is indicated. If the bone heals but skin temperature remains significantly elevated, or if there are bony changes associated with neurarthropathy, immobilization should continue until skin temperature is reduced and bony changes have stabilized.

Management of patients with active neurarthropathy is often an extremely long and frustrating process. The first problem can be making the diagnosis, because the swelling, discomfort, and increased skin temperature can continue for many months before bony changes are evident on radiograph. The differential diagnoses of increased blood flow associated with autonomic neuropathy, infection, or early Charcot neuroarthropathy are sometimes difficult to distinguish from one another. This mandates the approach that any patient with clinical symptoms and signs of possible early neurarthropathy (swelling, erythema, increased discomfort) should be treated with a total contact cast. There is no scientific evidence that early immobilization in a total contact cast will reduce the amount of bony destruction or even shorten the amount of time it takes for resolution of the active phase. However, clinical observation suggests that very few bony changes and little deformity occur once immobilization is begun. Bone destruction and fragmentation need to stabilize and the skin temperature should be within 2° to 3°C of the same sites on the other foot before casting is discontinued. After casting is complete, a brace must be worn for a period of time in patients with hindfoot Charcot and instability. Midfoot changes can be supported with custom-molded semirigid arch supports. These are made of two layers of different density Plastazote with a third layer of cork or special rubber for support.

Neurarthropathy may not be diagnosed until long after bony changes have begun and the foot has already become significantly deformed. In this case, the first decision must be whether the foot is still in an active phase with progressive bony changes occurring. This can be determined by a history of the patient's symptoms and comparison of recent and previous radiographs. If it is no longer active, treatment consists of prescribing appropriate footwear to accommodate the foot deformity and protect the skin from ulceration. However, if the process is still active, total contact casting is instituted with limitation of weight-bearing until the patient enters the consolidation phase of the disease. If there is dislocation or subluxation of joints in the foot, then surgical intervention to reconstruct the foot must be considered. Surgery should also be considered in any patient with deformity who fails to remain ulcer-free despite appropriate footwear and orthotic modifications or in patients with hindfoot deformity who are not amenable to brace treatment. Consideration must always be given to the contralateral foot while actively treating the foot with obvious disease. Although acute injury may only affect one foot, the underlying diabetic and neuropathic processes are found to involve both feet symmetrically. Bilateral involvement has been reported to occur in 5.9% to 39.3% of patients. Great caution must be exercised when selecting a form of nonweight-bearing since increasing load on the asymptomatic foot could theoretically increase its risk for developing neuroarthropathic changes. Both feet should be inspected during each examination of the patient, and appropriate tests (e.g., skin temperature) and radiographs obtained if there is any suspicion of early involvement of the contralateral foot. Finally, it should not be forgotten that any patient with neuropathy, particularly with neuroarthropathic involvement of one foot, should have the asymptomatic foot initially protected in an appropriate orthotic and shoe at the same time that treatment is begun on the symptomatic foot.

Rehabilitation of the Neuropathic Foot and Ankle

Once the acute treatment phase is complete, an equally difficult challenge begins. A program must be found that will protect the foot from further injury (ulcers or neuroarthropathy), be as functional as possible, and meet the individual's goals for cosmesis and quality of life.

Once a fracture is healed or the acute phase of the sprain or strain is over, attention is directed toward regaining as much strength, range of motion, and function as possible. One must be careful with stretching and the progression of strengthening exercises to avoid painless damage to the newly healed tissues. Neuropathy can affect balance, strength, and proprioception so that exercises must be tailored to individual patient's abilities. Because of the risk of developing neuroarthropathy following a fracture or soft tissue injury of the foot or ankle, the person directing the rehabilitation needs to be cognizant of recurrence of any of the unique early signs and symptoms in the diabetic. This requires monitoring skin temperature and swelling and observing for any alterations in the gait pattern or structure of the foot during physical therapy. Close communication between the physician and physical therapist is necessary to ensure continued progress without significant setbacks. A significant increase in pain, swelling, or skin temperature during rehabilitation warrants resumption of total contact casting.

Guidelines for Recovery

In the initial 2 to 3 weeks after immobilization has ended, the rehabilitation program should consist of active range of motion and cardiovascular exercise and gentle stretching with a slow return to weight-bearing activities. Swelling should be controlled. Traditional physical

Rehabilitation, Modalities, Trauma, Disease, and Pediatrics

therapy modalities may be used, including electrical stimulation, compression pumps, and Ace bandaging. The use of ice for persons with severe peripheral vascular disease is relatively contraindicated. Active range of motion for the ankle should be done in two to three sets of ten, 3 to 4 times per day and may be combined with ankle circles and alphabet exercises. These may be done in a whirlpool or pool. During this phase, repetitions can be increased by one additional set per week. Gentle stretching can be performed by the therapist or trainer, but no passive range of motion exercises should be done to avoid overstretching and injuring ligaments and muscles. Weight-bearing activities should be limited. If patients cannot or will not limit their ambulation or if swelling does not improve, the therapist should consult with the physician regarding the use of part-time immobilization. A cardiovascular training program should begin on a bicycle or in the pool. Bicycling should be done with lower resistance and higher speeds initially. Gentle stretching exercises should be followed by swimming in a warm water pool 3 times a week. Aquatic shoes, which are designed to be worn around the pool as well as in the water, should be used to prevent accidental damage to the foot from the occasional rough concrete or tile floors of the pool as well as to protect the feet from acquiring fungal and bacterial infections.

Once swelling is controlled and stretching exercises have begun, the patient may begin a strengthening program with increasing tolerance for weight-bearing activities. Theraband or surgical tubing is an excellent way to start strengthening the ankle musculature. Low resistance should be used for at least 1 week, and if no increase in swelling is noted, increasing resistance may follow. A sensible regimen may include increasing the resistance by 1 lb/per week, making sure that no swelling is present before advancing to the next stage. The use of isokinetic or closed chain exercise should not begin until the strength of the affected side is 75% that of the unaffected side. Closed chain exercises must be chosen carefully because diabetic neuropathy may affect balance, coordination, and proprioception. This fact must be taken into consideration when designing a exercise program. For example, the BAPS board may be difficult for the neuropathic individual to control, resulting in possible injury to the patient. The rehabilitation program should include balance and coordination exercises, but the therapist or trainer should realize that advanced balance and coordination exercises may not be appropriate. Single limb support or closed eye exercises are not indicated in these patients, since they lack the nervous pathways necessary to make significant functional gains in these areas. Intrinsic foot muscles, if not paralyzed by motor neuropathy, can be strengthened by using the toes to bunch up a towel on the floor or pick up marbles. In the final phase of therapy, passive range of motion exercises can advance to include mechanical modes (i.e., Cybex, Biodex) and self-stretching. If regaining range of motion is slow and mobilization is considered, begin with grade one and two only. If there is no swelling and improvement is not satisfactory, grade three mobilization can be used with caution.

The type of footwear, its insole, and the modifications necessary to protect the foot from ulceration are dependent upon the level of risk for ulceration. The lowest level of protection can simply be a well-fitting shoe with some plantar padding. The thicker the padding the more protection is afforded. A custom-molded shoe can be made with much more room for thicker insoles than is available in off-the-shelf shoes. Plugs of soft material can be built all the way through the outsole to provide more plantar pressure relief. Outsole modifications can also be used to reduce pressure and improve stability. A common outsole modification used to decrease forefoot pressure is the rigid rocker. A steel stay is placed in the shoe to make the shoe stiff. The outsole is modified so that from the midfoot on there is a gentle sloping with a tapered heel and outflaring for stability.

If a brace is needed, this must be provided before footwear is chosen. Motor neuropathy, neurarthropathy, or neurological deficits from a cerebrovascular accident may require the use of a brace. A molded plastic brace can be used in the neuropathic individual, but one must realize that the footbed is very hard and provides no cushioning. Therefore, in a patient with high risk for plantar ulceration, the foot plate should be padded. If plantar ulceration is a problem in someone who requires a brace, a double upright brace attached to the appropriately modified shoe may prove satisfactory. Neurarthropathy and recurrent heel ulceration require a patellar tendon–bearing brace, in an attempt to unload the foot.

Patients must assume responsibility for their daily and routine foot care. Essential patient responsibilities include proper nail and callus care, avoidance of barefoot walking, and diligent daily inspection. It is the caregivers' role to be sure this responsibility is clearly defined and followed. Denial and lack of appropriate diabetic education place even the most well-meaning patient at risk for complications, and continual support and reinforcement of the concepts of proper foot care are the health professional's most important tasks.

The Total Contact Cast

The total contact cast is an important modality in the treatment of the neuropathic individual. This differs from a typical cast in that there is little padding and the toes are covered (Fig. 10-8). This cast is indicated for healing ulcers and attempting to stabilize neurarthropathy.

There are contraindications to total contact casting. Significant infection (superficial or deep), inability to remain nonweight-bearing for the first 24 hours, very poor vascularity, avascular lesions, and gangrene are strict contraindications. Patient removal of the cast or failing to call regarding a broken, painful, or wet cast are examples of noncompliance that might make use of the total contact cast unadvisable. Also, if an ulcer produces excessive drainage so that the skin around the wound is becoming macerated or irritated from staying too wet, total contact casting may be inappropriate. However, this prob-

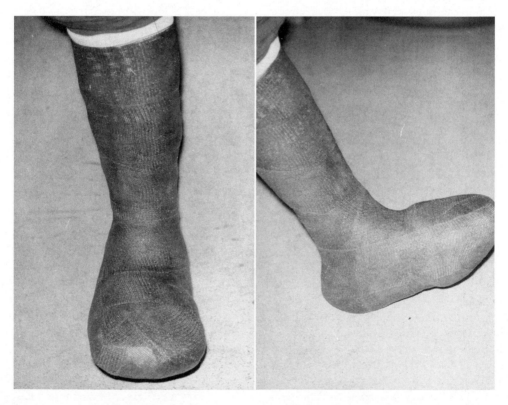

Fig. 10-8 An example of a total contact cast.

lem can usually be managed by increasing the frequency of cast changes.

The length of time a total contact cast should be on is dependent on several factors. Since neuropathy can allow for painless skin injury, total contact casting should be never be continued for more than 2 weeks before removal and thorough skin inspection. Presence of swelling and ulcer size and drainage may require that the cast be changed sooner than 2 weeks. In fact swelling may reduce so significantly in 24 hours that re-application of the cast is required within a few days of its initial placement. If the cast becomes damaged, wet, loose, painful, or foul-smelling, it must be changed without delay.

The first step in applying the total contact cast is washing and moisturizing the leg and foot and powdering between the toes. Then a 2-inch piece of cotton cast padding is woven between the toes. A piece of stockinette sewn or taped closed at one end is placed over the foot. Scifoam is cut and folded over the toes, then the edges are skived. A 1½-inch strip of ¼-inch adhesive felt is centered over the tibial crest. Cast padding is placed neatly around the leg and foot, overlapping the underlying piece by approximately 50%. Several additional pieces of cast padding are placed around the posterior heel, malleoli, and navicular. Plaster is placed over this and must overlap onto the Scifoam but does not need to completely cover the Scifoam. The type of plaster will affect the results. A smooth and creamy plaster, such as Gypsoma II or Orthowedge, should reduce the number of cast lesions. A final layer of fiberglass should be placed over the plaster and should cover the Scifoam. Either a reinforcing layer of fiberglass and cast boot or a walking heel can be applied to the bottom of the cast to allow for ambulation. Patients should be instructed in partial weight-bearing ambulation to begin 24 hours after cast application to allow for thorough drying.

Summary

Diabetes mellitus is a complex disease with chronic complications manifested in the feet.

Neuropathy and vascular insufficiency are the most common problems. Structurally the feet become stiff and weak, predisposing them to injury. Plantar insensitivity combined with neur-arthropathy results in the need for both acute and long-term treatment. Total contact casting combined with limited weight-bearing is a proven method of healing plantar ulcers. A well-thought-out physical therapy program is an important part of the recovery period. A multidisciplinary team approach including medical doctors, orthopedic and vascular surgeons, therapists, orthotists, and pedorthotists will ensure that diabetic patients receive the best possible care.

Bibliography

1. Bellavere F et al: Evidence of early impairment of parasympathetic reflexes in insulin dependent diabetics without autonomic symptoms, *Diabetes Metab* 11:152, 1985.
2. Burkhardt R et al: Is diabetic osteoporosis due to microangiopathy, *Lancet* 844, 1981.
3. Cavanaugh P: Personal communication, State College, PA, 1994.
4. Cundy TF, Edmonds ME, Walkins PJ: Osteopenia and metatarsal fractures in diabetic neuropathy, *Diabetic Med* 2:461, 1985.
5. Delridge L et al: The etiology of diabetic neuropathic ulceration of the foot, *Br J Surg* 72:1, 1985.
6. Edmonds ME: The diabetic foot: pathophysiology and treatment, *Clin Endocrinol Metab* 15:889, 1986.
7. Edmonds ME, Roberts VC, Watkins PJ: Blood flow in the diabetic neuropathic foot, *Diabetologia* 22:9, 1982.
8. Forgacs S, Salamon F: Bone changes in diabetes mellitus, *Isr J Med Sci* 8:782, 1972.
9. Harris JR, Brand PW: Patterns of disintegration of the tarsus in the anesthetic foot, *J Bone Joint Surg Br* 48B:4, 1966.
10. Hilsted J: Testing for autonomic neuropathy, *Ann Clin Res* 16:128, 1984.
11. Jacobs JE: Observations of neuropathic (Charcot) joints occurring in diabetes mellitus, *J Bone Joint Surg Br* 40A:1043, 1958.
12. Mayne N: The short term prognosis in diabetic neuropathy, *Diabetes* 17:270, 1968.
13. Stevens MJ, Roberts VC, Watkins PJ: Selective neuropathy and preserved vascular responses in the diabetic Charcot foot, *Diabetologia* 1992, in press.
14. Stokes IAF, Faris IB, Hutton WC: The neuropathic ulcer and loads on the foot in diabetic patients, *Acta Orthop Scand* 46:839, 1975.
15. Weiss RE, Reddi AH: Influence of experimental diabetes and insulin on matrix induced cartilage and differentiation, *Am J Physiol* 238:200, 1980.

11

Rehabilitation of Congenital and Developmental Conditions in Children

Betsy K. Donahoe

Kimberly A. Kuhnell

Mariann L. Strenk

There are numerous foot deformities that are present at birth or become apparent as the foot develops. The critical period of skeletal differentiation occurs during the embryonic period from 3 to 7 weeks after ovulation. This foot differentiation is divided into three phases: blastemal condensation, chondrification, and early joint formation. The immature embryonic foot may be influenced at any one of the above phases to produce a congenital foot anomaly. The fetus is also influenced by the intrauterine position. In the prenatal period, the legs are in a position of hip flexion, internal rotation, adduction, and knee extension from 8 to 12 weeks with the feet positioned in dorsiflexion and inversion. From 12 to 26 weeks, the hamstrings and external rotators begin to contract bringing the legs into a folded position. The feet progress from an in-verted position to one of eversion secondary to changes in the calcaneus and talus at about 16 weeks. At about 28 weeks, the feet are in a somewhat neutral position. Delay or arrested derotation of the feet may cause the feet to be plantarflexed and inverted in the equinovarus position at birth. When an infant is born, the normal foot has increased mobility, especially into dorsiflexion. The forefoot and hindfoot are in varus initially but gradually move into a more neutral position as the child develops. At about 6 to 8 years of age, the skeletal elements resemble those of the adult, with the foot becoming adult-sized at about 14 years of age for girls and 16 years for boys.[2]

This chapter details several congenital and developmental foot deformities commonly seen in the pediatric patient.

Congenital Deformities

Accessory Navicular
Pathophysiology

Common in the general population, the accessory navicular is one of the most frequently seen orthopedic foot conditions in children. The accessory navicular is an additional tarsal bone of the foot, which is situated on the medial plantar border of the navicular. This bone appears during early developmental life but does not ossify until 9 to 11 years of age. Rather than attaching to the main body of the navicular, the posterior tibialis tendon attaches to this accessory tarsal bone. Clinicians must differentiate between an accessory navicular and a sesamoid bone within the posterior tibialis tendon.

Clinical Features

The patient does not usually present until adolescence and often presents with pain over the tuberosity of the navicular. These symptoms tend to increase with weight-bearing activities. Upon evaluation, there is tenderness to palpation over the navicular with a prominence observed on the medial plantar border. The patient may have a significant posterior tibialis tendonitis or the beginning symptoms of this condition.

In order to diagnose by radiographic evaluation, one may see an enlarged cornuted tuberosity, or an accessory ossicle will be observed medially and proximally to the navicular bone on standing films. The clinician must be careful to rule out other causes of foot pain even though an accessory navicular may be present on X-ray.

Treatment Techniques

The most common nonoperative treatment is use of a foot orthosis to decrease pressure over the navicular combined with antiinflammatory medication. Another conservative treatment method is immobilization through casting. If symptoms do not cease with casting, lift use is initiated. Should symptoms continue, surgical intervention becomes appropriate.

Operative treatment may involve simple excision of the accessory bone with early weight-bearing or utilization of a modification of the Kidner procedure.[8] This procedure involves transplantation of the posterior tibialis to the undersurface of the navicular to redirect the muscle pull, thereby restoring the medial longitudinal arch. The patient is then treated with 4 weeks of casting, part of the time being nonweightbearing.

Postoperative physical therapy intervention includes gait training with an appropriate assistive device. At the time of cast removal, the patient may be instructed in a range of motion and strengthening program.

Congenital Clubfoot
Pathophysiology

Talipes equinovarus, commonly termed clubfoot, is considered the most common congenital foot deformity, and its incidence is comparable to that of congenital dislocation of the hip and myelomeningocele. Clubfoot is more common in boys than girls and occurs bilaterally in 50% of those affected.[1]

Many theories exist, both genetic and environmental, to explain the etiology of clubfoot. Clubfoot has shown to be transmitted by the following genetic patterns: autosomal dominant, autosomal recessive, X-linked transmission, and gross chromosomal abnormalities. Some other theories that exist to explain the occurrence of clubfoot include intrauterine mechanical compression; regional growth disturbance in the first weeks of fetal life; germ plasm defect in the talus causing plantarflexion and inversion of the talus with soft tissue changes; and primary soft tissue abnormalities within neuromuscular units causing secondary bony changes.

In a patient with a clubfoot, the ankle, midtarsal, and subtalar joints are all involved in the pathological process. As with the etiology of congenital clubfoot, the pathological anatomy is also complex and has stimulated much discussion. The chief abnormality is a deformity of the talus, which is smaller than normal. The talar head and neck of the talus are deviated medially, and the talus is in an equinus position. Medial displacement of the navicular and calcaneus occurs around the talus in a plantarward and medial direction. Contractures or anomalies of soft tissues exert further deforming forces that prevent spontaneous rearrangement of the bony malposition. The metatarsals may also be deformed by deviating at the tarsometatarsal joint, or the shafts of the metatarsals may be adducted. Contractures in the medial and lateral ligaments of the foot may also contribute to the deformity. Further contributing to a cavus deformity of the foot are the contracted flexor digitorum brevis, the abductor hallucis, and the plantar aponeurosis. In summary, the pathogenesis of a congenital clubfoot includes the following findings or theories: bony abnormalities, ligamentous contractures with fibrosis, neurogenic findings, collagen abnormalities, muscular weakness, and primary muscle imbalance.[1]

Clinical Features

It is important to assess the severity of a clubfoot at birth, although it is difficult to predict how the foot will respond. One thing for certain is that a true clubfoot will never be a normal foot. The clinical assessment must analyze the fixed deformities and range of motion as well as identify the tibia and hindfoot orientation, assess forefoot-hindfoot mobility and relationship, observe the amount of dorsiflexion, identify the absence or presence of forefoot supination, and obtain radiographic studies to identify bony abnormalities.

The following components must be present on clinical examination to receive the diagnosis of clubfoot: inversion and adduction of the forefoot; varus of the calcaneus; equinus position of the foot; contraction of the tissues on the medial side of the foot; underdeveloped and contracted calf muscles; and resistance to passive dorsiflexion. A rigid foot that cannot be brought into a dorsiflexed or everted position implies talipes equinovarus. Typically there is atrophy of the calf musculature and the involved foot is a half to one size smaller with respect to length and width. In a clubfoot, the toes are flexed and resist extension and there is usually an associated internal tibial torsion. Muscular imbalances exist, with the invertors being stronger than the evertors and the plantarflexors stronger than the dorsiflexors. There are also progressive soft tissue contractures in the clubfoot, which are more common on the medial and plantar surfaces. If

the patient is able to stand, weight-bearing occurs primarily on the base of the fifth metatarsal. If the deformity remains, the joints fuse spontaneously and degenerative changes occur.

The clinical examination is also important in making a differential diagnosis. The patient with metatarsus varus has a foot that resembles a clubfoot, but the heel is in valgus and is mobile. The postural clubfoot also resembles the congenital clubfoot; however, there is a significant difference. The clinician is able to fully correct the postural clubfoot to the anatomical position at birth or shortly thereafter. Clubfoot may also be seen in patients with arthrogryposis, myelomeningocele, and other neuromuscular and genetic disorders.

The clinical examination is important in the diagnosis of clubfoot, but radiographic examination is essential for accurate diagnosis. With the nonambulatory patient, anteroposterior and dorsiflexion lateral stress X-rays of both feet should be obtained. Standing anteroposterior and lateral X-rays are important in the diagnosis of an older patient. The radiographic studies are necessary to determine the shape and positional relationship of the tarsal bones. In a patient with a clubfoot the following will be observed on X-ray: talus is plantarflexed, anteriorly displaced, and rotated laterally along the longitudinal axis; calcaneus is inverted, laterally subluxed, and rotated in all three planes; navicular is medially and plantarwardly rotated and may articulate with the medial malleolus; and the cuboid is inferior to the navicular and cuneiforms.

Measurement of the talocalcaneal, tibiocalcaneal, and talometatarsal angles on X-rays also aid in the diagnosis of clubfoot. In the patient with a clubfoot, the talocalcaneal angle on the anteroposterior view progressively decreases with increasing heel varus. The talocalcaneal angle decreases with severity to an angle of zero on the dorsiflexed lateral view. The tibiocalcaneal angle on the lateral film is negative, which indicates equinus of the calcaneus in relationship to the tibia. In the patient with a clubfoot, the talo–first metatarsal angle is usually negative. This negative angle suggests forefoot adduction.[1] The above angle measurements and bony positions correlate with the clinical appearance of the foot.

Throughout treatment of a clubfoot, it is important to obtain adequate X-rays to be certain the foot is corrected not only clinically but radiographically. In a patient with a persistent clubfoot with rearfoot deformity, a computed tomography (CT) scan may assist in accurate diagnosis.

Treatment Techniques

A clubfoot is difficult to manage secondary to the variability and lack of common language used to describe the deformity. Treatment of clubfoot deformity is initiated immediately after birth; however, the prognosis is guarded due to atrophic, fibrosed, and contracted tissues and irreversible muscle imbalances. Preventing bony and articular deformity and minimizing fibrous contractures are the primary aims of clubfoot treatment.

The nonsurgical treatment of choice requires serial manipulation and corrective casting of the clubfoot. The cast is applied with a thin layer of cast padding so the contours of the foot can be molded while protecting the bony prominences. Once the cast has begun to set, the position should not be modified, to avoid wrinkles that may cause blisters or areas of skin breakdown. The order of correction is staged and includes the following: first correct forefoot adduction, then heel varus, and finally hindfoot equinus. In order to prevent a rocker-bottom deformity, the casting must be performed in stages. The cast should also include a flexed knee to control the heel position, and a bar may be incorporated into the casts to correct internal tibial torsion. Casting is typically continued for 3 to 6 months or until correction has been achieved. Once adequate correction is achieved, bivalved casting, night-time bracing, corrective shoes with a bar incorporated, and/or shoe inserts are used to prevent recurrence and maintain correction (Fig. 11-1). Physical therapy may be incorporated to provide a range of motion and strengthening program.

Surgical intervention is indicated if the clubfoot is not corrected with casting. The age at which surgery should be performed is a decision that varies among clinicians, as does the appropriate surgical procedure; however, most surgeons operate between 3 and 6 months of age to minimize secondary tarsal deformities. The type of surgical intervention and the staging of the operation are individualized and should be based on clinical, ergometric, radiological, and neurophysiological evaluation of the patient. A posteromedial release is indicated for a mild de-

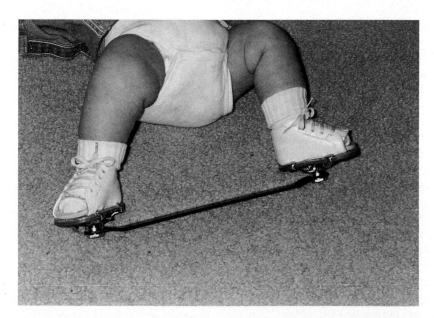

Fig. 11-1 Corrective shoes used with a 5-month-old patient with bilateral congenital clubfoot deformity.

formity without severe internal rotation of the calcaneus or need for an extensive posterolateral release. In a patient with a severe deformity, a procedure that takes into account the three-dimensional deformity of the subtalar joint is more appropriate. This allows for correction of the internal rotation deformity of the calcaneus and releases contractures of the posteromedial and posterolateral foot. Postoperative management of the above procedures involves casting for up to 4 months. The cast is changed at 2 weeks to achieve a greater amount of dorsiflexion and at 6 weeks to achieve full correction. An ankle-foot orthosis may be worn after the cast is removed to maintain correction. In a patient with a corrected forefoot deformity but residual hindfoot equinus, a tendo Achilles lengthening and posterior capsulotomy may be indicated. Postoperatively, these patients are casted for 6 weeks followed by 6 to 9 months' use of an ankle-foot orthosis. Another problem found in the clubfoot population is a dynamic metatarsus adductus. This typically occurs in older children who have had previous correction. The treatment of choice is to transfer the anterior tibialis to become an evertor of the foot.[1] Physical therapy intervention may be used to instruct the patient in peroneal and anterior tibialis strengthening exercises.

In the treated clubfoot, typically some degree of restriction remains in dorsiflexion, plantarflexion, and subtalar and midtarsal joint motion. The goal of treatment is a pliable, plantigrade and painless foot. However, in some treated clubfoot patients, this does not occur. Recurrence may result when there is insufficient repositioning of the talus, calcaneus, and navicular or failure to retain the tarsal bones in a corrected position. Treatment of residual or resistant clubfoot in the older child is quite difficult. There are no clear-cut guidelines for treatment, and the deformity may take many forms. The forefoot and hindfoot must be thoroughly evaluated to determine appropriate treatment. Soft tissue releases and osteotomies are the basic surgical procedures for resistant clubfoot. In a severe resistant clubfoot with metatarsus adductus, hindfoot varus, and equinus, a triple arthrodesis may be appropriate in the patient older than 10 years.

Congenital Metatarsus Adductus
Pathophysiology

Metatarsus adductus is a fairly common foot anomaly that consists of medial deviation of the forefoot in relation to the midfoot and hindfoot. Several theories, both static and dynamic, exist as to the cause of metatarsus adductus. These include abnormal insertion of the tibialis anterior and posterior muscles; absent medial cuneiforms; abnormal intrauterine pressure; and hyperactive adductor hallucis muscle in the dynamic type of deformity. Metartusus varus, skewfoot, and metatarsus adductus are confusing terms often used interchangeably but which mean different types of deformity.

Clinical Features

The foot deformity may be present at birth but is often not recognized until the patient is 3 months to 1 year of age. Patients most often presents with an intoeing gait and complaints that they often trip and fall. On physical examination, the following features are noted: the forefoot is in adduction; the lateral border of the foot is convex, with a prominence at the base of the fifth metatarsal and cuboid; the heel position may vary but usually presents in valgus; and internal tibial torsion is commonly present. Patients present with varying degrees of foot flexibility, and abnormal shoe wear may be evident. Older children or adults with an uncorrected metatarsus adductus occasionally have bunions and hallux valgus; however, they rarely present with complaints of pain.

Radiographic studies in weight-bearing may be helpful in confirming the diagnosis of metatarsus adductus. The X-ray findings will reveal adduction of the forefoot at the tarsometatarsal articulation on an anteroposterior view. The first metatarsal may also appear to be more adducted than the fifth. On the lateral view, there are no visible abnormalities.

Treatment Techniques

With a mild deformity, treatment is usually not necessary because they tend to correct on their own. If the deformity corrects with stimulation, exercises and stretching are initiated. The parents are instructed in a home stretching program, which consists of stabilizing the tarsal bones while bringing the forefoot into abduction (Fig. 11-2). If appropriate, the patient is instructed in active forefoot abduction. These patients may also be treated with a high-top, open-toe normal-last shoe.

Plaster casts are used to correct the deformity in patients with a rigid or severe metatarsus adductus or a foot that is not responsive to exercise or special shoes. The recommended total wearing time and frequency of cast changes vary among clinicians. Each cast is applied with progressive passive abduction of the forefoot against a stabilized heel or a heel in inversion if valgus is present. According to Bleck, casting has been found to be most successful if initiated before 8 months of age.[3]

Surgical options are not typically considered until conservative treatment measures fail and the patient continues to have pain, difficulty with shoe fitting, and to disapprove of the appearance of the foot. Between the ages of 2 and 6, tenotomies, capsulotomies, and ligamentous releases are the surgical options of choice. The procedure often used at this stage is the Heyman-Herndon procedure, which involves a tarso-metatarsal capsulotomy.[6] Patients with a fixed residual deformity and/or older children often undergo metatarsal osteotomies for correction. After surgical correction, children may be in-structed in gait training while immobilized. Range of motion and strengthening exercises are initiated after cast removal.

Congenital Vertical Talus
Pathophysiology

Congenital vertical talus is considered a rare childhood foot deformity; however, when present, it is often associated with other congenital deformities or neuromuscular disorders. This condition is also referred to as rocker-bottom foot, and the etiology of the primary isolated form is unknown. In a foot with a congenital vertical talus, the navicular articulates with the dorsal aspect of the neck of the talus, the proximal surface of the navicular is tilted plantarward, and the calcaneus is in an equinus position. As weight-bearing is initiated, the shape of the talus abnormally changes to resemble that of an hour glass, thus changing the articulating surfaces with the tibia. The calcaneus continues to maintain an equinus position but becomes displaced posteriorly.

Clinical Features

The newborn with a congenital vertical talus is easily diagnosed at birth secondary to the convex appearance of the foot. Clinical examination shows that the hindfoot is held in equinus and the heelcord and peroneal muscles are shortened.

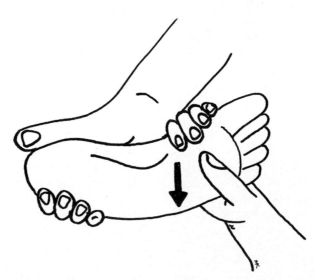

Fig. 11-2 Demonstration of stretch utilized for patients with congenital metatarsus adductus.

Rehabilitation, Modalities, Trauma, Disease, and Pediatrics

The following features are also seen on clinical examination: the head of the talus is palpable medially; the hindfoot is in a valgus position; the forefoot is abducted; and the midtarsal joint is in dorsiflexion. As the child begins to ambulate, calluses develop near the head of the talus on the medial aspect of the foot, the hindfoot is in marked valgus, and the child is unable to get the heel down. In more severe cases, balance may become decreased with the foot toeing out. The patient may begin complaining of pain in the early adolescent years as well as expressing difficulty with shoe wear.

On X-ray examination, a talonavicular dislocation is present with the calcaneus in fixed equinus and the anteroposterior talocalcaneal angle is abnormally increased. A lateral view in maximum plantarflexion demonstrates the fixed relationship between the talus and navicular.

Treatment Techniques

The choice of treatment is variable and dependent upon the severity of the deformity and the age of the patient. The initial treatment typically involves manipulation and casting, with cast changes usually twice a week; however, this usually only stretches the soft tissues rather than correcting the deformity.

Surgical treatment techniques tend to vary according to the age of the patient and the treating physician. The younger patient undergoes soft tissue releases and reduction with realignment of the subtalar and talonavicular joints. With a severe deformity in these children, an excision of the navicular may be necessary. School-age children are often treated with open reduction and soft tissue releases combined with extraarticular subtalar arthrodesis. Adolescents and adults are most effectively treated with a triple arthrodesis. Postsurgically, patients are treated initially in an above knee cast followed by pin removal if appropriate and further above and below knee casting. After cast removal, special shoe wear may be indicated.

Polydactyly
Pathophysiology

Polydactyly is one of the most frequently seen foot anomalies, and many of these patients

present with a bilateral deformity. This deformity is defined as the presence of more than five fingers or toes and in the foot may include supernumerary tarsal or metatarsal bones. The exact etiology is unclear; however, the most common cause is believed to be an autosomal dominant trait with variable expression. It may also be the result of an autosomal recessive trait, an X-linked recessive trait, or polygenic inheritance. Patients with polydactyly may also have another deformity such as hypoplasia of the tibia or associated syndrome.

Controversy exists about the most effective way to classify polydactyly. The Temtamy and McKusick classification system is one of the most widely used in describing polydactyly.[13] Preaxial polydactyly is defined as an extra or supernumerary digit on the medial aspect of the foot, and postaxial polydactyly, which is the most common type, involves the lateral aspect of the foot. Duplication of the fifth digit is also termed
postaxial polydactyly. Involvement of the second, third, or fourth digits is defined as central ray duplication. Classification of polydactyly may be helpful but is often criticized as being too general, confusing to apply, and providing limited value in clinical management.

Clinical Features

Polydactyly is easily recognized at birth if the child presents with an extra digit or digits. Duplication of tarsal or metatarsal bones may not be diagnosed until radiographic studies are obtained. A thorough medical history and physical exam are imperative to rule out associated conditions or syndromes. The osseous and musculotendinous structures must also be carefully evaluated to construct and initiate appropriate surgical treatments.

Treatment Techniques

Conservative treatment measures for polydactyly involve special shoe wear to accommodate the supernumerary digits; however, most patients present for surgical intervention.

Surgical treatment is indicated for comfortable shoe wear and/or cosmesis. Careful preoperative planning is important because of the uniqueness of each individual case. If the digit is composed only of skin and soft tissue, it is usually tied off or surgically excised at a very early age. With osseous involvement, surgery is typically delayed until the patient is 1 year old to allow for better definition of bony structures. Generally the most medial or lateral supernumerary digit is excised. With excision of an inner digit, correction of the intermetatarsal ligament needs to be performed to prevent splaying of the metatarsals. Bandaging and splinting postoperatively are necessary to maintain surgical correction. Surgical complications include splayfoot, hallux varus, and angulation deformities of the digits, all of which may be caused by musculotendinous imbalances.

Tarsal Coalition
Pathophysiology

Tarsal coalition is the fusion—bony, cartilaginous, or fibrous—of two or more bones in the midfoot or hindfoot. This deformity may be an isolated anomaly but is occasionally associated with a generalized syndrome. These coalitions may be either congenital or acquired and may have a genetic predisposition. There are multiple theories of the etiology, the most popular being failure of differentiation and segmentation of primitive mesenchyme.[5] Acquired coalitions, although less common in pediatric patients than adults, can be caused by the following: trauma, infection, arthritis, and neoplasms.

Tarsal coalitions are classified as either intraarticular or extraarticular. Extraarticular coalitions occur between two or more tarsal bones that do not normally articulate with each other, or the coalition is outside of the joint space of two tarsal bones that typically articulate. A calcaneonavicular coalition is the most common type of extraarticular coalition. Intraarticular coalitions occur within the joint space of two or more tarsal bones that typically articulate, and most frequently occur between the middle facets of the talocalcaneal joint, and frequently occur between the middle facets of the talus and calcaneus.

Clinical Features

The patient with a tarsal coalition will present with complaints of pain in the area of the coalition. The time at which symptoms initially become apparent is dependent upon ossification of the coalition, and quite often the patient is an adolescent. The onset is usually insidious and may be brought on by a twisting injury of the foot or an ankle sprain. In some patients, tarsal coalitions may be found accidentally with no complaints or symptoms. These may occur bilaterally or unilaterally.

On physical examination, the patient presents with varying degrees of pes planus, forefoot abduction, and calcaneal valgus in standing. If pain is severe, an abnormal gait pattern may also be observed. The patient's symptoms are worsened by activity and relieved by rest. Subtalar and midtarsal motion is markedly reduced or absent and is correlated with the onset of ossification of the coalition. The peroneal muscles may present as tight or infrequently spastic, causing pain with inversion.

The clinical diagnosis should be confirmed by radiographic evaluation. Anteroposterior, lateral, and oblique radiographs are usually diagnostic in calcaneonavicular coalitions. When the bar has not yet ossified, the diagnosis is implicated by an elongated process of the calcaneus or prolongation of the navicular. The talocalcaneal coalition is difficult to diagnose by plain X-ray secondary to overlap of the subtalar joint. Secondary bony changes may present on plain films, indicating the need for CT scanning. These changes include talar beaking; broadening or rounding of the lateral process of the talus; concave plantar surface of the talus; narrowing of the subtalar jo int; and inability to see the middle subtalar joint.

Treatment Techniques

Conservative treatment focuses on decreasing the motion of the painful joints as a means of attempting to alleviate pain. Orthotic devices and shoe modifications that increase the support to the medial side of the foot have been used. While under treatment, patients should avoid activities that increase their pain. A trial period of cast immobilization with restricted weight-bearing is another method of treatment. Immobilization is usually performed for at least 3 weeks. After cast removal, patients may be seen in physical therapy for ankle strengthening exercises, range of motion exercises to increase inversion, and techniques to decrease pain. Morgan and Crawford found that none of their patients, who were adolescent athletes, had lasting relief with conservative treatment.[10]

Surgery is indicated for those patients who have persistent pain and stiffness after a trial of conservative treatment. The type of surgery depends on the type of coalition, the occurrence of secondary degenerative changes, and the age and activity level of the patient. For calcaneonavicular coalitions, resection and interposition of the extensor digitorum brevis between the calcaneus and navicular is the treatment of choice, especially for the younger adolescent athlete. An above knee cast is worn for a short period of time, and physical therapy is then initiated for range of motion exercises. In the older adolescent, resection of the coalition may not completely relieve pain and limited motion may persist. Also, degenerative joint changes may be present. In these cases, a triple arthrodesis is frequently indicated. For talocalcaneal coalitions, there is more controversy over the best choice for surgical management. One option is to excise the coalition with fat interpositioning. After surgery, a cast is worn for a few weeks, and range of motion exercises are then initiated. This procedure is currently recommended only for those coalitions that are small and without existing articular degenerative changes. Excision of the coalition was shown to be successful in one study of adolescent athletes.[10] If the foot is in severe, rigid valgus, if the coalition is large, if degenerative changes are noted, or if symptoms of pain and limited motion persist, a triple arthrodesis is the recommended treatment.

Developmental Deformities

Flexible Flatfoot
Pathophysiology

Flexible flatfoot is a fairly common finding in the general population. The cause of this condition appears to be genetically determined and related to an abnormality in the internal arrangement of the tarsal bones, their relationship to one another, and laxity of the ligaments. All children until about 6 years of age exhibit some pronation, which tends to correct spontaneously with time.

Clinical Features

Flexible flatfoot is not a fixed deformity, and the foot should have a normal contour when the patient is not weight-bearing. Upon physical examination in weight-bearing, the heel is in valgus and the forefoot is abducted, with the longitudinal arch depressed or absent. The talus is plantarflexed, and its head can be palpated over the medial aspect of the foot. When the child weight-bears on the ball of the foot, the heel shifts into varus, confirming flexibility of the subtalar joint. Evaluation of the plantar aspect of the foot in older children reveals a callus pattern in the area of the longitudinal arch. In younger children, the foot is asymptomatic, but the older child may complain of pain with prolonged standing.

Routine radiographic evaluations are not necessary in all patients but may be helpful if treatment is warranted. On the lateral standing view, depression at the talonavicular and/or the naviculocuneiform joint will be noted to disrupt the normal straight-line relationship between the talus and the first metatarsal. Heel valgus is also assessed on the anteroposterior view. In the symptomatic patient, further radiographic views may be necessary to rule out other foot deformities or degenerative changes.

Treatment Techniques

Patients typically present with a painful flatfoot or with an asymptomatic foot and cosmetic concerns about its appearance from the patient or parents. Parents often insist on treatment for their child's condition because of the previous wide use of corrective orthopedic shoes for various foot deformities. No treatment is warranted if the patient presents with a mild deformity or without symptoms. If the child has a painful flatfoot or a severe flexible deformity, treatment is initiated on a trial basis. Treatment options include corrective shoes, shoe modifications to typical shoes, and a variety of orthotic inserts. Most clinicians feel that modifications should be used to support the foot and decrease symptoms rather than correct the existing deformity. In a recent study of children with flexible flatfeet, children 1 through 6 years of age were treated with a variety of conservative measures including standard-last leather shoes, shoe inserts, and shoe modifications. The results indicate the deformity improved over a 3-year time period, but the degree of improvement was not influenced by using a shoe insert or corrective shoes. The authors advised patients with typical flexible flatfeet to wear no shoes or soft, flexible shoes and occasionally recommended shoe inserts or modifications for those with a severely symptomatic flatfoot.[14]

A few patients will develop significant pain, limited motion, and disability from flexible flatfeet. A variety of procedures have been attempted with varying results. Which procedure is most effective depends upon several factors, including the degree of hindfoot valgus, the area of sagging of the longitudinal arch, and the degree of medial deviation of the talar axis. Tachdjian has described procedures for each type of deformity.[12] Gait training may be initiated for ambulation while the patient is in a cast. After cast removal, strengthening and range of motion exercises may be indicated. The exercise program is typically dependent on the type of surgery performed.

Idiopathic Toe-walking
Pathophysiology

A child identified as an idiopathic toe-walker is an otherwise normal child without evidence of abnormal tone, sensory, or reflex changes. The child primarily walks on the toes, although a heel-toe pattern may be present at times. By 1½ years of age, a child typically develops a heel-toe gait pattern, and a mature gait pattern is established by 3 years of age. Intermittent toe-walking may be normal until 7 years of age, although persistent toe-walking beyond 7 is not. Toe-walking, when not linked to an associated condition, may be due to a congenitally short tendocalcaneus, congenital contracture of the triceps surae, or to habit. Some clinicians have found a positive family history and learning disabilities to be associated with toe-walking.[9]

Clinical Features

A careful evaluation, including a history of when toe-walking began and the amount of time the child spends on the toes, is important. On clinical examination, passive range of motion of the heelcord with the knee extended will be limited to varying degrees, and active motion in this position may also be limited. Reflexes and gait pattern are also important to evaluate to make a differential diagnosis. If reflexes are hyperactive in a toe-walker, they are suggestive of a neurological condition.

A recent study collected data on gait patterns of idiopathic toe-walkers and spastic diplegics. Although both groups lacked a heel strike at initial contact, two distinct gait patterns were found. In the toe-walkers, the primary gait deviation was abnormal ankle motion, with moderate to severe plantarflexion at stance. Other abnormalities in this group included increased external rotation of the foot and increased knee extension in stance, both of which are compensation mechanisms for the decreased dorsiflexion. The spastic diplegic patients exhibited a repeatable gait pattern with minimal deviation from normal. In these patients, absence of a heel strike is due to sustained knee flexion at terminal swing and initial contact. The patient is unable to fully extend the knee secondary to tightness or increased tone in the hamstrings.[7]

The use of dynamic electromyography as a diagnostic indicator is controversial.

Treatment Techniques

For the younger child with a small limitation in passive dorsiflexion and occasional toe-walking, observation and/or passive heelcord

stretching performed several times daily is recommended. If the child is older or presents
with a fixed contracture, serial casting is appropriate. The casts are changed weekly or
biweekly, attempting to bring the foot into
progressively more dorsiflexion, and may remain in place for a period of 2 months. Ankle
exercises to strengthen the ankle dorsiflexors
and stretching of the heelcord are often initiated after cast removal (Fig. 11-3). If a child
reverts to toe-walking and does not have a
limitation in passive ankle dorsiflexion, an ar-
ticulated ankle-foot orthosis may be an effective
treatment tool.

If conservative treatment has failed or if the
child is not appropriate for serial casting, percutaneous heelcord lengthening is advised. After
surgery, a cast is applied for a few weeks. Ankle
range of motion and strengthening exercises may
be initiated after cast removal.

Juvenile Arthritic Foot
Pathophysiology

Juvenile rheumatoid arthritis (JRA) is a disease
that occurs before 16 years of age, defined as arthritis and synovitis in one or more joints for a
minimum period of 3 months. The disease is
classified by its method of presentation. These
categories include monoarticular (involvement
of one joint), pauciarticular (involvement of two
to four joints), polyarticular (involvement of five
or more joints), and presentation as a systemic
illness. Peak incidence of JRA is at 1 to 3 years
of age, and it is more prevalent among females.
Most children will enter into remission; however, a percentage will develop persistent,
chronic illness. The cause of the disease remains
unknown.

The skeleton of the pediatric foot is immature
and malleable; therefore, arthritis in the foot and
ankle can result in growth alterations and bony

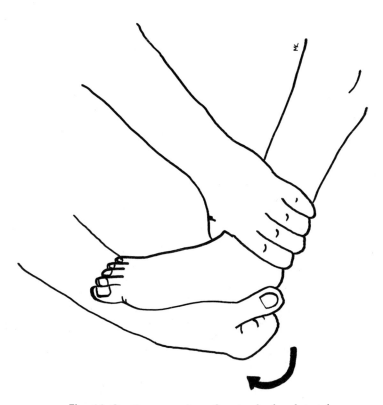

Fig. 11-3 Demonstration of passive heelcord stretch.

destruction. Frequently the ankle is an early site of synovial proliferation and inflammation, which can result in intraarticular and periarticular tissue fibrosis and shortening. As the disease process progresses, osteoporosis commonly occurs. Bone demineralization is related to the inflammatory process, but other factors, such as muscular wasting and poor nutrition, may exacerbate this problem. Development of growth disturbances is related to local and systemic irritation, which may result in fusion or epiphyseal closure. Because of the thick joint cartilage typical in children, bony erosion generally indicates long-standing or virulent disease. This severe joint damage is often accompanied by ankylosis. Weight-bearing stressors through the ankle and foot influence the direction of deformity and ultimately the degree of functional deficiency.

Clinical Features

Possible foot and ankle deformities resulting from JRA are numerous. Gastroc-soleus contracture due to equinus positioning is a common manifestation, which can progress to a fixed deformity. Involvement of the subtalar joint frequently results in pronation but could present as supination, contingent upon the weight-bearing forces over the affected joint. Hindfoot varus often accompanies pronation. Tarsal joint involvement most often leads to pes planovalgus. Hallux rigidus, hallux valgus, and hammertoe deformities are all fairly common and may be accompanied by splaying of the forefoot (Fig. 11-4).

Children with involvement of the foot and/or ankle often demonstrate pain and muscle spasm, which is influenced by weight-bearing. Atrophy of the gastroc-soleus musculature is not unusual. Limitations in mobility are often demonstrated on range of motion assessment, as well as during gait.

Treatment Techniques

Treatment of the JRA foot and ankle is dependent upon the stage of the disease process and includes both local and systemic intervention. Typical medications include a variety of antiinflammatory drugs. Ideally, treatment is initiated soon after diagnosis and before any muscular

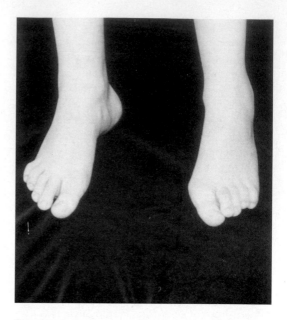

Fig. 11-4 A 15-year-old female with polyarticular juvenile rheumatoid arthritis (diagnosed at age 4 months) who presents with left hallux valgus and early indication for potential toe clawing deformity. Bilateral cavus deformities are also demonstrated.

contractures have developed. Superficial heat modalities are utilized to reduce pain and muscle spasm. However, deep heat, such as ultrasound, is contraindicated secondary to possible aggravation of inflammation and tissue destruction, as well as the potential for epiphyseal plate damage.[11]

A physical therapy program is useful in this early stage to focus on maintenance of full functional joint mobility and strength, as well as to prevent deformity. Positioning of the ankle in neutral alignment when at rest is accomplished via an ankle-foot orthosis or a resting posterior shell splint. This prohibits the tendency toward equinus posturing and decreases the potential development of a fixed contracture. In addition, an ankle-foot orthosis may be utilized during gait to provide support against abnormal stressors and maintain optimal joint alignment. However, if joint involvement is mild, a flexible arch support may be effective and will allow a less restricted gait pattern, thereby decreasing the compensatory stressors on other lower extremity joints.

For children with more progressive disease involvement, the focus of treatment intervention shifts to correction of present deformity. In addition to passive stretching exercise, muscle contracture may be addressed via serial casting or splinting. Intraarticular corticosteroid injections can be used during an acute flare-up to provide temporary reduction of inflammation. Relief of associated pain might then permit participation in a physical therapy program designed to eliminate contractures and provide optimal functional positioning. Following gains in mobility, implementation of a strengthening program is indicated to assist in maintaining muscle length.

Surgical intervention on the foot and ankle is rare secondary to a generally good response to more conservative treatment. Synovectomies were utilized in the past but are no longer a frequent choice because of limited successful results. Soft tissue releases, such as a tendo Achilles lengthening, may be considered to address a fixed deformity. Osteotomies may provide correction of a hindfoot deformity, but the results are generally not reliable. In the case of a painful, fixed hindfoot, a triple arthrodesis may correct the deformity. Arthroplasty has been used only infrequently, with unpredictable results and a high rate of complications.

Cerebral Palsy Foot
Pathophysiology

A variety of different foot deformities are seen in children with cerebral palsy (CP). Different classifications of CP include spastic (increased muscle tone); athetoid (slow, irregular, involuntary muscular contractions); ataxic (failure or irregularity of muscular coordination with voluntary muscle contraction); hypotonic (decreased muscle tone); hyperkinetic (increased muscular movement); and dystonic (impaired or disordered muscle tone). Depending on the site and extent of the lesion, the resulting neurological deficit affects specific areas of the body: hemiplegia (affecting one half of the body); diplegia (affecting similar parts on both sides of the body); and quadriplegia (affecting all four extremities and usually the trunk) (Fig. 11-5). Various degrees of involvement may occur. The motor deficit affects coordination of posture and move-

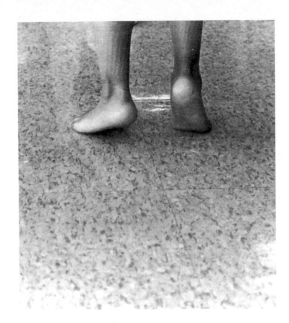

Fig. 11-5 A 2½-year-old male with spastic diplegia and secondary equinus deformity.

ment as well as qualities and distribution of postural tone. Due to a limited movement repertoire, secondary impairments in the musculoskeletal system are likely and produce changes in joint mobility, alignment, and muscle lengths.

Clinical Features

Equinus is the most common foot and ankle deformity in children with CP. The primary cause of the equinus deformity is imbalance between ankle plantarflexors and dorsiflexors. The muscular imbalance may be caused by overactivity of the ankle plantarflexors, adaptive shortening of spastic musculature, and growth and developmental differences. As with idiopathic toe-walking, children with equinus deformity secondary to CP ambulate on the balls of their feet with an absent heel strike during gait. They typically demonstrate decreased range of motion in ankle dorsiflexion as well as hamstring tightness. Their gait pattern is highly repeatable from cycle to cycle. Another common foot and ankle deformity seen in children with CP is spastic pes varus. These children ambulate with the majority of weight-bearing through the lateral borders of their feet. Dynamic varus deformities are most often due to spasticity of the posterior tibialis or the anterior tibialis muscles. Spastic pes valgus is another foot deformity associated with the CP patient and is frequently seen with spastic diplegia. These children weight-bear through the medial borders of their feet, which results in deforming stressors on the medial longitudinal arch. In the patient with hypotonic involvement of the lower extremities, a pronated flatfoot may be apparent.

Treatment Techniques

A variety of nonoperative treatment options exist for the previously mentioned CP foot deformities. The child may be treated with passive and/or active ankle exercises to increase range of motion and control of the ankle. In conjunction with range of motion exercises, therapeutic techniques, such as neurodevelopmental treatment (NDT), are also used to improve function at the ankle. Other options, including casting and splinting, may be incorporated in the treatment plan.

If conservative treatment fails or the deformity is too severe for conservative treatment measures, surgical intervention is necessary. In some

patients with deforming forces about the foot and ankle, tendon transfers and releases are appropriate to correct the deformity. For the more rigid foot or with the older child, osteotomies or a triple arthrodesis may be indicated. A variety of surgical techniques for the CP patient are outlined in the orthopedic literature.[4] Following surgery, splints and range of motion exercises may be used to maintain the correction and prevent further deformities (Fig. 11-6). In patients that undergo tendon transfers, muscle retraining and strengthening may be appropriate.

Acknowledgment

We would like to acknowledge Marilyn Geier for her contribution to this chapter. Her expertise regarding the cerebral palsied patient is greatly appreciated. Marilyn is a staff physical therapist at Children's Hospital Medical Center in Cincinnati, Ohio.

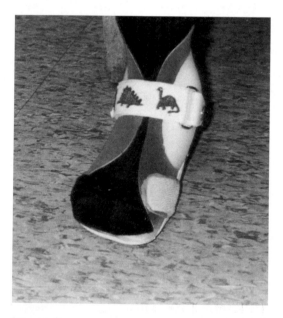

Fig. 11-6 Corrective splint commonly used with foot deformities in the cerebral palsy patient.

Bibliography

1. Beaty JH: Congenital anomalies of the lower and upper extremities. In Canale ST, Beaty JH, editors: *Pediatric operative orthopedics,* St Louis, 1991, Mosby–Year Book.
2. Bernhardt DB: Prenatal and postnatal growth and development of the foot and ankle, *Phys Ther* 68:1831, 1988.
3. Bleck EE: Metatarsus adductus: classification and relationship to outcomes of treatment, *J Pediatr Orthop* 3:2, 1983.
4. Green NE: Cerebral palsy. In Canale ST, Beaty JH, editors: *Pediatric operative orthopedics,* St Louis, 1991, Mosby–Year Book.
5. Harris BJ: Anomalous structures in the developing human foot (abstract), *Anat Rec* 121:399, 1955.
6. Heyman CH, Herndon CR, Strong JM: Mobilization of the tarsometatarsal and intermetatarsal joints for the correction of resistant adduction of the forepart of the foot in congenital clubfoot or congenital metatarsus varus, *J Bone Joint Surg* (Am) 40:299, 1958.
7. Hicks R, Durnick N, Gage JR: Differentiation of idiopathic toe walking and cerebral palsy, *J Pediatr Orthop* 8:160, 1988.
8. Kidner FC: The prehallux (accessory scaphoid) in its relation to flatfoot, *J Bone Joint Surg (Am)* 11:831, 1929.
9. Meehan P: Other conditions of the foot. In Morrissy RT, editor: *Lovell and Winter's pediatric orthopedics,* Philadelphia, 1990, JB Lippincott.
10. Morgan RC Jr, Crawford AH: Surgical management of tarsal coalition in adolescent athletes, *Foot Ankle* 7:183, 1986.

Rehabilitation, Modalities, Trauma, Disease, and Pediatrics

11. Scull SA: Physical and occupational therapy for children with rheumatic diseases, *Pediatr Clin North Am* 33:1053, 1986.
12. Tachdjian MO: The foot and leg. In Tachdjian MO, *Pediatric orthopedics,* Philadelphia, 1990, WB Saunders.
13. Temtamy SA, McKusick VA: The genetics of hand malformations, *Birth Defects* 14:364, 1978.
14. Wenger DR et al: Corrective shoes and inserts as treatments for flexible flatfoot in infants and children, *J Bone Joint Surg* (Am) 71:800, 1989.

12

Rehabilitating Pediatric Conditions Using Casting and Splinting

Betsy K. Donahoe

Kimberly A. Kuhnell

Mariann L. Strenk

Orthotic appliances play an important role in the rehabilitative treatment of the pediatric foot and ankle. Their benefits are not only related to prevention of deformity and instability but also include improvement in the gait pattern and functional mobility skills. The terms *orthosis* and *splint* are somewhat interchangeable but may be used to indicate a variety of treatment options. Generally, an orthotic device is considered to be one that has been fabricated, usually by a certified orthotist, of low-density, high-thermo-setting plastic. Typical fabrication of an orthosis is based on a plaster cast impression of the lower extremity. Appliances fabricated by a physical therapist are also referred to as orthotic devices, such as the ankle-foot orthosis (AFO); however, in this grouping the terminology may be considered interchangeable with the descriptor *splint*.[1] Splints fabricated by a physical therapist are most often made of low-density, low-thermosetting plastic via direct molding over the lower extremity.

Determination of the method of appliance fabrication is based on many considerations. Options fabricated by a physical therapist are frequently used for an interim period of time while a child is being evaluated for an appropriate, more long-term orthotist-fabricated orthosis. These devices can also be ideal for a child demonstrating rapid status changes or growth, because to a certain degree they are easily modified. Disadvantages of such models fabricated by a physical therapist include low durability and the tendency to shrink or melt down. Also, bulky splint structure may require an increase in shoe size.

In this chapter, a variety of appliances typically fabricated by a physical therapist are addressed and described. Serial casting, a treatment technique utilized to gain range of motion, is also explored.

Serial Casting

Rationale

Serial casting has been demonstrated to be an effective method of treatment in the reduction of contracture in muscle and connective tissues. Adaptive muscle lengthening is a physiologically active process that can be achieved through a progressive series of casts. During this process, lengthening occurs specifically via the longitudinal addition of sarcomeres. Casting promotes a prolonged decrease of hypertonicity, enabling progression toward optimal positioning, which may then facilitate functional motoric improvements.

Indications for Use

The primary indication for serial casting is contracture reduction, and the technique should only be implemented when the deformity is not fixed. A reduction of hypertonicity should be achieveable with handling techniques in order to achieve maximal responsiveness to casting. In addition, persistent tonic reflexes in the foot are an indication for this procedure. Diagnoses for which this intervention can be beneficial include traumatic brain injury, cerebral palsy, and juvenile rheumatoid arthritis.

In certain cases, use of a series of bivalved casts is preferred. One reason for this option is significant potential for skin irritation requiring intermittent cast removal for visual inspection. Also, bivalving permits removal of the cast for the physical therapy program, including range of motion and strengthening exercises (Fig. 12-1). Overall, however, this variance may lead to less successful long-term results because of difficulty in securing optimal fit.

Technique

Prior to casting, all bony prominences on the ankle and foot are covered with foam. Cotton padding is then applied to the entire surface to be casted. Following these skin integrity protection measures, neutral alignment of the subtalar joint is secured. The ankle is then molded in its comfortable end range of dorsiflexion. The cast may be fabricated from either plaster or fiberglass material, based on its desired properties. Some forms of plaster may be soaked off quickly in emergency situations, making it attractive to an outpatient population. Also, the heaviness of plaster may promote active muscle cocontraction and decreased hypertonicity throughout the lower extremity. A lighter fiberglass cast may be preferred if muscle weakness is profound and the weight of the cast could interfere with control of movement. The benefits of fiberglass also include more rapid setting of the cast, allowing return to weight-bearing sooner.

The first cast is changed after 3 to 7 days, at which time the ankle is ranged and subsequently recast at its new end range of dorsiflexion.

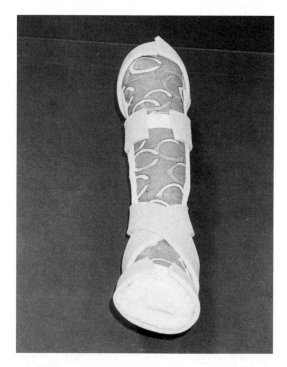

Fig. 12-1 Bivalved serial cast constructed of plaster and covered with fiberglass, used to increase range of motion at the ankle and knee.

This process is repeated every 5 to 10 days contingent on progressive gains in mobility.

Outcome

The effectiveness of serial casting to gain ankle mobility and improve foot alignment has been documented for many patient populations, including traumatic brain injury, cerebral palsy, and juvenile rheumatoid arthritis. Long-term results of this intervention with a cerebral palsied population indicate gradual reaccommodation to a shorter muscle length, generally within 5 months after treatment.[3]

Soft Foot Orthosis

Rationale

The purpose of using soft foot orthotics is to balance the foot biomechanically and support the arches, calcaneus, and plantar surface of the toes. Such support may provide optimal stability to the foot and thereby minimize or reduce potentially deforming stressors.

Indications for Use

The utilization of a soft foot orthosis is indicated when abnormal biomechanical alignment of the foot is present, resulting in functional limitations or gait deviations; however, additional medial and/or lateral support is not necessary. Populations that may benefit from this device include those with moderate cerebral palsy, those with mild hemiplegia, and idiopathic toe-walkers.

Technique

These orthotics can be made out of medium-density pelite (3 and 5 mm), 1½-inch zonas tape, and latex enamel paint. A tracing of the foot is drawn on the pelite, and the outline of the metatarsal heads and calcaneal pad are cut out with a sharp knife. The longitudinal and peroneal arches are built up with layers of pelite, and the device is covered entirely with zonas tape. It is then painted with latex paint to increase its durability.

Another method of fabricating this orthotic involves casting the foot in the deformity-correcting position. This technique is mainly utilized when forefoot or hindfoot deformities are also present.

Outcome

Clinically, soft foot orthotics are a useful tool in the management of the above patient types; however, research on the utilization of orthotics has generally been limited, and studies are recommended to produce objective outcomes on the use of soft foot orthotics with foot deformities.

Supramalleolar Orthosis

Rationale

The supramalleolar orthosis (SMO) is generally representative of various devices (Fig. 12-2). Technically, it may be considered an AFO since it crosses the ankle joint. The SMO supports the subtalar and midtarsal joints in neutral alignment,

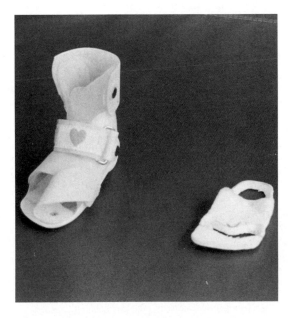

Fig. 12-2 Supramalleolar orthosis of dynamic type *(left)* and soft foot orthosis *(right)*.

thus providing control and stability in an external manner. It has been postulated that neutral or midline orientation around major body joints may be the optimal orientation around which functional movements take place. The SMO permits movement in the sagittal plane while prohibiting frontal plane instability from being expressed. Accommodations for forefoot and hindfoot deformities may be accomplished via fabrication of a sole plate. The combination of orthotic support of neutral alignment and freedom of ankle dorsiflexion/plantarflexion may allow the foot and ankle to be utilized in active balancing.

Indications for Use

The implementation of an SMO is indicated when instability and poor alignment of the subtalar and midtarsal joints are present, but minimal to no restriction of ankle dorsiflexion/plantarflexion is desired. An SMO molded to the natural contours of the foot's arches may be preferred when joint instability is the primary factor; however, when instability and excessive hypertonus are present and interfering with the quality of movement and gait, a SMO fabricated with a custom-contoured sole plate may be indicated. A sole plate provides support and stabilization to the dynamic arches of the foot. This type of SMO is sometimes described as a dynamic AFO, or DAFO. Variations of the SMO with a sole plate are based on different trim lines and serve unique purposes, including the following: the standard variety allows free ankle dorsiflexion/plantarflexion with strong medial/lateral support; the plantarflexion stop model restricts equinus posturing while providing free ankle dorsiflexion and medial/lateral stability; and the anterior stop style permits plantarflexion at the ankle and provides knee extension assist while providing medial/lateral support (also called a short floor-reaction AFO).

Patient populations that may benefit from the implementation of the SMO include children with moderate to severe hypotonia and marked ankle/foot instability; children with excessive hypertonia and ankle/foot instability; and children with dynamic varus or valgus foot deformities with mild to severe hypertonus. Diagnoses may include cerebral palsy, myelomeningocele, arthrogryposis, muscular dystrophy, traumatic brain injury, and cerebrovascular accident.

In addition, other factors may create indications for a particular SMO model. The SMO with a plantarflexion stop may be preferred over an AFO for cosmetic reasons. The flexible plastic utilized in the SMO with a sole plate may be better tolerated by children with sensitive skin or increased risk for development of pressure areas.

Technique

The simple SMO model is fabricated of a low-density, low-thermosetting plastic. Measurements for the plastic are taken from midcalf to the toes and circumferentially around the heel and metatarsal heads. The plastic is softened in a warm water bath until malleable. The foot and ankle are prepared for splint fabrication with application of foam padding to bony prominences and coverage with two layers of stockinette to accommodate for splint shrinkage. If tolerated, the child is positioned in prone and the plastic is pulled around the ankle and foot and pinched anteriorly. The ankle is then dorsiflexed to approximately 5 degrees, and neutral subtalar joint alignment is secured. The forefoot should not be permitted to abduct. The natural arches of the foot are contoured into the posterior portion. Trim lines for the SMO include coverage of the malleoli. The posterior trim line is made about1 inch above the calcaneus. On the foot portion, trim lines are dependent upon presence of deformity. Posting at the calcaneus or forefoot may prohibit rocking and accommodate existing forefoot deviations. Straps are typically not necessary to secure the SMO to the foot, because this is generally accomplished by the child's shoe.

The SMO with a sole plate typically involves the combined skills of a physical therapist and an orthotist, and its fabrication can be divided into two phases. In the first phase, the patient's foot is outlined and significant landmarks are identified. The drawing of the foot is transferred onto plywood. The metatarsal head and calcaneal pad area are routed out. The arches of the foot and neutral alignment of the metatarsal joints are built onto the sole plate once the outline of the foot has been cut out with a jigsaw. The patient's foot is always kept in subtalar neutral during this process. In addition to this method, a sole plate may be produced on a triwall cardboard base, using casting plaster or modeling clay as build-up. The method of production is generally based on subjective preference. Once the fabrication is complete, the sole plate is casted onto the patient's foot to produce a negative mold of the foot and ankle. From this form, the product is ultimately produced, usually by an orthotist, generally as the second phase of fabrication. The cast is filled with plaster and a positive mold is made. Appropriate modifications are made, and a polypropylene material is pulled over the positive mold. The trim lines are then marked and cut. The orthotic wraps around the medial and lateral aspects of the foot, and the anterior trim line almost meets down the center of the dorsum of the foot. The posterior trim line may be trimmed to approximately 1 inch above the superior calcaneus when free plantarflexion is desired, or it may extend 2 or 3 inches above the malleoli when a plantarflexion stop is indicated. Velcro straps are placed to secure the orthosis to the foot.

Outcome

The SMO has been widely used in the physical therapy clinic for the past 15 years in the management of the foot and ankle, particularly with the cerebral palsied population; however, there are limited studies related to the use of this device.

Inframalleolar Orthosis

Rationale

The inframalleolar orthosis provides alignment of the subtalar and midtarsal joints and support to the arches with a minimal external structure; therefore, stability of the foot and ankle may be achieved while the greatest possible degree of free mobility is maintained.

Indications for Use

In general, an inframalleolar orthosis may be indicated in mild cases of joint instability and poor alignment, where external ankle support would be excessive. Populations that may benefit from the use of this device include those with flexible pes valgus or ligamentous laxity that allows subtalar joint deviation. Also, the inframalleolar orthosis may be indicated for postsurgical support of the foot. Diagnostic groups that may utilize this unit are similar to those outlined for an SMO, except that the degree of foot and ankle deformity is less.

Technique

The fabrication of the inframalleolar orthotic is identical to that of the SMO, with the differentiation involving its trim lines. This model is trimmed just below the malleoli, with a posterior line approximately 1 inch above the superior calcaneus. Posting at the calcaneus and forefoot may be added as indicated. As with the SMO, this device is held onto the foot by the shoe and generally does not require securing straps.

Outcome

Clinically, use of inframalleolar orthoses has resulted in a decrease in structural deviations and improvement in joint stability.[1] Data on the effectiveness of this device with a specific patient population are currently not available.

Ankle-Foot Orthosis

Rationale

The traditional AFO can be utilized to effectively alleviate potential deformities. The primary reason for employing this device is to ensure optimal joint alignment and thereby maintain normal functional muscle length across the joints of the foot and ankle. Support and protection of bony surfaces, cartilage, and soft tissue can be achieved by this intervention. In addition to providing structural stability, the AFO can also serve to maintain functional positioning during gait when normal active muscle forces are reduced or absent.

Indications for Use

There are several variations of the AFO, and implementation of a specific type is dependent upon the functional status of the joints and the goals of intervention. In all cases it is necessary that the equinus positioning not be a fixed deformity.

A solid AFO is most commonly indicated for prohibiting equinus posturing, with subsequent muscle shortening, and maintaining neutral positioning of the joints of the foot. In a nonweight-bearing role, this splint can be implemented to maintain ankle range of motion, usually to neutral. This device provides more of a custom fit than a resting splint, and a neutral subtalar joint alignment can be achieved and maintained. A solid AFO may also be indicated in weight-bearing. It is utilized to provide support and alignment against deforming forces and abnormal muscle tension at the foot and ankle. In addition, the splint may protect against abnormal knee joint alignment to some degree. With this stabilization, a typically nonambulatory child can utilize static standing as a means of achieving the physiological benefits of weight-bearing. In ambulatory children, a solid AFO is beneficial in providing postoperative protection against tissue overlengthening. Also, the static posture may be used to simulate ankle cocontraction during the early development of ambulation skills.[1] Diagnostic populations that may benefit from this device, particularly in the early recovery stages, include those with traumatic brain injury, cerebrovascular accident, peripheral nerve injury, cerebral palsy, and postoperative patients when indicated.

A hinged AFO allows the child to utilize ankle dorsiflexion through stance and thereby achieve a more normal gait pattern. Therefore, passive ankle dorsiflexion of 5 to 10 degrees, with maintenance of neutral foot alignment, is mandatory for this AFO. In addition to enabling a less deviated gait pattern, the hinged splint permits ankle dorsiflexion in transitional movement and decreased restriction of normal motor patterns. As with the solid AFO, this device may reduce genu recurvatum in stance to a variable degree. A hinged AFO is typically utilized as a progression from the solid version. It is beneficial for the child who has begun to develop some degree of effective control at the ankle. Patient populations that may be indicated for this device include those with cerebral palsy or later stages of posttraumatic brain injury.

Technique

The AFO is fabricated from a low-thermosetting plastic material with controlled stretch properties. The child is first sized for an appropriate piece of material. Measurements are taken from the popliteal crease to the toes and circumferentially around the calf musculature, heel, and metatarsal heads. The material is marked and cut from these measurements and heated in a warm water bath. Bony prominences are padded with a foam material, and the surface to be splinted is covered with a stockinette. Two layers of stockinette are recommended to accommodate splint shrinkage which can occur as the plastic cools. If tolerated, the child is positioned in prone, and the plastic material is draped over the lower extremity from the calf to the toes while the ankle is permitted to plantarflex (Fig. 12-3). Once the material has been pulled closed anteriorly, the knee is flexed while the ankle is simultaneously dorsiflexed to approximately 5 degrees. The calcaneus is held in a position of neutrality while the material is molded to produce a clear calcaneal outline. The forefoot is then rotated perpendicular to the tibia, unless this motion is restricted, and then the forefoot should remain inverted. Molding should be done along the longitudinal arches of the foot. When the material has begun to cool, the splint should be removed and desired trim lines cut. Padding should be transferred to the splint and velcro straps added across the proximal calf and in a figure-eight pattern about the ankle. Posting at the calcaneus and/or medial metatarsal heads may be necessary to achieve a stable base and prohibit rocking.

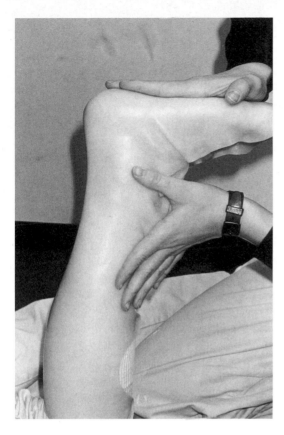

Fig. 12-3 Ankle-foot orthosis being molded to a patient positioned in prone.

When fabricating a hinged AFO, the method is essentially the same as with the solid version, except that the two components of the splint are molded separately and then assembled as a unit. The foot piece is measured from the Achilles tendon to the toes and circumferentially at the heel and the metatarsal heads. The calf piece is measured from the popliteal crease to the Achilles tendon and circumferentially at the proximal calf. The first portion to be molded is the foot component, and the application technique is identical to that for the ankle-foot region of the solid AFO. After fabrication and subsequent trimming, the malleoli and heel portions of the plastic are covered lightly with lotion or petroleum jelly and placed on the child's foot. Then the calf piece is molded with the ankle positioned in approximately 5 degrees of dorsiflex-ion. Once this piece has been trimmed, the components are aligned and a screw is punched through the malleoli portion of the splint. Straps are applied at the proximal and distal calf and across the instep.

Outcome

The AFO is generally considered an effective positioning device for preventing equinus deformity, although its success is reduced in children with significant lower extremity hypertonicity.[1] Stabilization and joint protection in weight-bearing are easily gained and maintained with ongoing splint utilization, provided that optimal custom fit is achieved. The choice of a solid vs. a hinged splint is based on the clinician's evaluation and indications outlined previously in this chapter.

Posterior Resting Splint

Rationale

The posterior resting splint for the ankle and foot is utilized to maintain range of motion within a comfortable range as well as normal functional muscle length across the ankle joint. Other primary purposes include support and protection of bony surfaces, cartilage, and soft tissue.

Indications for Use

There are numerous diagnostic populations with which the posterior resting splint is used to provide protection and prevent loss of joint mobility. These include postoperative patients, those with trauma, juvenile rheumatoid arthritis, lower extremity burns, foot and/or ankle wounds, and those who lack active foot and ankle movement (Fig. 12-4). A resting splint is not to be used for weight-bearing activities; therefore, the patient should also be provided with an assistive device to maintain nonweight-bearing for ambulation purposes. With this type of splint, it is difficult to achieve neutral subtalar joint positioning. The resting splint may also include a knee component to provide protection

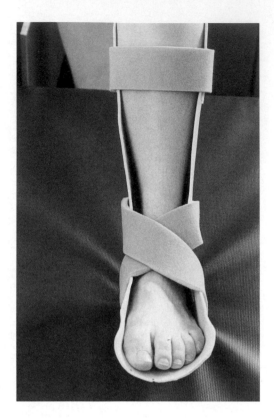

Fig. 12-4 Posterior resting splint, used to provide joint protection and maintain ankle dorsiflexion.

across the knee joint. This type of posterior splint may be indicated for hemophiliac patients with an acute bleed.

Technique

A thorough evaluation is performed before splint fabrication is begun and includes the following: active and passive range of motion, presence of swelling, muscle tone, skin integrity, sensation, skin color, and functional skills as appropriate.

After the evaluation, the patient is measured from the popliteal crease to the toes and from the heel to the toes. Circumferential measurements are taken at the proximal calf, heel, and metatarsal heads. These measurements are then transferred to a piece of low-thermosetting plastic that does not stretch. The position of the patient varies according to the therapist's preference. After being placed in a warm water bath, the plastic is molded to the foot and ankle

with the foot in the desired position until the plastic cools. It is helpful to cut a triangular dart in the plastic at the level of the heel on each side to allow the foot piece to be formed without producing folds in the plastic. If the patient's skin is sensitive or if there are areas of potential skin breakdown, padding may be added. Velcro straps are applied at the proximal calf and in a figure-eight across the ankle to secure the splint. Elastic wraps may also be used to hold the splint in place. In patients who require long-term splint use, the splint should be checked occasionally to accommodate growth of the child's foot.

Outcome

The posterior resting splint is considered an effective protection device used to maintain ankle range of motion. The use of a resting splint is often combined with a range of motion exercise program. With ongoing splint utilization, the joints are protected.

Hallux Valgus Orthosis

Rationale

Hallux valgus is a deformity found frequently in children and adolescents (Fig. 12-5). Patients may experience occasional discomfort over the medial prominence of the metatarsal head, and many are concerned with the appearance of the deformity. The hallux valgus orthosis, developed by Groiso, is used to prevent progression of the deformity and in some cases to correct it.[2]

Indications for Use

The hallux valgus splint is used in children varying in age from 1 month through the adolescent years. The patient either has a deformity clinically obvious or noted on radiographs or requests treatment due to the unsightly appearance of the foot.

Technique

The patient's midfoot and forefoot are measured, and circumferential measurements are

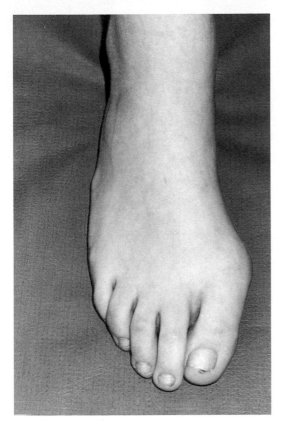

Fig. 12-5 A 10-year-old female with hallux valgus deformity.

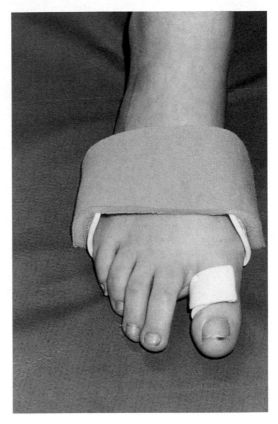

Fig. 12-6 Hallux valgus orthosis applied to patient in Fig. 12-5. Note correction of the valgus deformity.

taken at the metatarsal heads and the first toe. A pattern is initially drawn on lightweight paper and contains the following components: a flange about half the width of the foot at the level of the metatarsal heads and a flange to accommodate the first toe. The pattern is then transferred to a low-thermosetting plastic without properties of stretch. The splinting material is softened in a warm water bath, and the larger flange is molded to the foot. Before the distal flange is molded, it is folded to double the thickness, providing increased durability at the level of the first toe. While the splint cools, pressure is applied in a medial direction on the first phalange to provide a stretch of the soft tissues. A Velcro strap is applied to the splint to secure it to the foot (Fig. 12-6). The splint is typically worn at night and may be covered by a sock to prevent slippage. The splint is adjusted as needed to achieve neutral positioning of the first phalange. While

being treated with the splint, the child is also instructed to perform active toe abduction exercises and passive medial mobilization of the first metatarsophalangeal joint.

Outcome

The patient with a hallux valgus deformity may be treated conservatively with a hallux valgus orthosis combined with range of motion exercises. The splint may be worn until bone maturation to prevent progression or recurrence of the deformity. In the patients treated by Groiso, splint use delayed progression of the deformity and in some patients the deformity was completely corrected.[2]

Acknowledgement

Marilyn Geier served as a consultant and contributed her knowledge regarding soft foot orthosis and dynamic ankle-foot orthosis.

Bibliography

1. Cusick B: *Casts and splints: their changing role in the management of foot deformity*, instructional course material, Cardinal Hill Hospital, Lexington, KY, 1988.
2. Groiso J: Juvenile hallux valgus: a conservative approach to treatment, *J Bone Joint Surg* 74:1367, 1992.
3. Watt J: A prospective study of inhibitive casting as an adjunct for cerebral-palsied children, *Dev Med Child Neurol,* 2:480-488, 1986.

Rehabilitation of the Athlete's Foot and Ankle

13

Rehabilitation Strategies and Protocols for the Athlete

Pamela Davis

Donald E. Baxter

Anna Pati

The Physical Therapy Perspective

The science of physical therapy for the foot and ankle, like athletic footwear, has become more sophisticated with the increased popularity of aerobic calisthenics, walking, jogging, and running. The treatment of associated injuries has served to develop physical therapy rehabilitation of the foot and ankle into a specialty area of its own. Several fine texts and courses[18,27,44] have refined physical therapy expertise in this area and outline well the biomechanical issues of concern. Physical therapists view the foot-ankle complex as *the* interface of the human being with the environmental ground forces. In athletics the magnitude and direction of ground forces vary with the sport. The athlete's foot-ankle complex must be able to function at the level of the demands placed on it; otherwise the athlete is at risk for injury or the development of overuse syndromes. Activities such as running, jumping, dodging, skiing, skating, and dancing exert extraordinary forces on the ligaments, muscles, and joints. The biomechanical accommodation of the foot determines the extent and pattern of these forces as they are transmitted to the more proximal joints. Ideally, attention to the athlete's ankle and foot should begin early in preseason training before intense competition begins.

Evaluation for Injury Prevention

Screening

The physical therapist provides valuable information as a participant in preseason screening programs. Evaluation of the athlete involves identifying risk factors that predispose to injury, especially as they relate to specific tasks demanded by the athlete's sport. Specific areas that the physical therapist evaluates include strength and range of motion (ROM), postural alignment, soft tissue mobility and compliance, muscle balance, gait variations, activity and stress patterns, and support needs. The therapist identifies and addresses deficiencies in all of these areas to prevent potential problems in play or performance.

Postural Alignment

Bony alignment, particularly of the subtalar joint, integrity of the arches, and static and dynamic weight-bearing posture are considered. Analysis of alignment faults to differentiate problems of the skeleton from those of soft tissue and muscular imbalance directs the focus of the treatment program. Identifying postural alignment variations, such as hindfoot varus or valgus, that put the foot-ankle complex at risk for injury facilitates preventive intervention. Mild deviations in alignment of the foot are compensated for with footwear adjustments or orthotics. The goal is to promote normal functional alignment and motion, thus preventing injury.

Mobility

Beyond joint ROM, mobility issues encompass joint play and soft tissue characteristics such as tightness of the musculotendinous units, degree of ligamentous laxity, and fascial compliance. Soft tissue characteristics have increasingly been implicated as an important factor in musculoskeletal dysfunction of the foot-ankle complex. For example, left uncorrected, a tight heel cord can compromise performance technique and ankle stability in an ice skater, or predispose to plantar fasciitis in a runner.[48] Another example is the athlete with a flat foot tendency that is accentuated by tight peroneal and triceps surae muscles and a weak anterior tibialis. Soft tissue tightness and muscle imbalance are often correctable by muscle strengthening and stretching.

Accessory joint play of the intermetatarsal, metatarsophalangeal (MTP), and interphalangeal joints enhances toe and arch mobility and encourages intrinsic muscle action. The woman athlete who works in high-heeled shoes that hyperextend the MTP joints all day acquires adaptive changes of decreased MTP joint plantar tilt and glide and intrinsic muscle weakness. Lack of joint play predisposes the athlete to injury; therefore the physical therapist attempts to reverse the adaptations to chronic hyperextension by designing a home program consisting of stretching, Mennel's joint manipulation techniques,[65] and specific strengthening exercises.

When hypermobility is present, preventive measures such as taping may be indicated. Taping supports the very supple feet of young gymnasts and dancers to prevent injury, discourage hypermobility, and possibly retard degenerative changes to prolong the athletic career. To prevent weakness caused by external support, an exercise program that enhances natural support mechanisms should accompany taping programs.

Flexibility of the arches and plantar fascia is frequently an issue. Evaluation may suggest the need for an arch support, metatarsal pad, or other shoe insert. In the presence of tightness, very high arches, or limited toe mobility, stretching exercises for the toes and heel cord may be indicated.

Muscle Function and Balance

A simple manual muscle test of the major groups of the foot screens for muscle imbalances or deficiencies. Muscles should be tested for strength in the primary movement as well as in synergistic motions. Once muscle imbalance or weakness is identified, the ability of the muscle action to correct or minimize malalignments should be assessed and therapeutic programs designed accordingly.

The most common and clinically significant deficiency involves weakness of the ankle evertors, which predisposes to and results from ankle sprains. Weakness of the peroneal muscles is particularly troublesome in sports involving uneven terrain, sudden starts and stops, up-on-toes activity, quick direction changes, or jumping. The stirrup muscles of the ankle must react instantly to stabilize the ankle and to support and protect the ligaments.

The intrinsic muscles function in toe flexion, depression, and abduction. Assessment of the foot's intrinsic muscle strength often reveals deconditioned intrinsic muscles. Deficiency of toe

Rehabilitation of the Athlete's Foot and Ankle

abduction and depression rarely creates but commonly perpetuates faulty alignment and predisposes to bunions. Deconditioning of the intrinsic muscles occurs in those who rarely go barefoot and also results from noncompliant footwear. High heels, men's dress shoes, and pointed-toed shoes tend to crowd the toes and provide little room for their free movement. Wide shoes or shoes with an adequate toe box allow spreading of the forefoot and simple toe curl exercises, which promote function, comfort, and health for the foot. A regular exercise program that increases mobility and corrects minor deficits of strength that cause muscle imbalance is a wise investment of time that results in injury prevention.

Gait

In evaluating the athlete's gait, the physical therapist looks beyond normal ambulation and assesses the alignment of the proximal joints (e.g., hip rotation, tibial torsion), weight distribution and transfer during stance, and the takeoff and landing position of the foot. During the evaluation, simulation of the most typical ankle and foot maneuvers of the sport reveals deficiencies that would not otherwise be discovered. Footwear biases takeoff and stabilizes landing; therefore a complete assessment of gait includes an evaluation of the athlete's shoes. Important features of the shoes are compliance at the MTP joint area and adequacy of the heel height, heel cushion, and heel counter.

Activity and Stress Patterns

Anticipating the stresses and demands of the sport on the ankle and foot enhances the evaluation. Just as in recent years work simulation and work hardening have become part of the assessment and rehabilitation of injured workers, evaluation using sport action simulation alerts the therapist to fitness deficits and training needs of the athlete. Simulation equipment such as the NordicTrack for cross-country skiing, the Heiden board for speed skating (Fig. 13-1), and the Fitter for downhill skiing (Fig. 13-2) are recommended.

In many sports the patterns of muscle tightness and resulting problems can be anticipated. Long-distance runners typically have tight hip flexors and triceps surae, which predispose to back pain and plantar fasciitis,[48] respectively.

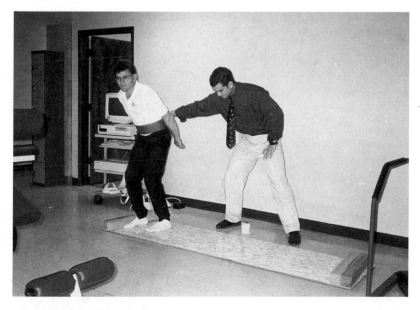

Fig. 13-1   Although designed to simulate speed skating, the Heiden board may be used to add variety to a general ankle rehabilitation program.

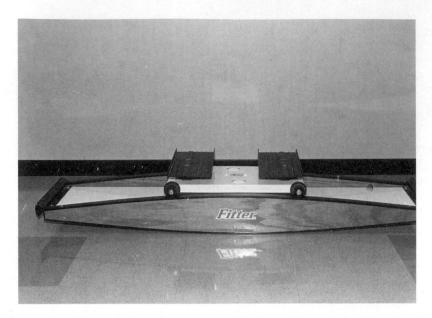

Fig. 13-2 The Fitter, designed to simulate downhill skiing, is often used in general rehabilitation programs to increase agility and coordination (Fitter International, Inc. #321, 1021 10th Avenue SW, Calgary, Alberta, Canada T2R 0B7).

Gymnasts with tight hip flexors compensate with increased lumbar lordosis, which causes additional stress on the pars interarticularis, predisposing to a pars stress fracture. Ballet dancers who have limited external rotation of the hip are at risk for medial knee strain. Athletes who sustain lateral forces while on the planted foot, as in rugby, football, or soccer, require additional strength in the peroneal muscles to retain balance and prevent ankle injury.

Support

The need for foot support depends on the demands of the sport and the athlete's inherent stability and postural alignment. Based on these factors, the physical therapist recommends the amount and type of external support indicated. Supports are invaluable to allow healing and prevent additional injury during rehabilitation; however, less support is probably better for prevention. Physical therapists emphasize development of inherent stability through well-directed training to achieve adequate strength, coordination, balance, and endurance. The minimum ex-

ternal support needed for protection against anticipated stresses should be used. Preventive supports can range from a proper shoe fit to taping to specifications for a custom flexible, semirigid, or rigid orthosis. Often, commercially available shoe inserts are adequate. Dr. Scholl's Flexosoles, which incorporate a metatarsal pad and an arch support into an insole, are useful in a variety of situations. Most prophylactic supports address arch or subtalar joint alignment problems, but tendencies toward bunions, hammertoes, and quiescent heel spurs also respond well to minor supportive interventions.

Training

Following preseason screening, the training regimen incorporates exercises and occasionally modalities (as described later in the chapter) to assure tolerance of the foot and ankle to the activity level demanded by the sport. Cool-down massage, stretching, and icing minimize soreness by enhancing circulation for removal of fluid and metabolic wastes. Gradual increase in work load and moderation of work intensity during pre-

Rehabilitation of the Athlete's Foot and Ankle

season training and within the season prevent overuse syndromes.

Injury

In many instances the physical therapist's first evaluation of the athlete's ankle and foot is after an injury or surgical intervention. Evaluation and rehabilitation of the injured athlete include the elements outlined previously and an additional consideration: inflammation and edema, not uncommon following injury or surgery, must be resolved. Assessment of tissue tension for the presence of excess fluid by palpation and circumference measurements reveals increased thickness of the tissues. The presence of inflammation impairs function, comfort, and ROM. The foot-ankle complex is in a dependent position and remote from major lymphatic drainage and central circulation; therefore it benefits from fluid mobilization techniques and external compression and support. Ace wraps and sleeves, sequential compression, compression boots and splints, cold with compression (see section on Cryotherapy), and deep stroking and kneading massage are used to remove edema. Reduction of edema increases ROM and relieves discomfort.

Principles of Rehabilitation

Prior to designing a rehabilitation program, the therapist must evaluate the athlete's attributes, the characteristics of the injury (acute vs. chronic), and the functional demands of the particular sport. Subsequently the therapist designs a program that addresses four components of rehabilitation: facilitation of healing and recovery, identification and correction of tissues that may have predisposed to injury or that could jeopardize recovery, restoration of optimal function, and successful return of the athlete to play. All athletes, whether gymnasts, football players, runners, or ballet dancers, have unique adaptations of their body habitus to the demands of their particular sport. Physical adaptations facilitate high-level performance but may predispose the athlete to overuse syndromes or particular acute injuries.

Rehabilitation Strategies

Rehabilitation strategies for overuse syndromes and dysfunction of the foot-ankle complex differ from rehabilitation programs for the acutely injured or postoperative situation. Rehabilitation of dysfunction is active and aggressive, deemphasizing modalities and emphasizing therapeutic exercise, stretching, muscle reeducation, and modification of performance techniques. Chronic overuse problems require modification of the athlete's physical characteristics by stretching and strengthening, and modification of biomechanics by changing techniques of performance or modifying shoes or other equipment. When chronic inflammation is present, the use of modalities, antiinflammatory medication, cross-training, and relative rest are indicated.

Rehabilitation of the acutely injured or postoperative foot or ankle condition requires time and protection for healing, then emphasizes reduction of edema, minimization of pain, and support to prevent reinjury. Eventually graduated exercise programs to condition the athlete for expedient return to play are indicated. Modalities to alleviate pain and decrease swelling are an important part of the rehabilitation programs for acute injuries. Explicit directions regarding exercise and activity progression are often necessary to guide the ambitious athlete who is eager to return to play.

Return to Play

The ultimate goal of the physician, therapist, and athletic trainer is to return the athlete safely to play and competition as soon as possible. To design the most effective rehabilitation for an athlete, one focuses not only on the athlete's physiological deficits but also on the specific demands of the sport. A rehabilitation program designed to prepare the athlete to face the unique requirements of the sport makes use of the "specific adaptation to imposed demand principle."[3,28] The demands of ballet dancing *en pointe, demi pointe,* and performing *relevé* (moving from foot-flat to *pointe*) predispose the ballerina to os trigonum impingement,[59] stenosing tenosynovitis,[41] cuboid subluxation,[60] and other conditions of the foot and ankle. Retraining the athlete to the demands of the sport gives the athlete confidence and affirms to the therapist and physician that the athlete is ready to perform at an increased intensity level. As mentioned before, devices that stimulate the specific demands of sports activities such as the Fitter, the Heiden board, and the NordicTrack are useful for rehabilitation as well as training. The BAPS board, rocker board, and balance disk (Fig. 13-3) incorporate balance and coordination demands that will be encountered in sport. Creative exercises designed to increase the functional demands of the entire lower extremity in a controlled environment also advance the rehabilitation program (Fig. 13-4). As the athlete is phased back into sport, it is necessary to fine-tune the rehabilitation program, modifying performance technique and troubleshooting to prevent recurrent injury. Home exercise programs are adjusted and integrated to complement training schedules.

Rehabilitation Protocols

Lateral Ankle Sprain

Ankle sprains are one of the most common injuries of the athletic population. The vast majority are mild and do not result in chronic instability; however, all ankle sprains should be considered potentially disabling to the athlete. With this in mind, an appropriate evaluation of the ankle to determine the severity of the sprain and delineate associated pathology is warranted. After determining the extent of injury to the lateral ligaments, the appropriate treatment regimen and progression of the rehabilitation program can be initiated. Grade I and II injuries have partial tears of the anterior talofibular ligament (ATFL) or calcaneofibular ligament (CFL) or both. Grade III injuries have a complete tear of either one or both of the lateral ligaments.

Jackson[45] has outlined a three-phase program for the rehabilitation of ankle sprains: (1) limit extension of injury, (2) restore motion, (3) restore agility and endurance. The first phase requires the use of ice, elevation, and compression to decrease swelling and relieve pain. The ankle should be protected with the use of crutches and by wrapping or splinting the ankle. Grade III injuries require 6 weeks of immobilization[30,79] to allow the ligaments to heal. Smith and Reischl[78] suggest immobilizing the ankle in the maximum amount of dorsiflexion tolerated, and Drez et al[30] suggest immobilization in dorsiflexion and slight eversion to reapproximate the torn ends of the ATFL. Isometric exercises of the anterior tibialis and peroneal muscles are encouraged during the period of casting to decrease muscle atrophy.[71]

The second phase begins when the athlete with a Grade I or II injury is comfortable bearing weight or when the athlete with a Grade III injury comes out of the cast. ROM exercises that emphasize stretching the Achilles tendon[79] and gentle strengthening exercises emphasizing the peroneal and anterior tibialis muscles[36,79] are mainstays of the second phase. Surgical tubing or Thera-Band is helpful in providing resistance to the evertors and dorsiflexors and requires both concentric and eccentric muscle contractions. Ice is preferred over contrast baths and heat to reduce swelling in the subacute period following ankle sprains.[20] The athlete is advanced to the third phase when ROM is normal and unassisted ambulation is not painful.

The third phase concentrates on functional neuromuscular retraining and increasing strength and endurance. Balance board exercises are used to promote coordination and proprioceptive conditioning.[82,87] Progressive resistance strengthening exercises emphasizing the peroneal and anterior tibialis muscles[79] using surgical tubing or Thera-Band are continued. Graduated functional conditioning begins with brisk walking and progresses to jogging, straight running, figure-eight running, cutting, and other sport-specific maneuvers. The use of ultrasound may be helpful to decrease tenderness over the ligaments.[79]

Return to play is dependent on the ability of the athlete to perform sport-specific activities with confidence in the ankle and without discomfort. Athletes with a Grade III injury should not go back to competition for 1 month after

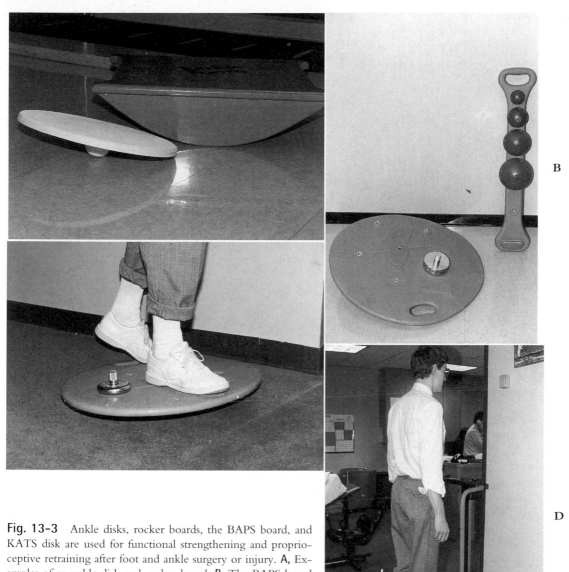

Fig. 13-3 Ankle disks, rocker boards, the BAPS board, and KATS disk are used for functional strengthening and proprioceptive retraining after foot and ankle surgery or injury. **A,** Examples of an ankle disk and rocker board. **B,** The BAPS board and accessories, including weights and different sizes of half spheres. **C,** Patient using the BAPS board to rehabilitate injured right ankle. **D,** The KATS disc has an electronic data-collecting system for objective documentation of improvement.

the cast is removed, and the ankle should be taped for at least 3 to 6 months.[30] Splinting the ankle with an Air-Stirrup (Aircast Inc., PO Box 709, Summit NJ 07902) is an acceptable alternative to taping.[85]

Plantar Fasciitis

Plantar fasciitis is a relatively common problem, especially in running athletes. The athlete with heel pain due to plantar fasciitis presents a problem because of the associated prolonged

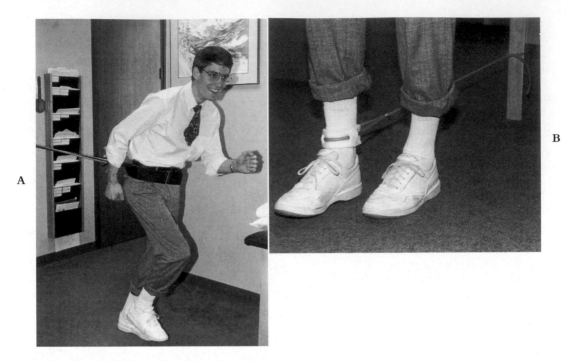

Fig. 13-4 Creative exercises designed to increase functional demands of the lower extremity in a controlled environment advance the rehabilitation program. **A,** Controlled resisted running in place is an excellent method of gradually returning to sports activities. **B,** This patient is working on increasing postural stability of the left ankle. He swings the right foot against resistance of the surgical tubing while maintaining balance on the left leg, which requires cocontraction and coordination of all the leg muscles.

morbidity, which necessitates absence from competition. Kibler et al[48] have found that athletes with plantar fasciitis have decreased dorsiflexion ROM and decreased plantarflexion strength. These deficits may cause or contribute to the development of plantar fasciitis by creating a weak link in the system of the posterior calf, ankle, and foot.[48,93] The pathological lesion, as seen in patients who ultimately have surgery, is local inflammation and fibrosis of the plantar fascia with areas of mucinoid degeneration.[51] While no specific treatment has been proven to be most effective, a comprehensive treatment plan may return the athlete to competition as expediently as possible.

The mainstay of treatment is relative rest, including reduction of mileage, reduction of speed work, and alternating activities (cross-training). In runners, maintenance of cardiovascular fitness should be achieved by bicycling, swimming, or running in an aquatherapy pool during the most symptomatic period. Stretching the Achilles tendon corrects the abnormal biomechanics of the calf, ankle, and foot linkage system caused by a tight Achilles tendon. The dorsiflexion ROM achieved by stretching can be maintained through the night by the use of night splints.[94] If the athlete has a pronated foot, orthotics such as the UC-BL orthosis[13] may be helpful. Heel lifts, cushions, and heel cups may also be helpful.

Nonsteroidal antiinflammatory medication and ice after activity decreases inflammation of the plantar fascia insertion. Deep heating modalities such as ultrasound or shortwave diathermy increase the circulation and thereby promote healing of the involved tissues. Occasional administration of corticosteroids by injection or

Rehabilitation of the Athlete's Foot and Ankle

phonopheresis may be considered; however, corticosteroids should be used sparingly because of the risk of causing fat pad atrophy and predisposing the plantar fascia to rupture.[1,50]

Shin Splints

Shin splints are associated with high impact aerobics, treadmill use, and running. Because shin splints involve muscle strain and concomitant swelling, rest and icing are indicated. Transcutaneous electrical nerve stimulation (TENS) is useful in relieving acute discomfort. Myofascial release techniques that facilitate soft tissue mobilization and reduce edema are more helpful and tolerated better than massage. In the subacute or recurrent stages, deep heat and mobilization of the fibula are effective. Tibialis anterior muscle strength and endurance, if deficient, should be built gradually with the balance disk, BAPS board, and free weights or Thera-Band progressive resistance exercises. Activity levels and training terrain may need to be altered to allow recovery. Needless to say, predisposing factors and training errors should be identified and corrected.

Tendinitis/Tendinosis

Rigorous, high-intensity training schedules predispose the athlete to the vicious cycle of overuse or overload injury. The flexor hallucis longus tendon is at risk for overload in ballet dancers.[41] Running and jumping athletes are predisposed to Achilles tendon overload and degeneration. Evaluation of the athlete with tendinitis or tendinosis includes screening for associated conditions such as inflexibility, weakness of the involved muscle, and strength imbalance so that the rehabilitation program can be directed toward resolving these deficits.

The rehabilitation program consists of three phases[47]: acute, recovery, and maintenance. The acute phase focuses on prevention of additional tissue injury and diminishing the symptoms. Protection and rest of the injured tissues are mandatory. Nonsteroidal antiinflammatory drugs and physical therapy modalities are most helpful in the acute phase to decrease tissue inflammation. Ice is suggested for acutely inflamed, painful tendinitis to achieve pain relief and decrease edema. In the recovery phase, appropriate loading of the muscle is initiated. Gentle strengthening and ROM exercises are begun. Finally, functional exercises are started to achieve sports–specific muscle reeducation. If normal ROM is difficult to achieve, warming the tissues with diathermy or ultrasound prior to exercise is helpful to achieve maximal benefit from stretching.[56] The maintenance phase focuses on maintaining strength and flexibility restored by the acute and recovery phases of the rehabilitation program so that overload of the tendons does not recur. A maintenance program of strengthening and stretching is designed to prevent the recurrence of deficits associated with the tendinosis or tendinitis. Plyometric exercises and sports-specific activities emphasizing proper biomechanics are begun.

Postoperative Rehabilitation Programs

Following surgery, a period of rest or inactivity is necessary for soft tissue healing to take place. The active rehabilitation program may begin very early for procedures such as tendon sheath releases for stenosing tenosynovitis or the removal of an os trigonum, but in cases that require bone or ligament healing, a period of immobilization is necessary to allow for healing. Generally, tendons and ligaments require 6 weeks to heal, but maximum tensile strength may not be achieved for a year. Skin and subcutaneous tissue is healed sufficiently to allow suture removal at 2 weeks. During the time of immobilization, isometric exercises[71] and electrical muscle stimulation[4,37] maintain muscle tone and limit disuse atrophy.

Operative scars on the foot and ankle can produce adhesions to underlying tendons and nerves because of the paucity of subcutaneous fat. Symptomatic scars respond well to friction massage, which restores soft tissue mobility and compliance over tendon sheaths and bony prominences. Compression in the form of elastic supports (which can be obtained off the shelf or custom fabricated) is particularly useful for retarding hypertrophic scarring.

The rehabilitation program for lateral ligament

reconstruction follows the program already outlined for Grade III lateral ligament sprains. After the cast is removed, phase two of the program is initiated to regain ROM, and progression to phase three for functional strengthening is rapid. Similarly, the postoperative rehabilitation of the athlete who has had debridement of the Achilles tendon or release of the flexor hallucis longus tendon sheath follows the program outlined for tendinitis and tendinosis.

Os Trigonum Excision

The dancer who has symptomatic posterior ankle impingement due to the presence of a large or fractured os trigonum may elect to have this accessory bone excised.[59] Postoperative goals include early recovery of complete dorsiflexion and achievement of increased plantarflexion. Aggressive rehabilitation is necessary for the dancer to achieve maximal results from the procedure. Common problems that inhibit full ROM include pain and swelling, so TENS for pain control and ice and elevation for reduction of edema are used during the first 3 to 4 days after surgery. Functional muscle imbalance may inhibit return to dance or cause secondary overload of other structures. Most dancers have very little difficulty regaining ROM and function by rehabilitating themselves with a home program of stretching and strengthening exercises. Occasionally physical therapy is necessary to facilitate expedient return to the stage. Limited ROM must be corrected first. Therapeutic heat modalities such as hydrocollator moist heat packs, ultrasound, or shortwave diathermy are used to warm the tissues prior to stretching and so diminish pain. The Malleotrain (Bauerfeind USA, Inc., 811 Livingston Court, Marietta, GA 30067) ankle brace is helpful to reduce swelling around the ankle. The Malleotrain has viscoelastic pads contoured to fit around the malleoli sewn into an elastic support. Its use during activity promotes intermittent compression of the soft tissues around the ankle, which facilitates lymphatic drainage to decrease swelling. Manual therapy with joint mobilization is helpful to regain the normal joint play necessary to achieve full active ROM. Postoperatively the calf muscles, particularly the peroneal and anterior and posterior tibialis muscles, are weakened by disuse. Thera-Band and ankle disk exercises are useful tools to strengthen the muscles and facilitate neuromuscular reeducation and coordination. Ice decreases edema and inflammation after stretching and exercise sessions. In addition to working with a physical therapist in the therapy department, the dancer should be given a home program consisting of stretching and strengthening exercises to be performed several times daily.

Therapeutic Exercise

Rehabilitation of the athlete requires restoration of flexibility, strength, and endurance prior to return to competition. Athletes are motivated to recover to the preinjury level of performance as quickly as possible, increasing the potential for reinjury. Careful monitoring of the exercise progression and intensity of workout sessions is an important function of the physician, physical therapist, and athletic trainer. The exercise program should be individualized and efficient, requiring performance of the minimum number of different exercises to achieve each goal. Selection of the types of exercises, frequency, and intensity is based on the severity of the functional deficit associated with the athlete's condition. The program prescribed should be tailored to meet the goals of the athlete while preventing injury during the recovery period. Early in the rehabilitation program, strengthening exercises of low intensity need to be performed several times daily; however, as strength is recovered and the intensity of the rehabilitation program increases, decreasing the frequency of the workouts to allow recovery is necessary. Stretching exercises should be performed throughout the day to increase or regain flexibility that was lost during a period of imposed immobilization. When a desired level of flexibility is achieved, stretching exercises should become a daily routine.

The biomechanics of ankle function change in weight-bearing vs. nonweight-bearing situations. The kinetics of a weight-bearing extremity are referred to as "closed chain." "Open-chain" kinetics refer to the nonweight-bearing extremity.[27] Consequently, the incorporation of each has been emphasized in therapeutic exercise regimes. Passive ROM, the most elementary form of exercise, gives an indication of the joint play, tracking, compliance, and mobility of the joints. Active assistive ROM exercises are useful to retrain motion execution in cardinal and diagonal planes. Mobilization to regain accessory joint motions is also incorporated. Active ROM requires independent muscle action and incorporates muscle reeducation when mild manual resistance and facilitory techniques are added. Classic programs of foot and toe exercises always prove helpful. These use towels and marbles to develop strength, tone, and coordination of the intrinsic and extrinsic muscles. Proprioceptive neuromuscular facilitation patterns, balance disks, and BAPS boards integrate activity of the foot and ankle with the proximal joints. These drills should be done in stocking feet as well as in regular and athletic footwear.

Stretching

Stretching programs are designed to achieve prevention of injury or to regain normal ROM and flexibility during recovery from an injury or surgery. A decrease in ankle injuries has been seen following the institution of stretching programs.[12,62,67] McClusky et al[62] observed that the incidence of severe ankle sprains was decreased after a program of Achilles tendon stretching was integrated into the conditioning program for athletes.

Following a period of immobilization, musculotendinous units and joint capsules and ligaments are contracted. Therapeutic stretching is required to regain normal ROM and flexibility and allow normal functioning of the limb. Stretching should be performed in a smooth, slow, controlled manner to avoid injury to the muscle or tendon.

A successful technique for stretching is the contract–relax technique of proprioceptive neuromuscular facilitation.[91] Two athletes work together to perform this stretching exercise. After slowly stretching the muscle to the limits of motion, the athlete being stretched performs a 5-to 10-second isometric contraction against resistance provided by the partner. When the stretching athlete relaxes, the partner elongates the muscle slowly until a stretching sensation is felt by the athlete being stretched. This sequence is repeated 3 times for each muscle group being stretched. Sady et al[73] found this method of stretching more effective than either ballistic stretching (rapid ROM exercises) or static stretching exercises. Pain should not be elicited during stretching. Pain causes a protective reflex contraction of the muscle being stretched. The contract–relax method is particularly helpful to increase flexibility of the hamstrings.

The heel cord wedge is an excellent tool for stretching the Achilles tendon (Fig. 13-5). The wedge may be used in at least two ways.[62] First the wedge is placed with the vertical side against the wall, and the athlete stands facing the wall with feet pigeon-toed and directed up the incline. Then the athlete leans into the wall, increasing the stretch on the heel cord. Second, the wedge is turned so that the apex is against the wall. The athlete stands with back against the wall and feet directed up the incline for a longer, sustained stretch. Another useful tool for stretching the heel cord and plantar fascia together is the Pro-Stretch (Fig. 13-6). Of course, stretching the heel cord can also be accomplished without any special equipment by standing on level ground and leaning the body toward a wall or standing with the ball of the foot on a step and allowing the heel to lower. While doing any of these exercises, the athlete should intermittently bend the knees slightly to achieve additional stretch of the soleus.

Joint Mobilization

Classic joint mobilization addresses the accessory motions of the 30 major synovial joints in the foot and ankle that dissipate ground forces. In kicking a soccer or football, the ligaments and joints of the tarsals and metatarsals dissipate impact. Accessory movements, termed *joint play*, are not volitional but accompany voluntary movements or occur passively in response to the ground or other forces. The amount of joint play within a joint is a function of ligament and soft tissue compliance as well as bony configuration.

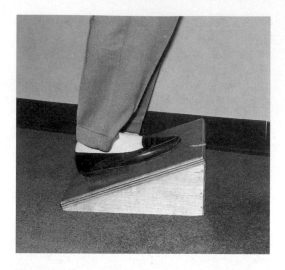

Fig. 13-5 The heel cord wedge supports the foot from heel to toe, allowing sustained stretch of the Achilles tendon.

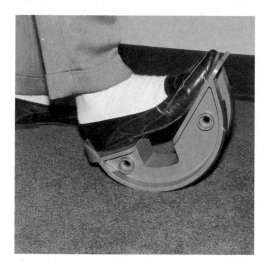

Fig. 13-6 Athletes accomplish simultaneous stretch of the plantar fascia and Achilles tendon with the Pro-Stretch (Flexible Fitness, 82 Birch Avenue, Little Silver, NJ 07739).

Ligament injuries of the foot and ankle result in hypermobility and pathologically increased joint play. An example is the increased amount of anterior glide of the talus on the tibia demonstrated by the positive anterior drawer test in the case of a torn ATFL. The accessory motions of the neighboring joints also develop pat-

terns of hypermobility or hypomobility, which may or may not be functional compensations. Muscle tightness, inflammation, and edema can restrict accessory motions and thus decrease ROM.

Mobilization techniques involve the oscillating and gliding movements of the joints in the planes of the accessory motions. The range of oscillations and gliding is graded but is always within the physiological limits of the joint. While treatment of hypomobility often ameliorates a neighboring hypermobility problem, stabilization of hypermobile joints may also be indicated. Taping and/or shoe supports are also used to address hypermobility.

Strengthening

Muscle strengthening is achieved by performing concentric or eccentric contractions against resistance or by isometric contractions. These terms refer to the muscle length produced by the contraction. A concentric contraction causes muscle shortening and is exemplified by the biceps during a pull-up. An eccentric contraction of the biceps, in which the muscle lengthens while maintaining tension, occurs during the descent from a pull-up. During an isometric contraction, the muscle does not change in length. Because there is no motion produced, isometric exercises may be performed while the injured athlete is still immobilized to minimize atrophy.[71] Eccentric contractions produce more force than either concentric or isometric contractions; therefore, eccentric contractions have a greater potential for producing muscle soreness and even injury.[84]

A program of progressive resistance exercises for strengthening muscles weakened by disuse was developed by DeLorme in the late forties.[25,26] DeLorme's program used increasing work loads to increase muscle strength, a principle that had been known for ages but that had not previously been applied in an organized therapeutic manner. Today modifications of his program are used throughout the medical community for rehabilitation and throughout the sports world to enhance performance.

When rehabilitating the foot and ankle, weights tend to be cumbersome. Thera-Band or

Thera-Band tubing is a useful tool for providing progressive resistance to the peroneal and anterior tibialis muscles (Fig. 13-7). Thera-Band is a rubberband type of material that comes in seven different levels of resistance to provide minimal to moderate resistance. The athlete should be given the heaviest weight Thera-Band that can be taken through the muscle's full excursion for 10 repetitions. Work load for the exercises is increased by increasing the number of repetitions and progressing to heavier Thera-Band.

The resistance and buoyancy of water may be used to allow an athlete to continue fitness training while rehabilitating a foot or ankle injury, particularly a stress fracture. Runners can be suspended in a pool by a buoyancy belt and run in the water with resistance provided by hand and foot paddles. Resistance is increased by increasing the size of paddles being used.

Proprioceptive Retraining

Proprioception, the sense of joint position, is altered by injury, immobilization, and non-weight-bearing. Nerve receptors for proprioception are located in tendons, muscle, ligaments, and joint capsules and prevent excessive excursion of joints and musculotendinous units by causing reflex muscle contraction. Although normal proprioception may be permanently altered by injury to one component of the proprioceptive mechanism, rehabilitation of the other components allows compensation. Neglecting proprioceptive retraining in the rehabilitation program leaves the athlete at increased risk for injury. The foot and ankle must regain the sense of joint alignment and spatial orientation to meet the demands of jumping, cutting, and running on uneven surfaces. Exercises that emphasize proprioceptive retraining include walking on the heels, toes, and medial and lateral borders of the foot, as well as walking backward and side to side. The BAPS board, ankle disk, and rocker board are excellent tools that require proprioceptive sense for the athlete to maintain balance. Proprioceptive retraining progresses to weight shifting and counterbalancing with the use of external forces and cues (see Fig. 13-4). Using computer technology and paired force plates, athletes can be cued to perform side to side, forward, backward, and diagonal movements to improve agility and reaction time while simulating sports participation (Fig. 13-8). Of course, the final test of proprioceptive awareness is actual participation in sports in an uncontrolled environment.

Plyometric Exercises

Plyometrics, a concept gaining popularity in sports rehabilitation, refers to exercises and drills based on the science of the stretch reflex. Jumping and springing activities prestretch the muscle, enabling greater force generation via neuromuscular integration of the myotatic stretch reflex. These plyometric exercises load the muscle tendon unit with a lengthening force requiring an eccentric contraction, which immediately precedes a concentric contraction. Several authors have shown that a short-range quick stretch accompanied by an eccentric muscle contraction immediately preceding a concentric contraction of the same muscle increases the force produced by the concentric contraction.[6,9,14] The storage of energy by the natural elastic properties of muscles also contributes to the production of a stronger muscle response. In addition to increasing the force of muscle contraction, plyometric exercises may improve muscle performance through enhancing neuromuscular coordination.[90]

Sled on track equipment such as the Plyotrac and Pilates board have been specially designed to make use of the plyometric concept. Simple trampoline activities provide plyometric trainingto the foot and ankle muscles. Exercises progress from the trampoline to skipping rope, stair hopping, one-legged hops, vertical jumping, and broad jumping. The intensity of each drill is increased as fitness increases to develop speed and reduce reaction time.

Comprehensive Guide to the Modalities

Physical therapy modalities are used to decrease edema, relieve pain, decrease muscle spasm, reeducate and strengthen muscles, and

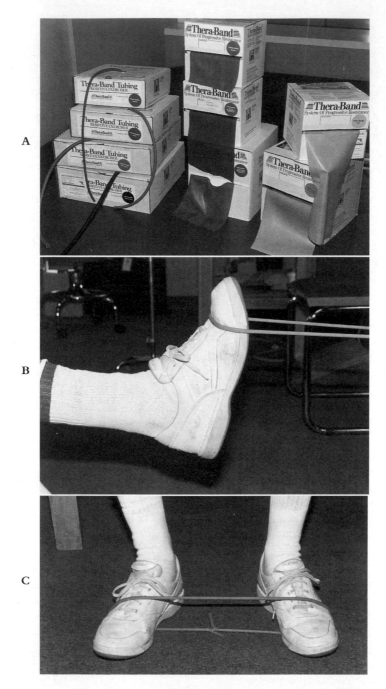

Fig. 13-7 **A,** Thera-Band and Thera-Band tubing are available in several weights that offer progressive resistance. **B,** Strengthening ankle and toe extensors using Thera-Band tubing. **C,** Peroneal muscle strengthening with Thera-Band tubing. (Hygenic Corp., 1245 Home Avenue, Akron, OH 44310).

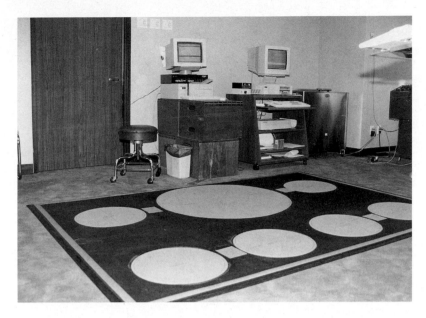

Fig. 13-8 Video Traq is a computer display system that cues the athlete to move from one force plate to another while the computer records performance data such as reaction time, stabilization time, and transit speed (Impulse Technology, Inc., 30612 Salem Drive, Bay Village, OH 44140).

deliver topical medications. Modalities are categorized as cold (cryotherapy), therapeutic heat (thermotherapy), and electricity (electrotherapy). The literature lacks well-designed scientific studies documenting the effectiveness of each modality for specific indications. Therefore, the choice of which modality to use for each indication is often empirical and depends on the therapist's preference and patient response. Table 13-1 summarizes general guidelines for the application of therapeutic modalities. In this section, the commonly used modalities are discussed in terms of their indications, physiological and therapeutic effects, actual prescription and application, and contraindications.

Cryotherapy

In the treatment of sports injuries, cold is applied to relieve pain, to reduce swelling and hemorrhage, and to decrease inflammatory infiltrates. Application of ice results in an almost immediate drop in skin temperature followed by a drop in the temperature of the subcutaneous fat. If the thickness of the subcutaneous fat is less than 1 cm, underlying muscle cools within 10 minutes; however, if the subcutaneous fat is 2 cm thick, there is very little cooling of the underlying tissue.[53] The application of cold decreases the formation of edema by reflex vasoconstriction, which decreases blood flow through injured capillaries.

Hocutt et al[43] outlined four sensory and physiological stages that occur during ice application. The sensation of cold during the first and second stages progresses from cold to burning or aching. In the third stage local anesthesia occurs, interrupting the pain–muscle spasm cycle, which relieves pain beyond the actual period of ice application. During the fourth stage of cold application, there is an increase in deep tissue vasodilitation without a concomitant increase in metabolism, which theoretically allows clearance of metabolites and injury debris. Ice should be applied for at least 15 minutes to achieve these physiological effects.

Cold is applied by immersion in ice water baths or ice whirlpools or directly with ice packs and ice massage. Ice massage relieves pain and allows gentle stretching of muscles in spasm. In

Table 13-1 General Guidelines of Indications for the Application of Therapeutic Modalities

Modality	Acute Edema	Chronic Edema	Muscle Spasm	Acute Pain	Chronic Pain	Soft Tissue Tightness
Cold immersion	✓	✓		✓		
Ice pack	✓	✓	✓	✓		
Ice massage	✓		✓	✓	✓	
Hot packs			✓		✓	✓
Whirlpool			✓		✓	✓
Shortwave diathermy		✓	✓		✓	✓
Ultrasound		✓	✓			✓
Electrical muscle stimulation	✓	✓	✓			
TENS				✓	✓	
Interferential stimulation	✓	✓		✓	✓	

TENS = transcutaneous electrical nerve stimulation.

the treatment of foot and ankle problems, ice massage is indicated for cooling of a localized area or when ice is indicated but the athlete cannot tolerate immersion of the entire foot. For acute injury, treatment frequency of 1 to 3 times a day for the first 3 days after injury has been recommended.[20,43,45]

Cold may be applied in combination with mild compression by using the Cryo/Cuff (Fig. 13-9). The Cryo/Cuff is inflated with cold water after being applied to the injured or postoperative foot and ankle. The pressure exerted by the inflated cuff is proportional to the elevation of the reservoir of water. A pressure of 20 mmHg is exerted by elevating the reservoir 10 inches above the Cryo/Cuff.

Contrast treatments of heat alternating with cold have been promoted to decrease swelling in the subacute and chronic stage of injury. Theoretically, the mechanism responsible for decreasing swelling is the pumping action that results from alternating vasodilatation and vasoconstriction due to alternating heat and cold.[19] The effectiveness of contrast bath treatments has not been well documented scientifically. Cote et al[20] compared the effects of cold, heat, and contrast bath treatments in the postacute phase of rehabilitation of ankle sprains. They found that heat and contrast treatments produced an increase in swelling and recommended cold as the most appropriate modality for the treatment of edema during the subacute postinjury period.

Complications of ice application include frostbite and nerve palsy. Nerve palsy is rare and can be prevented by limiting the duration of treatment to less than 20 to 30 minutes and protecting superficial nerves from pressure or compression during the application of ice.[7,29]

Contraindications to cryotherapy include Raynaud's phenomenon, cold urticaria, cold agglutinin disease, and paroxysmal cold hemoglobinuria.[11] Relative contraindications include patient intolerance of the discomfort associated with the burning or aching sensation during the application of cold, and certain rheumatic diseases in which cold causes increased joint stiffness.[43]

Rehabilitation of the Athlete's Foot and Ankle

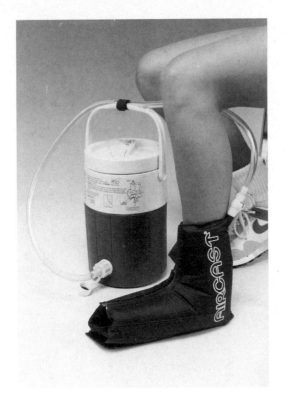

Fig. 13-9 The Cryo/Cuff apparatus (Aircast, Inc., PO Box 709, Summit, NJ 07902-0709).

Therapeutic Heat

Therapeutic heat is indicated in the treatment of injuries after the acute period is over and when residual joint stiffness and chronic pain are present. The heating modalities decrease muscle spasm and pain, warm the soft tissues prior to stretching and ROM exercises, and increase circulation to a specific area. The physiological effects of heat include vasodilation, clearance of inflammatory infiltrates, and increased metabolic rate of the warmed tissues.[54] A major benefit of heat may be simply that it feels good.[69]

Heat is commonly used for pain relief. The mechanism by which a therapeutic analgesic effect is achieved is unknown, but it has been documented that heat increases the pain threshold.[52] Heat may act as a counterirritant in the gate theory of pain,[64] in which pain impulses are inhibited by counterirritant impulses.

Clinicians observe that therapeutic heat decreases muscle spasms. Although the exact mechanisms are unknown, the muscle spindle is probably involved in decreasing muscle spasms.[54] Direct heating of the muscle spindle and its secondary nerve endings causes decreased activity, which may decrease muscle tone. When heated, the Golgi tendon organ increases its inhibitory activity and may also enhance muscle relaxation. Additionally, heating the skin directly affects the gamma fibers of the muscle spindles, causing a decrease in spindle excitability and sensitivity to stretch.[54]

Contraindications to heat therapy include insensate skin or underlying tissues, an obtunded patient, or heat-induced urticaria. Whirlpool therapy should not be used while a surgical wound is still healing. Generally, if acute edema is present, heat modalities should not be used. Heating increases blood flow and capillary permeability, potentially increasing edema.

Superficial Heat

Superficial heat penetrates only the skin and subcutaneous fat. At tissue depths below 2 cm, temperature drop-off is rapid because subcutaneous fat is an excellent insulator; therefore, the underlying muscle is not heated effectively.[54] In the hand and foot, the temperature of the ligaments and capsules of the small joints increases with the application of superficial heating modalities because of the proximity of these structures to the skin and because of the relatively thin layer of subcutaneous fat. Superficial heating modalities commonly used in sports rehabilitation are hydrocollator packs and hydrotherapy (whirlpool).

Hot Packs

Hydrocollator packs or hot packs consist of silicate gel in cotton canvas bags (Fig. 13-10). The packs are kept in a tank of water with the temperature set at 71° to 80°C. The silicate gel in the pack absorbs a large amount of water, which has a high heat-carrying capacity. For application, the hot packs are wrapped in several dry cotton terry cloth towels and applied for 20 to 30 minutes. Maximum skin temperature is

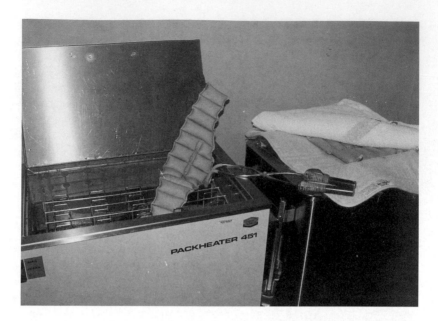

Fig. 13-10 Hydrocollator packs used for applying moist heat, a form of superficial heat (Chattanooga Corp., 101 Memorial Drive, PO Box 4287, Chattanooga, TN 37405).

reached at approximately 8 minutes after application.[54]

Whirlpool

Whirlpools make use of agitated water to achieve heating. Tanks of various sizes are available. For therapy of the foot, ankle, and lower leg, an extremity tank is used, which allows immersion of the lower extremity to above the knee. To prevent overheating or burns, the water temperature should not exceed 46°C for extremity immersion. Treatment for 20 to 30 minutes is suggested.

Indications for whirlpool therapy include joint stiffness and muscle soreness. Whirlpool may be used to facilitate callus removal by softening the skin. Whirlpool should not be used in the presence of acute swelling.

Deep Heat

Examples of commonly used deep heating modalities include shortwave diathermy and ultrasound. Deep heating modalities cause a rise in temperature of fat, muscle, and connective tissue well below the skin. With deep heating mo-

dalities, temperature rise in the deep tissues results from the conversion of energy into heat by the resistance of the tissues to the passage of the energy delivered by the modality. Tissue temperature of 40° to 45°C is aimed for to achieve therapeutic effects.[54]

Shortwave Diathermy

Shortwave diathermy uses high-frequency electromagnetic fields to produce heat at a depth of as much as 3 to 5 cm (Fig. 13-11). Energy transfer to the patient is either by the electrostatic (condenser) field method or the electromagnetic (induction) field method. In the electrostatic field method, the patient is placed between two electrodes and becomes part of the electrical circuit. The tissues that are most resistant to the current flow (skin and fat) tend to be heated preferentially by the electrostatic field method. Since skin is heated, the patient has a sensation of warmth during the treatment. Appropriate placement of the pad or air space plate electrodes is important to prevent overheating and avoid skin burns. In the electromagnetic field method, the patient is placed in a magnetic

Rehabilitation of the Athlete's Foot and Ankle

sweat, which concentrates heat, or too long a treatment time.

In addition to contraindications for heat in general, shortwave diathermy is contraindicated in the presence of metal implants that are within the range of the energy created by the electromagnetic or electrostatic fields. Metal concentrates the energy from the diathermy unit and causes rapid overheating and possible tissue necrosis. Metal should not contact the skin in or near the treatment area. Shortwave diathermy should not be used over an open growth plate in children, because heating the physis may cause the growth rate to increase or decrease. Electronic devices such as hearing aides, any transistorized units such as radios or stereos, TENS units, and electronic watches should be removed from the treatment area.

Ultrasound

Ultrasound makes use of acoustical vibrations to cause heating of deep tissues. Ultrasound units used for therapeutic heating of musculoskeletal tissues generate sound waves at a frequency of approximately 1,000,000 Hz (1.0 mHz), which achieves tissue warming up to 5 cm deep.[54,86] Homogeneous tissues, such as fat, are not heated; rather, they conduct ultrasound directly to the underlying tissues, which are heated.

Ultrasound has both thermal and nonthermal effects. Most research suggests that the clinically useful effects of ultrasound are due to the tissue temperature rise caused by the absorption and conversion of ultrasonic energy to heat[16] rather than the nonthermal effects. The thermal effects produced by ultrasound are similar to those produced by other heating modalities except that tissues at greater depths can be selectively heated. Exposure to ultrasound increases tendon extensibility. Lehmann et al[55] showed that if a constant load was applied to a tendon that had been heated to 45°C, the tension in the tendon would rapidly decrease. They also noted that the greater the load applied, the greater the residual elongation. However, if the same loads were applied to tissues at normal temperatures, no residual elongation occurred. The therapeutic implication is that tissues should be stretched during or immediately after heating to achieve greater

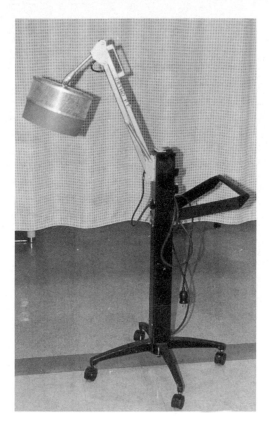

Fig. 13-11 Shortwave diathermy machine (Mettler Electronics Corp., 1333 South Claudina Street, Anaheim, CA 92805).

field and is not a part of the circuit. The magnetic field is created by induction coils (cable or drum electrodes). Tissues with high electrolyte content (blood and muscle) are heated preferentially by the induction method through vibration and distortion of the molecules. It is important to remember that because the skin is not heated, the patient will not have as much of a sensation of warmth with the electromagnetic field method of applying heat. The specifics of how to apply each type of shortwave diathermy are beyond the scope of this chapter. A duration of 20 to 30 minutes is recommended.

Complications of shortwave diathermy include burns of the skin and subcutaneous fat necrosis from overheating. Overheating occurs as a result of improper electrode or coil placement, patient movement, collection of moisture or elongation of the tissues and to maintain the effects of stretching.

Nonthermal effects of ultrasound in therapeutic dosages are mechanical and have been termed the *micromassage effect*.[28] The acoustic vibrations cause streaming of fluids in the ultrasonic field, which increases the gradient of concentration of ions and other materials across cell walls. Thus the rate of diffusion is accelerated. The streaming phenomenon and resultant increase in diffusion rate are the basis for phonophoresis, which is discussed in the next section. Streaming may also be one of the mechanisms by which ultrasound enhances tissue regeneration.[31,32]

The indications for ultrasound are similar to those for other heat modalities. Ultrasound is specifically indicated when heating of deep tissues is necessary. In the treatment of foot and ankle problems, ultrasound may be useful for plantar fasciitis, tendinitis, and joint capsule tightness because myofascial interfaces, tendon sheaths, ligaments, and joints can be selectively heated.[54] Ultrasound aids in the treatment of adhesions that cause limited ROM[8,72] and has also been advocated in the treatment of stump neuromas[72] and reflex sympathetic dystrophy.[68] Ul-

trasound has been used for the treatment of plantar warts; the results have been reported as beneficial by some[15,46,88] and of no benefit by others.[10]

For the application of ultrasound, a liquid or semiliquid coupler must be used between the transducer and patient because ultrasonic energy is almost entirely absorbed by gases in the atmosphere (Fig. 13-12). When applying ultrasound to a flat surface such as the lateral compartment of the lower leg, an aqueous gel or lotion is used as a coupling agent. When applying ultrasound to uneven surfaces of the foot, the transducer and foot are immersed in water, which is the coupling agent. The amount of ultrasound delivered to the patient is referred to as the *intensity* of ultrasound and is measured in watts per square centimeter (W/cm^2). Greater intensities result in greater penetrance and heating of the tissues. When treating superficial tissues of the foot, intensities of 0.1 to 1.0 W/cm^2 are adequate. The intensity of the treatment is adjusted by monitoring the patient's sensation. A sensation of mild warmth is aimed for if mild heating is the goal. Overheating of the periosteum causes a deep aching or piercing sensation and should be

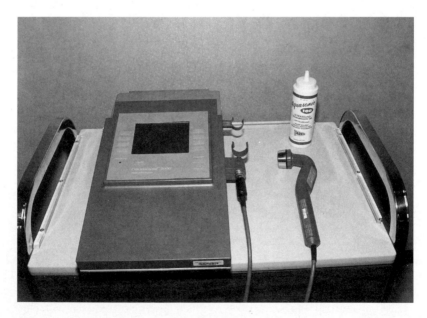

Fig. 13-12 Omnisound 3000 portable ultrasound unit (Physio Technology, Inc., 1505 SW 42nd Street, Topeka KS 66609).

Rehabilitation of the Athlete's Foot and Ankle

avoided. Treatment duration of 5 to 10 minutes, depending on the size of the area being treated, is suggested.

Contraindications for ultrasound are the same as those for heat in general. Metal implants are not a contraindication to ultrasound[56]; however, implants containing plastics contraindicate the use of ultrasound because the plastic may be selectively heated to the point of damage. Ultrasound should not be applied to areas of fluid collection or open growth plates.[89]

Phonophoresis

Phonophoresis is the use of ultrasound to deliver antiinflammatory and/or local anesthetic directly into tissues below the skin without the discomfort of an injection. The nonthermal effects of ultrasound, including streaming of extracellular fluids, increased diffusion rates, and increased permeability of membranes to ions, are responsible for the movement of large molecules through the tissues. The following medications have been used in phonophoresis[49,75]: 1% to 10% hydrocortisone cream, dexamethasone and 2% lidocaine gel, 10% salicylate. Medication driven into the tissues by ultrasound can be recovered from as deep as 10 cm below the skin.[39] There is a small risk of causing discomfort due to periosteal overheating during phonophoresis, but there is no risk of burning the skin.

Electrotherapy

Electrotherapy involves the use of electricity to achieve therapeutic goals. In rehabilitation, electrotherapy includes TENS for pain reduction, high-voltage stimulation or interferential current for edema reduction and muscle retraining, and low-voltage direct current for delivering medication with iontophoresis (described below). Other uses of electricity in medicine are promotion of bone and soft tissue healing.

Contraindications to the use of electricity include pacemakers and cardiac arrhythmias.[38] Electrodes should not be placed on abnormal skin, because the skin impedance to the electrical current may be increased (psoriasis with plaques) or decreased (second-degree burn), which changes the necessary current intensity and predisposes the skin to being burned, espe-cially when direct current is being used. Deep venous thrombosis contraindicates the use of electrical stimulation of sufficient amplitude to cause muscle contraction, because of the risk of causing a thrombus to embolize.

Electrical Muscle Stimulation

Clinical uses for electrical muscle stimulation include disuse atrophy, reflex inhibition of muscles, muscle spasm, strength deficits, and pain. Disuse atrophy occurs with immobilization or decreased activity. Both physical and physiological changes occur in atrophied muscles. Muscles that are not used lose bulk, which is evidenced by their decrease in cross-sectional area.[33,74] Additionally, there is a selective atrophy of Type I muscle fibers and a decrease in the amount of oxidative enzymes.[40] Electrical muscle stimulation limits the loss of muscle mass[4,34,83,95] and minimizes the physiological changes.[34,83]

Electrical muscle stimulation for muscle reeducation interrupts the central reflex inhibition of a muscle that occurs after an injury or surgery. Most of the research on muscle reeducation with electrical stimulation has focused on the quadriceps[4,21,34] in which reflex inhibition is a well-recognized problem. Areas of potential application in foot and ankle rehabilitation include reeducation of the peroneal muscles after ankle ligament injury or reconstruction and the gastrocsoleus after hindfoot injury or surgery. Muscular contractions produced by electrical muscle stimulation reduce edema by the pumping action of the muscle increasing flow through venous and lymphatic channels.

Many electrical stimulation machines have been developed; however, none has been proven superior to the others.[28] Machines that produce high-voltage current are popular because of their versatility[2] (Fig. 13-13). High-voltage stimulators use alternating or pulsed direct current to deliver up to 500 V in short-pulse durations of less than 100 msec. These devices achieve a strong, comfortable muscle contraction because the short pulse duration minimizes stimulation of nerve fibers that transmit pain. Specific recommendations for type of current, intensity, and waveform characteristics to achieve maximal

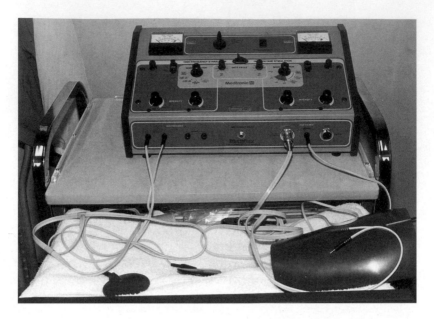

Fig. 13-13 Electrical stimulation machine (Medtronic, Inc., PO Box 1250, Minneapolis, MN 55440).

benefit of electrical muscle stimulation when used for each indication have been published elsewhere.[2,69] Generally, electrical muscle stimulation treatment times are 15 to 30 minutes, and treatment may be repeated 2 to 5 times daily depending on the goals of treatment.

Transcutaneous Electrical Nerve Stimulation

The use of electrotherapy for pain relief flourished following the publication of Melzak and Wall's[64] gait control theory of pain. The sensation of pain is carried from the periphery to the spinal cord by slow, unmyelinated nerve fibers. From the spinal cord, long tracts such as the spinothalamic tract transmit the pain stimulus to the brain. Light touch and proprioception are carried to the central nervous system by fast, myelinated nerve fibers. The gait control theory proposes that stimulating the fast, myelinated cutaneous nerve fibers blocks the transmission of pain from the spinal cord to the brain by segmental inhibition in the substantia gelatinosa at the spinal gate. Thus, the conscious perception of pain is diminished.

A second mechanism of pain modulation is based on the endogenous opiates called endorphins and enkephalins.[80,81] Endorphins are long-chain peptides with a 2- to 3-hour half-life that are secreted by the pituitary gland. Enkephalins are 5-amino acid chains produced in the spinal cord that have a very short half-life. Electricity can be used to achieve pain relief by the gait theory using high-frequency TENS or by stimulating the secretion of endorphins using low-frequency TENS (Table 13-2).

Clinical studies have shown that TENS used for postoperative pain relief decreases the amount of narcotic analgesia required and decreases the hospital stay.[5,77] TENS also successfully controls chronic pain such as that associated with the lower back,[35,57,63] osteoarthritis,[76] and rheumatoid arthritis.[58]

TENS units are small battery-powered units that have adjustable current intensity, pulse frequency, and pulse duration for different modes of application (Fig. 13-14). To date, no specific waveform of the electrical current has proved to be superior in terms of achieving analgesia. Most machines produce a balanced biphasic waveform to avoid skin irritation.

High-frequency TENS achieves pain relief by stimulating the large myelinated nerve fibers that close the spinal gait to the transmission of noxious stimuli to the brain. The analgesic effects of

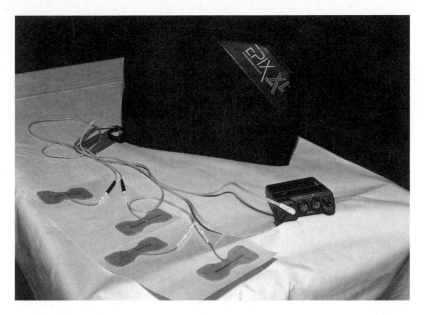

Fig. 13-14 Transcutaneous electrical nerve stimulation (TENS) unit used for the management of acute and chronic pain (Empi, Inc., 1275 Grey Fox Road, St. Paul, MN 55112).

Table 13-2	Characteristics of Low-Frequency vs. High-Frequency TENS	
	High-Frequency TENS	Low-Frequency TENS
Mechanism of action	Spinal gait	Endorphins, enkephlins
Pulse frequency	50-100 Hz	1-4 Hz
Pulse duration	20-60 ms	20-30 ms
Amplitude	Pins and needles paresthesia	Muscle contraction
Treatment duration	30 min to 24 hr/day	30-45 min
Duration of analgesia	During treatment only	3 hr to 3 days

TENS = transcutaneous electrical nerve stimulation.

high-frequency TENS are not inhibited by naloxone, an opiate antagonist, so the endogenous opiate mechanism of pain relief is unlikely. Suggested settings for the TENS unit are a pulse frequency of 50 to 100 Hz, pulse duration of 20 to 60 ms, and pulse amplitude sufficient to provide a comfortable "pins and needles" paresthesia without muscle contraction. Accommodation to the stimulus commonly occurs during a treatment session, necessitating frequent alteration of the pulse duration and pulse amplitude to provide continued analgesic benefits. The electrodes may be placed adjacent to the site of pain or in the same segmental dermatome or myotome as the painful stimulus. Treatment duration may be 30 minutes to 24 hours/day. With high-frequency TENS, a rapid onset of pain relief occurs, but analgesia is not maintained beyond the treatment session; therefore, many patients use the modality 24 hours/day.

Low-frequency TENS achieves prolonged pain relief by indirectly stimulating the release of endorphins from the pituitary gland. The analgesic effect of TENS applied in this mode is inhibited by naloxone.[61] Suggested settings for the TENS unit are a pulse rate of 1 to 4 Hz, pulse duration of 20 to 30 ms, and pulse amplitude high enough to create a visible but comfortable muscle contraction. Electrodes should be placed in a segmentally related myotome of the painful stimulus, over a motor nerve or motor point, or over acupuncture points. The suggested treatment regimin is 30 to 45 minutes daily. With low-frequency TENS, the analgesic effect is delayed 30 to 45 minutes, but the duration of pain relief may be several hours to several days.[58]

Interferential Current Therapy

Interferential current therapy is used to promote analgesia, stimulate muscle contraction, and reduce edema. Two biphasic pulsed currents of 3500 to 5000 Hz are delivered to the tissues via two sets of electrodes. The currents are superimposed in the tissues, resulting in a third current, the interference current. The amplitude and frequency of the interference current is dependent on the characteristics of two initial currents. When the two currents are completely in phase, the amplitude of the interference current is the amplitude of the two primary currents added together. The frequency of the interference current, known as the *beat,* is the frequency at which the two primary currents become completely in phase and ranges from 0.5 to 200 beats per second depending on the difference in frequency of the initial currents. The medium frequency of the primary currents delivered has the advantage of causing less skin nociceptor stimulation so that higher voltage may be used. The greater the voltage delivered, the greater the penetrance of the current.

Interferential therapy may be used similarly to TENS to modulate pain by exploiting the gait theory of pain or by stimulating the release of endogenous opiates. A frequency of 100 Hz stimulates the large-diameter myelinated fibers to close the gait, whereas a frequency of 15 Hz stimulates the release of endogenous opiates.[23] Electrode placement is adjusted to concentrate the perceived interference current in the area of the painful stimulus.

Muscle stimulation by interferential current, unlike other forms of electrical muscle stimulation, causes an asynchronous muscle contraction similar to that of a voluntary muscle contraction. The advantage of an asynchronous contraction is that the muscle does not fatigue as rapidly as it does with a synchronous contraction. Interferential current frequency of 40 to 80 Hz is used to stimulate skeletal muscle contractions.[24]

Interferential current therapy achieves reduction of chronic edema by first stimulating with a current frequency of 10 Hz to promote vasodilitation, then stimulating with a frequency of 100 Hz to achieve muscle contraction to pump the fluid away. There may also be a direct effect on the cell membrane that reduces the escape of extracellular fluid. Acute edema is treated by only stimulating to achieve a muscle contraction; vasodilatation is omitted. Most reports of edema reduction by interferential therapy are anecdotal[17]; however, edema has been cited in textbooks as an indication for the use of interferential therapy.[22,92]

Iontophoresis

An iontophoresis unit uses low-voltage direct current to drive medication into the tissues (Fig. 13-15). Iontophoresis is advocated for calcific tendinitis[70] and other inflammatory conditions.[42] Salicylates, lidocaine, and steroids are the medications most commonly used. When administering salicylates by iontophoresis, the negative electrode is used as the active electrode and is placed on the area being treated. Hydrocortisone, which is an alkaline molecule (positively charged), requires the positive electrode to be used as the active electrode. Chemical effects of the electrical current occur under the electrodes. The alkaline reaction under the negative electrode is more irritating than the acidic reaction under the positive electrode and can be minimized by using a larger negative electrode. Placement of both positive and negative electrode should be changed every 5 minutes during the treatment.[75] Iontophoresis treatment

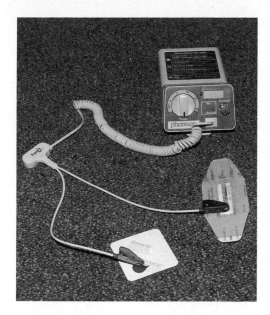

Fig. 13-15 Portable electrical stimulator used for iontophoresis (Iomed, Inc., 1290 West 2320 South, Salt Lake City, UT 84119).

times of 10 to 20 minutes are necessary, and treatment may be repeated daily. Medication is delivered directly to the involved tissues, eliminating the discomfort of an injection. However, the depth of penetration of the medication is at best 1 cm,[66] and the risk of skin irritation or burns is significant. Generally, phonophoresis is safer, more commonly used, and achieves greater penetrance of medications.

Writing the Physical Therapy Prescription

Traditionally the prescription for physical therapy includes suggestions and guidelines for a treatment plan. Every prescription should include the patient's diagnosis, precautions, and usually treatment frequency and duration. When the skill and competence of the therapist are known, an "evaluate and treat" order gives the therapist the freedom to apply his or her best skills. After evaluating the patient and initiating the treatment requested, a report of the assessment, goals, and treatment plan is submitted by the therapist for physician input and approval.

Bibliography

1. Ahstrom JP: Spontaneous rupture of the plantar fascia, *Am J Sports Med* 16:306, 1988.
2. Alon G: High voltage stimulation, a monograph, Chattanooga, Tenn, Chattanooga Corp.
3. Anderson MA: Postinjury rehabilitation in the runner, *Techniques Orthop* 5:64, 1990.
4. Ardvisson I: Prevention of quadriceps wasting after immobilization: an evaluation of the effect of electrical stimulation, *Orthopedics* 9:1519, 1986.
5. Arvidsson I, Eriksson E: Postoperative TENS pain relief after knee surgery: objective evaluation, *Orthopedics* 9:1346, 1986.
6. Asmussen E, Bonde-Peterson F: Storage of elastic energy in skeletal muscles in man, *Acta Physiol Scand* 9:385, 1974.
7. Basset FH et al: Cryotherapy-induced nerve injury, *Am J Sports Med* 20:516, 1992.
8. Bierman W: Ultrasound in the treatment of scars, *Arch Phys Med* 34:209, 1954.
9. Bosco C, Komi PV: Potentiation of the mechanical behavior of the human skeletal muscle through prestretching, *Acta Physiol Scand* 106:467, 1979.
10. Braatz JH, McAlister BR, Broaddus MD: Ultrasound and plantar warts: a double blind study, *Mil Med* 139:199, 1974.
11. Braunwald E et al, editors: *Harrison's principles of internal medicine,* ed 11, New York, 1987, McGraw-Hill.
12. Cahill BR: Chronic orthopedic problems in the young athlete, *J Sports Med* 3:36, 1973.
13. Campbell JW, Inman VT: Treatment of plantar fasciitis and calcaneal spurs with the UC-BL shoe insert, *Clin Orthop* 103:57, 1974.
14. Cavagna G, Saibene F, Margaria R: Effect of negative work on the amount of positive work performed by an isolated muscle, *J Appl Physiol* 20:157, 1965.
15. Cherup N, Urban J, Bender LF: Treatment of plantar warts with ultrasound, *Arch Phys Med Rehabil* 44:602, 1963.
16. Coakley WT: Biophysical effects of ultrasound at therapeutic intensities, *Physiotherapy* 64:166, 1978.
17. Coats GC: Interferential current therapy, *Br J Sports Med* 24:87, 1990.
18. *Comprehensive review of the foot and ankle,* course syllabus, Dallas, 1990, University of Texas Southwestern Medical School.
19. Cooper DL, Fair J: Contrast baths and pressure treatment for ankle sprains, *Physician Sports Med* 7:143, 1979.
20. Cote DJ et al: Comparison of three treatment procedures for minimizing ankle sprain swelling, *Phys Ther* 68:1072, 1988.
21. Currier DP, Lehman J, Lightfoot P: Electrical stimulation in exercise of the quadriceps femoris muscle, *Phys Ther* 59:158, 1979.

22. De Domineco G: *New dimensions in interferential therapy: a theoretical and clinical guide,* Lindfield, Australia, 1987, Reid Medical Books.

23. De Domineco G: Pain relief with interferential therapy, *Aust J Physiother* 28:14, 1982.

24. De Domineco G, Strauss GR: Motor stimulation with interferential currents, *Aust J Physiother* 31:225, 1985.

25. DeLorme TL: Restoration of muscle power with heavy resistance exercise, *J Bone Joint Surg* 27:645, 1945.

26. DeLorme TL, Watkins AL: Technics of progressive resistance exercise, *J Bone Joint Surg* 29:263, 1948.

27. Donatelli R, Wolf SL: *The biomechanics of the foot and ankle,* Philadelphia, 1990, FA Davis.

28. Drez D, editor: *Therapeutic modalities for sports injuries,* Chicago, 1989, Yearbook Medical Publishers.

29. Drez D, Faust DC, Evans JP: Cryotherapy and nerve palsy, *Am J Sports Med* 9:256, 1981.

30. Drez D et al: Nonoperative treatment of double lateral ligament tears of the ankle, *Am J Sports Med* 10:197, 1982.

31. Dyson M, Pond JB: The effect of pulsed ultrasound on tissue regeneration, *Physiotherapy* 56:136, 1970.

32. Dyson M et al: The stimulation of tissue regeneration by means of ultrasound, *Clin Sci* 35:273, 1968.

33. Edstrom L: Selective atrophy of red muscle fibers in the quadriceps in long-standing knee-joint dysfunction, *J Neurol Sci* 11:551, 1970.

34. Eriksson E et al: Effects of electrical stimulation on human skeletal muscle, *Int J Sports Med* 2:18, 1981.

35. Fried T, Johnson R, McCracken W: Transcutaneous electrical nerve stimulation: its role in the control of chronic pain, *Arch Phys Med Rehabil* 65:228, 1984.

36. Glick JM, Gordon RB, Nishimoto D: The prevention and treatment of ankle injuries, *Am J Sports Med* 4:136, 1976.

37. Gould N et al: Transcutaneous muscle stimulation as a method to retard disuse atrophy, *Clin Orthop* 164:215, 1982.

38. Griffin JE, Karselis TC: Nerve and muscle stimulating currents. In *Physical agents for physical therapists,* ed 3, Springfield, Ill, 1988, Charles C Thomas.

39. Griffin JE, Karselis TC: Ultrasonic energy. In *Physical agents for physical therapists,* ed 3, Springfield, Ill, 1988, Charles C Thomas.

40. Haggmark T et al: Fiber type area and metabolic potential of the thigh muscle in man after knee surgery and immobilization, *Int J Sports Med* 2:12, 1981.

41. Hamilton WG: Stenosing tenosynovitis of the flexor hallucis longus tendon and posterior impingement upon the os trigonum in ballet dancers, *Foot Ankle* 3:74, 1983.

42. Harris PR: Iontophoresis: clinical research in musculoskeletal inflammatory conditions, *J Orthop Sports Phys Ther* 4:109, 1982.

43. Hocutt JE et al: Cryotherapy in ankle sprains, *Am J Sports Med* 10:316, 1982.

44. Hoke BR, Lefever-Button S: When the feet hit the ground, take the next step, course notes, Toledo, 1990, American Physical Therapy Rehabilitation Network.

45. Jackson DW, Ashley RL, Powell JW: Ankle sprains in young athletes: relation of severity and disability, *Clin Orthop* 101:201, 1974.

46. Kent H: Plantar wart treatment with ultrasound, *Arch Phys Med Rehabil* 40:15, 1959.

47. Kibler WB, Chandler TJ, Pace BK: Principles in rehabilitation after chronic tendon injuries, *Clin Sports Med* 11:661, 1992.

48. Kibler WB, Goldberg C, Chandler TJ: Functional biomechanical deficits in running athletes with plantar fasciitis, *Am J Sports Med* 19:66, 1991.

49. Kleinkort JA, Wood F: Phonophoresis with one percent versus 10 percent hydrocortisone, *Phys Ther* 55:1320, 1975.

50. Leach R, Jones R, Silva T: Rupture of the plantar fascia in athletes, *J Bone Joint Surg* 60-A:537, 1978.

51. Leach RE, Seavey MS, Salter DK: Results of surgery in athletes with plantar fasciitis, *Foot Ankle* 7:156, 1986.

52. Lehmann JF, Brunner GD, Stow RW: Pain threshold measurements after therapeutic application of ultrasound, microwaves and infrared, *Arch Phys Med Rehabil* 39:560, 1958.

53. Lehmann JF, DeLateur BJ: Cryotherapy. In Lehmann JF, editor: *Therapeutic heat and cold,* ed 4, Baltimore, 1990, Williams & Wilkins.

54. Lehmann JF, DeLateur BJ: Therapeutic heat. In Lehmann JF, editor: *Therapeutic heat and cold,* ed 4, Baltimore, 1990, Williams & Wilkins.

55. Lehmann JF et al: Effect of therapeutic temperatures on tendon extensibility, *Arch Phys Med Rehabil* 51:481, 1970.

56. Lehmann JF et al: Influence of surgical metal implants on the distribution of the intensity in the ultrasonic field, *Arch Phys Med Rehabil* 39:756, 1958.

57. Lundberg T: The pain suppressive effect of vibratory stimulation and transcutaneous electrical nerve stimulation compared to aspirin, *Brain Res* 294:210, 1984.

58. Mannheimer C, Lund S, Carlsson CA: The effect of transcutaneous electrical nerve stimulation on joint pain in patients with rheumatoid arthritis, *Scand J Rheumatol* 7:13, 1978.

59. Marotta JJ, Michelli LJ: Os trigonum impingement in dancers, *Am J Sports Med* 20:533, 1992.

60. Marshall P, Hamilton WG: Cuboid subluxation in ballet dancers, *Am J Sports Med* 20:169, 1992.

61. Mayer DJ, Price DD, Rafii A: Antagonism of acupuncture analgesia in man by the narcotic antagonic naloxone, *Brain Res* 121:368, 1977.

62. McClusky GM, Blackburn TA, Lewis T: Prevention of ankle sprains, *Am J Sports Med* 4:151, 1976.

63. Melzak R, Vetere P, Finch L: Transcutaneous electrical nerve stimulation for low back pain: a comparison of TENS and massage for pain and range of motion, *Phys Ther* 63:489, 1983.

64. Melzak R, Wall PD: Pain mechanisms: a new theory, *Science* 150:971, 1965.

65. Menell JM: *Joint pain, diagnosis and treatment using manipulative techniques,* Boston, 1964, Little, Brown.

66. Murray W et al: The iontophoresis of C_{21} esterified glucocorticoids: preliminary report, *Phys Ther* 43:579, 1963.

67. O'Sullivan MP: Indians stretch for strength, *Physician Sports Med* 7:109, 1975.

68. Portwood MM, Lieberman JS, Taylor RG: Ultrasound treatment of reflex sympathetic dystrophy, *Arch Phys Med Rehabil* 68:116, 1987.

69. Prentice WE: *Therapeutic modalities in sports medicine,* St Louis, 1986, Times Mirror/Mosby College Publishing.

70. Psaki CE et al: Acetic acid ionization: a study to determine the absorptive effects upon calcific tendonitis of the shoulder, *Phys Ther Rev* 35:84, 1955.

71. Rozier CK, Elder JD, Brown M: Prevention of atrophy by isometric exercise of a casted leg, *J Sports Med* 19:191, 1979.

72. Rubin D, Kuitert J: Use of ultrasound vibration energy in treatment of pain arising from phantom limbs, scars, and neuromas, *Arch Phys Med Rehabil* 36:445, 1955.

73. Sady SP, Wortman M, Blanke D: Flexibility training: ballistic, static or proprioceptive neuromuscular facilitation? *Arch Phys Med Rehabil* 63:261, 1982.

74. Sargeant AJ et al: Function and structural changes after disuse of human muscle, *Clin Sci Mol Med* 52:337, 1977.

75. Schroeder MA: Physical modalities for foot pain. In Hunt GC, editor: *Physical therapy of the foot and ankle,* New York, 1988, Churchill Livingstone.

76. Smith CR, Lewith GT, Machin D: Transcutaneous electrical nerve stimulation and osteoarthritic pain, *Physiotherapy* 69:266, 1983.

77. Smith MJ, Hutchins RC, Hehenberger D: Transcutaneous neural stimulation use in postoperative knee rehabilitation, *Am J Sports Med* 11:75, 1983.

78. Smith RW, Reischl SF: The influence of dorsiflexion in the treatment of severe ankle sprains: an anatomical study, *Foot Ankle* 9:28, 1988.

79. Smith RW, Reischl SF: Treatment of ankle sprains in young athletes, *Am J Sports Med* 14:465, 1986.

80. Snyder SH: Brain peptides as neurotransmitters, *Science* 209:976, 1980.

81. Snyder SH: Opiate receptors and internal opiates, *N Engl J Med* 296:266, 1977.

82. Soderberg GL et al: Electromyographic activity of selected leg musculature in subjects with normal and chronically sprained ankles performing on a BAPS® board, *Phys Ther* 71:514, 1991.

83. Stanish WD et al: The effects of immobilization and electrical stimulation of muscle glycogen and myofibrillar ATPase, *Can Appl Sport Sci* 7:267, 1892.

84. Strauber WT et al: Extracellular matrix disruption and pain after eccentric muscle action, *J Appl Physiol* 69:868, 1990.

85. Stover CN: AirStirrup management of ankle injuries in the athlete, *Am J Sports Med* 8:360, 1980.

86. Summer W, Patrick M: *Ultrasonic therapy,* New York, 1964, Elsevier.

87. Tropp H, Askling C: Effects of ankle disc training on muscular strength and postural control, *Clin Biomech* 3:88, 1988.

88. Vaughn DT: Direct method versus underwater method in treatment of plantar warts with ultrasound, *Arch Phys Med Rehabil* 44:602, 1963.

89. Vaughen JL, Bender LF: Effects of ultrasound on growing bone, *Arch Phys Med Rehabil* 46:158, 1959.

90. Voight ML, Draovitch P: Plyometrics. In Albert M, editor: *Eccentric muscle training in sports and orthopedics,* New York, 1991, Churchill Livingstone.

91. Voss DE, Ionta MK, Myers BJ: *Proprioceptive neuromuscular facilitation,* ed 3, Philadelphia, 1985, Harper & Row.

92. Wadsworth H, Chanmugam APP: *Electrophysical agents in physiotherapy,* ed 2, Marrickville, Australia, 1983, Science Press.

93. Waller JF, Maddalo A: The foot and ankle linkage system. In Nicholas JA, Hersham EB, editors: *The lower extremity and spine in sports medicine,* St Louis, 1986, CV Mosby.

94. Wapner KL, Sharkey PF: The use of night splints for treatment of recalcitrant plantar fasciitis, *Foot Ankle* 12:135, 1991.

95. Wigerstad-Lossing I et al: Effects of electrical muscle stimulation combined with voluntary contractions after knee ligament surgery, *Med Sci Sports Exerc* 20:93, 1988.

14

Athletic Shoewear: Practical and Biomechanical Considerations

Paul S. Cooper

G. James Sammarco

The past two decades have seen an accelerated interest in fitness and conditioning in this country. Running became extremely popular in the 1970s, to an estimated peak of 30 million participants, or 1 out of every 10 Americans. Tennis, previously reserved for the select few, soon followed, as did other court sports including basketball, racquetball, and squash. The country's rapidly growing interest in soccer has contributed to a worldwide estimate of over 60 million participants by the International Soccer Federation. Biomechanical research on the shoe and the shoe-surface interface has only recently grown out of its infancy, as demonstrated by the sparse literature (only five publications on sports footwear and even fewer on playing surfaces) prior to 1976.[29] Spurred by increasing consumer awareness and demand and by improved technology in materials and production, the athletic shoe market has grown to over an $11 billion dollar industry, including sport-specific and cross-training shoes and apparel. The purpose of this chapter is to discuss orthopedic and biome-chanical aspects of athletic footware in order to allow the team physician, athletic trainer, physical therapist, coach, and orthopedic surgeon to make informed decisions about how to minimize injuries while maximizing the athlete's performance using the appropriate footware.

Any discussion of athletic footwear requires an understanding of the kinetics and kinematics of a specific sport. Running has been the most well-studied event and typifies many of the considerations involved in sport shoe design.

The gait cycle has traditionally been divided into stance and swing phases. A cycle is defined as all events occurring from heel strike on one foot to the following ipsilateral heel strike. Stride length is the distance covered in a single cycle and includes two steps. The average walking cycle of 5.63 km/hr or 120 steps/min has a gait cycle time of 1 second.[25] The stance phase comprises 60% of the gait cycle and includes heel strike, foot flat (occurring at 15%), and heel rise (at 30%), terminating at toe-off. The remaining 40% of the cycle is the swing phase, partitioned into acceleration, toe clearance, and deceleration phases. The walking cycle has two double limb support events, at the initial 12% and final 15% of stance phase.

The running gait is not a replication of the walking cycle. At a 5-minute-mile pace, total cycle time diminishes to 0.6 seconds, with the stance phase decreasing to 0.2 seconds, or now 33% of the cycle.[25] An increase in the swing phase and an added float phase replace the double limb support event.

The kinetics of the lower extremity in gait are a complex sequence of events involving the hip; knee; ankle; subtalar, transverse tarsal, and metatarsophalangeal joints; and the pelvis. Beginning at heel strike, foot pronation occurs in conjunction with hip extension, knee flexion, and ankle dorsiflexion to absorb forces on the order of 2 to 3 times body weight while running.[5,6] The lower extremity rotates passively internally in conjunction with hindfoot pronation, and the transverse tarsal joint axes align to unlock the midtarsal joints to further absorb the initial shock. Maximum pronation occurs at 150 ms at a walking pace but drops to 30 ms while running, with a peak angular velocity at 15 ms, thus creating excessive loads on bone and soft tissues in the hindfoot. Runners who hyperpronate, or demonstrate excessive magnitude and duration of pronation, may create excessive repetitive overload. Later in the stance phase, when the center of gravity moves rapidly forward over the foot, external rotation of the stance limb is associated with inversion of the subtalar joint. This serves to create a stable and rigid tarsal construct in preparation for toe-off.

Ground reaction forces at heel strike while walking range from 85% to 110% of body weight. Mann estimated that a 150-pound individual absorbs 63.5 tons per foot when walking a mile. The vertical force increases to 110 tons per foot when running the same mile.[24] It is thus apparent that even minor biomechanical aberrations in the foot's ability to properly dissipate forces may create overload and result in injury. Foot shear forces are present fore and aft, as well as in the medial and lateral planes. Fore shear reaches 20% of body weight at heel strike followed by aft shear of 20% body weight at 50%

of the gait cycle. A medially directed shear is also noted at heel strike, quickly changing to a laterally directed shear force until toe-off.

Evaluation of center of pressure force patterns by Cavenaugh shows rearfoot strikers' initial contact along the lateral border of the heel with subsequent rapid migration medially and anteriorly.[5] At 50 ms into the stance phase, the center of pressure is at the midshoe level. Progression from this point to toe-off demonstrates no medial-lateral migration, with the forefoot region representing two thirds of the contact phase. Cavenaugh also notes variability in distribution of pressure patterns within the same individuals depending on speed and side tested.

Shoe Design and Construction

In order to make an informed decision about appropriate sport-specific shoewear, an understanding of the basic elements and construction techniques is essential. The structural components of the athletic shoe are broadly divided into the upper and the sole. The upper, or the part of the shoe above the insole, covers the dorsum and sides of the foot and is often constructed of up to twenty components.[22] The upper consists of a toe box, vamp, quarter, throat, tongue, and heel counter and is attached to the sole of the shoe. The toe box is the roofed area that covers the toes, and it should be at least 1½ inches deep to allow for proper toe motion.[21,26] The vamp covers the forefoot and is usually constructed of a single piece to avoid irritation from seams. The vamp is often continuous with the quarter, or posterior panel of the upper, and is frequently reinforced with leather. It is termed the *saddle* if it joins the shank of the upper for added support and stability. The counter is the posterior part of the quarter, molded to the heel, and is very important in securing and stabilizing the hindfoot. While the shape of the counter remains constant, its length can vary considerably. Many shoe manufacturers market a long medial counter that extends into the medial longitudinal arch as an antipronation feature.[22] Foxing consists of strips of material that encircle the upper and sole, adding additional medial-lateral support, and is used primarily in court shoes. Typically, the upper has been made of either leather or canvas, but synthetic materials, including nylon mesh, offer breathability with lightweight durability.

The sole of the shoe consists of three layers: the innersole or sockliner, the midsole, and the outersole. The insole provides a platform for the foot to interact with the shoe, and separates the upper from the midsole. The outersole, usually constructed of injection-molded polyurethane, polyvinyl chloride (PVC) compound, or ethylene vinyl acetate (EVA), is molded independent of the midsole and assists in shock absorption and perspiration absorption. It also contributes to stability of the foot. The insole may be removed easily to allow for the insertion of orthotics.

Perhaps no area of athletic shoe design has received as much attention as the midsole, the portion between the upper and the outer sole. Designed initially for running shoes, the midsole provides for cushioning, stability, heel elevation, rockering, and toe spring (Fig. 14-1). It was made of heavy sponge rubber until Brooks Shoes introduced EVA to their running shoes in the 1970s. EVA has the advantages of lighter weight, improved shock absorption, and stability but has

been shown to deform over time and loses up to 30% of its cushioning effect at 500 miles of wear. One technique of compression molding adds durability to EVA. Another material, polyurethane (PU), has become popular because of its enhanced durability and shock absorption. While heavier, PU has demonstrated versatility in construction of midsoles and outersoles and can be formed as a unit. Combinations of EVA and PU have been used and offer the advantages of both. Multidensity midsoles, with firmer material on the medial side, and anatomically contoured midsoles are newer attempts to use the midsole for hindfoot control, especially in the overpronater. Newer generation midsoles include the gas-filled chambered AirSole by Nike, the Asics silicone gel packet, the Brooks Hydroflow, and the KangaROOs interlocking coil fabric. Shock attenuation has been shown to be inversely related to stability; thus the continued attempts by the shoe manufacturers to find an ideal midsole material.

The outersole provides a protective layer of material between the midsole and the ground. The characteristics of the outersole material should include durability, flexibility, and traction properties. Traditional outersoles have been made of rubber and its various forms, either solid

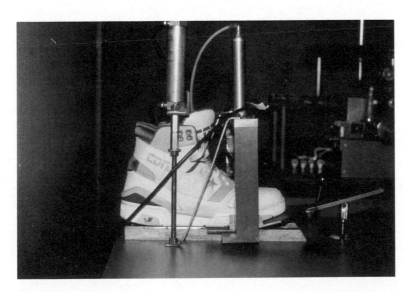

Fig. 14-1 Material impact tester used to determine the shock attenuation properties of materials and whole shoe components in the hindfoot and forefoot regions. (Courtesy Converse, Inc., North Reading, Mass.)

Athletic Shoewear: Practical and Biomechanical Considerations   Chapter 14

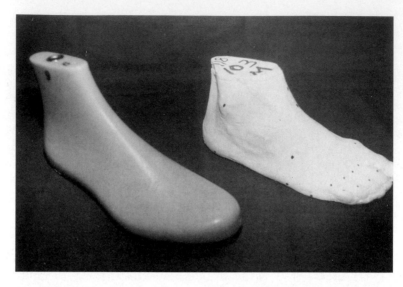

Fig. 14-2 Example of standard last *(left)* and plaster anatomical last *(right)* used to mold the shoe and determine its shape. (Courtesy Converse, Inc., North Reading, Mass.)

or blown. Carbon rubber has the advantages of extreme durability with resistance to abrasions. Styrene butadiene rubber (SBR), a synthetic rubber polymer, is often used in tennis and basketball shoes because of its superior traction properties. EVA elastimers are used in combination with other materials due to its poor abrasion properties. PU, with the ability to be formed into a one-piece-unit sole, is often used on cleated shoes.

The tread pattern on the outersoles determines the flexibility path, toe break, and pivoting points of the athletic shoe and is constantly modified by the shoe manufacturers. The waffle or nub pattern originally designed to improve traction in off-road runners was seen to contribute to shock attenuation on concrete surfaces. In addition, this pattern was shown to be not as durable as full-surface outersoles.[5] The herringbone pattern, while popular, often fills with debris during off-road running. On grass surfaces, tennis shoes with a deep herringbone or nub sole patterns offer the best traction, whereas smooth-soled shoes are used on clay surfaces.[7] Multicomposite outersoles offer added durability in heavily worn areas, including the toe drag and pivot points.

Shoe construction is based on the last, a three-dimensional form from which the shoe is shaped. The last determines the shape, size, fit, and style of the shoe[26] (Fig. 14-2). The shape of the last may be straight from heel to toe, which has been marketed by the shoe companies for athletes having pes planus or those who tend to over-pronate and require a medial-longitudinal support. The curved inward last is designed for the athlete with a cavus or metatarsus adductus foot. Recent interest in lasts for women has led to the incorporation of a narrower instep and forefoot with a thinner heel.[22]

Slip lasting construction uses a continuous wrap of the upper and is sewn closed on the underside of the last, which is "slipped" onto the midsole or outersole. This technique offers a maximum degree of flexibility while reducing the weight of the shoe. In *board lasting,* the upper is pulled over the last, which is then sewn or cemented to the innersole board. The midsole is then cemented to this inner board (Fig. 14-3). This technique is commonly utilized in athletic shoewear and offers stability and rigidity to the shoe in both torsion and flexion. Combined lasting involves the use of an inner board to the toe break level, thus providing for forefoot flexibility without loss of hindfoot stability. Other variations include transverse slits in the

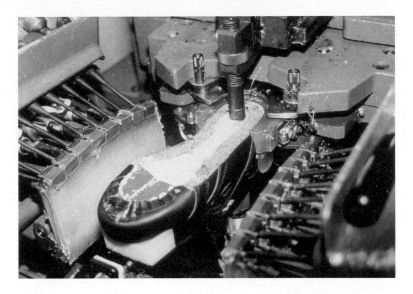

Fig. 14-3 Process of lasting where the shoe upper is attached to the insole board. (Courtesy Converse, Inc., North Reading, Mass.)

board or removal of the center of the board at the metatarsal break in order to gain forefoot flexibility.

The Running Shoe

An estimated 20 to 40 million Americans are involved in some form of running, with approximately 50% to 70% sustaining injury requiring medical treatment.[11] Common forefoot injuries include metatarsalgia, stress fractures, sesamoiditis, meuromata, and blistering. Hindfoot and lower extremity injuries may consist of plantar fasciitis, knee injuries, posterior tibial compartment syndrome, and Achilles tendinitis. Avoidance of these overload-related injuries while improving performance is the focus of design research in running shoewear, leading to the commercial availability of over 200 variations of the running shoe. More than 80% of runners are rearfoot strikers, which results in loads of 200% to 300% of body weight. Therefore, cushioning through the midsole is of paramount importance. Optimal hardness for a midsole should have such durability that the material offers similar shock

absorption before and after 1000 km of use.[15,16] Current materials in use, however, including EVA, PU, and combinations thereof, sustain losses of cushioning capacity of 20% to 30% by 800 km of use.[25] A high degree of flexibility within the forefoot of a running shoe is essential to allow a minimum of 30 degrees of metatarsal-phalangeal joint extension, thus reducing muscle fatigue (Fig. 14-4).

Both weight and hardness of the shoe sole may affect the performance of the shoe. Frederick reported that 100 g of excess weight per foot increases energy demands by 1% or adds 1 to 2 minutes in a marathon race.[14a] Stability of the hindfoot in limiting the degree of pronation at heel strike is another important consideration when designing the running shoe. Clark recommended an angle flare sole of less than 30 degrees and sole hardness of 25 to 45 shore A durometer to decrease the pronation moment.[10] Frederick noted that a significant reduction in maximum pronation occurred when a straight last, added medial support, or a wider heelbase was instituted. Jorgensen studied 11 athletes for the effect of a firm heel counter in heel strike running and noted a 2.4% decrease in V_{O_2} along with decreased activity in the triceps and quad-

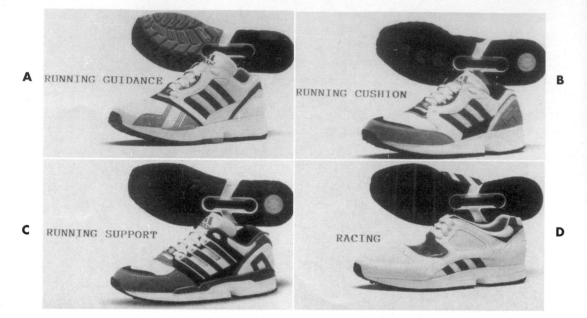

Fig. 14-4 Examples of running shoes. **A,** Note the large midsole, foxing around the toe box, and prominent heel counter. **B, C,** Antipronation control from the extended heel counter medially. **D,** Racing shoe with less midsole, grooved outersole for enhanced forefoot flexibility.

riceps.[18] Shoe designers control rearfoot motion through the use of extended or reinforced medial counters of thermoplastic material, or by using foxing or multidensity midsoles.[21] Both Bates and Stacoff et al have reported on the reduction of maximum pronation by increasing heel height, while Clarke, unable to confirm these findings, reported the reduction of maximum velocity of pronation.[1,10,39]

Many running shoe manufacturers now offer increased levels of individualization in shoewear. Adidas currently markets an Equipment Support Shoe, which is a heavy, sturdy shoe for the large runner with excessive pronation. The heel counter is extremely rigid, and the midsole consists of PU. The company also offers the Torsion Integral, which is designed for the mild overpronator and is lighter, with an EVA midsole. Care must be taken to scrutinize the design parameters of the shoe or injuries may result. Cases have been reported of torn peroneal tendons in runners who incorrectly use a shoe designed for overpronators.

The Court Shoe

Court sports, unlike running, involve noncyclical motions, including rapid lateral movements and sudden acceleration and deceleration. In addition, sports such as basketball and volleyball require rapid pivoting and jumping events. Ground reaction forces have been estimated at from 3.5 to 4.3 times body weight on forefoot landing and up to 6 times body weight in the less typical heel or footflat position, therefore necessitating additional cushioning in the heel and forefoot compared to the running shoe. Restriction of supinatory or lateral movements in the court shoe to prevent lateral ligament and tendon injuries has been the subject of recent studies. Segesser and colleagues recommend shoe construction with the lever arm shifted laterally to prevent a supinatory movement.[35,36] Firm heel counters and stiffened shafts prevent lateral movement without compromising flexion and extension in the shoe. Thick soles, while providing cushion, also extend the supinatory lever arm; therefore, a flatter shoe is recommended. Stussi evaluated three landing positions of the foot in breaking, which consists of a rapid lateral move in court sports.[41] By measuring ground forces, contact coordinates, and peroneus and soleus muscle activity, he concluded that a foot landing position on the lateral edge of the forefoot with tibial internal rotation has a high risk of injury and should be considered in designing the racquet court shoe.

Outersoles are generally flat, with contour-molded footbeds and unit shells for stability during rapid changes in direction. Foxing and extended firm heel counters offer additional stability to the ankle and hindfoot. Uppers are constructed of breathable leather and/or synthetic materials. Adequate toe boxes allow dorsiflexion of the metatarsophalangeal joints and offer additional support at the tarsometatarsal joints. Velcro straps at the midshoe or ankle serve to unify the upper into a more rigid construct.

The growth of tennis as a sport has paralleled that of running, with the shoe continuing to evolve. Unlike the running shoe, tennis shoe design must take into account landing on the ball of the foot, rather than the heel, and quick changes of the center of gravity. The various playing surfaces and their frictional properties have yielded significant differences in the frequency of injuries reported. Clay and synthetic sand have a much lower injury rate than synthetic surfaces and asphault.[30] Translational friction, as seen with sliding, supination, and lateral movements, is an important factor. Tennis shoe design should reflect the importance of supination, heel and ball cushioning, and rotational friction. Shoes are built with reinforced lateral supports in the saddle along with firm heel counters and wide toe boxes to prevent subungual hematomas. The sole is flat, with reinforcement for toe drag, and has a pivot point under the ball of the foot (Fig. 14-5). Tread patterns reflect the surface played on: the radial design is

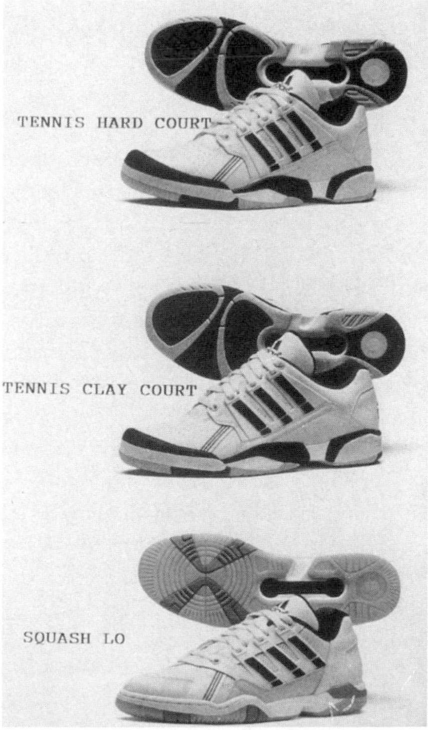

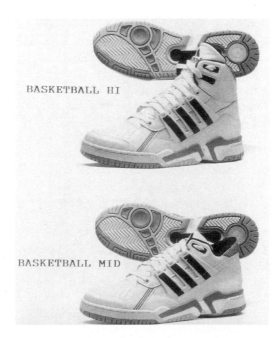

Fig. 14-5 Examples of court shoes. Note reinforced heel counter for medial-lateral stability, and pivot point in the forefoot.

Fig. 14-6 Basketball shoes. Note extensive reinforcement on the high-top shoe for additional ankle support. (Courtesy Converse, Inc.)

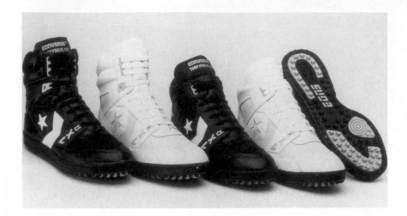

Fig. 14-7 Examples of Turf football shoes. (Courtesy Converse, Inc., North Reading, Mass.).

all purpose, the herringbone pattern is for grass or clay, and pillared soles are best for hard surfaces.[9,21] Unlike running shoes, a cushioned insole attenuates shock, lest a softer midsole decrease ankle stability. With lateral and deceleration motions, midcut level uppers give additional support.

The basketball shoe, in addition to requirements of other court shoes, incorporates a high top for lateral ankle support. Stacoff et al reported that high-top shoes significantly resisted supination motion with lateral movement, with maximum supination angles of 2 degrees occurring in the first 50 ms of contact.[39] The high top also serves to increase proprioceptive feedback for prevention of inversion injuries, by early firing of the peronei and stabilization against injury. The sprain frequency in one study was reported to drop by threefold when comparing high-top to low-cut shoes.[33] Added stability in the upper has been produced by some shoe companies through various external support straps, inner boots, and internal bladders (Fig. 14-6). The basketball outsole is constructed of unit shell soles made of rubber or multidensity materials to provide both cushion and support. While softer sole constructions have been shown to be superior on artificial floors, PU material has proven safer on hardwood, especially if the floor is dirty. The soles also have pivot points and tread patterns that allow for forefoot flexibility and propulsion. As in other types of shoewear, the midsole in basketball shoes incorporates various materials and air cells to allow for cushioning and energy return.

The Field Shoe

Field-specific sport shoes are designed for the individual sports: football, soccer, baseball, and golf. The field sport shoe requires greater durability than other athletic shoes. Uppers are constructed almost universally of leather, although plastic, nylon, or canvas are occasionally used.[42] Firm heel counters are essential and are often reinforced on the outside.[9] Soles are typically constructed of rubber, PU, PVC, or nylon and may either accommodate replaceable studs or be unit molded. Stud and cleat patterns are variable and sport-specific.

Football has been responsible for some of the highest rates of injuries, particularly in the lower extremity. This is due to the high level of contact involved and the shoe-surface interface. Shoes containing a few long cleats allow for excessive foot traction, with an increased load through the ankle and knee. Soccer-style shoes, with wider and more numerous cleats, decrease foot fixation by increasing the total cleat tip surface area by over threefold (Fig. 14-7). Recommendations based on studies of high school players have been instituted and include requirements of no less than 14 cleats, a cleat tip diameter of ½ inch, and maximum cleat length of ⅜

Rehabilitation of the Athlete's Foot and Ankle

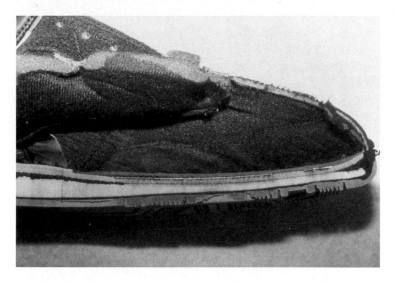

Fig. 14-8 Sagittal cut through football shoe. Note steel shank in forefoot to prevent hyperextension injuries to the hallux.

inch. Release coefficients of football shoe-surface interface have indicated that the molded sole soccer-style shoe is safe on all natural and artificial surface types but that the sole material should vary with surface type. Soft rubber soles have been shown to have an unacceptably high release coefficient on Astro-turf.[42]

Hyperextension and abduction of the first metatarsophalangeal joint, or "turf toe," is a common injury among football players, especially with the soccer-style shoe on Astro-turf.[3] The sprain of the plantar capsular ligament and the medial collateral ligament has been attributed to the high level of flexibility at the metatarsal break of the shoe. Rates of injury have decreased with the addition of a firmer sole or addition of a steel shank extending to the toes (Fig. 14-8).

Soccer involves a combination of running, kicking, and multidirectional movements and is played both outside on natural grass and indoors. The following considerations apply to choosing a soccer shoe. The upper should be lightweight and fit snugly for improved tactile input with the ball. A narrow, multistudded sole with tight last is ideal for hard ground, whereas detachable studs of varying length are recommended for softer turf or wet ground[9,35] (Fig. 14-9). Rubber studs are best for superior fixation on snow, while

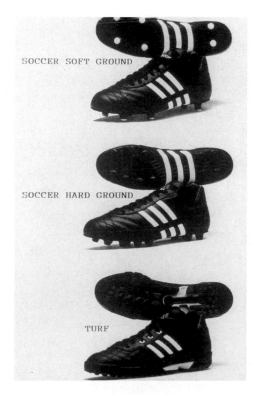

Fig. 14-9 Examples of soccer-style shoes for various surfaces. (Courtesy Converse, Inc.)

indoor soccer is played in a flat-soled shoe with a unit shell. Soccer shoe designs must address the reported accelerated degenerative osseous changes in the ankle, midfoot, and forefoot due to repetitive microtrauma and macrotrauma. The ball-shoe collision energy can range from 300 to 600 KPA if the ball is wet. Studs placed at the hallux metatarsal phalangeal joint level concentrate peak forces and may lead to avascular necrosis or stress fractures of the metatarsal. Increased flexibility in the toe box may cause excessive loading at the metatarsophalangeal joints. Indoor playing surfaces subject the foot and knee to excessive loads, predisposing joint ligaments, articular cartilage, and the Achilles tendon to injury. Two thirds of all soccer-related injuries have been related to the conflicting requirements of high translational forces (from rapid changes in motion) and low rotational characteristics of shoe-surface interaction.[14]

In addition to the movement requirements seen in other field sports, baseball involves the complex movements associated with batting and throwing, which result in weight transfer through a stable lower extremity platform.[9] Uppers have special lace modifications with a turned-over tongue, and a U-throat. Soles are made of nylon mold with standard steel cleat split formation of three in front and two in the heel. (Fig. 14-10). Astro-turf multistudded shoes are used by outfielders on synthetic surfaces.

Although golf is one of the most widespread sports in the world, with over 120 million regular players, attention to design characteristics of the golf shoe has been sparse until recently. Design must take into account two distinct functions, as both a walking shoe and a platform for the complex movements involved during drives and other strokes.[35] Primary motions during the golf swing include side to side in a frontal plane and more rotation than seen in other athletic events.[43] Kinetic events of the swing have recognized positions and patterns of shear and vertical forces, which influence stability, force production, and resistance to slippage with the swing. The alterations made with respect to golf shoe design include replacing raised heels with a continuous heel wedge, altering the cleat pattern, and a valgus heel wedge insert. An asymmetrical design is used for the right and left shoes to reflect their different functions.[35,43] Uppers are typically leather or plastic with an apron to protect the laces. Soles are often of waterproof PU, with spikes for traction on grass surfaces.

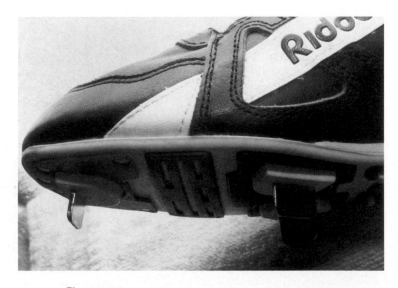

Fig. 14-10 Typical cleat pattern seen in baseball shoes.

Rehabilitation of the Athlete's Foot and Ankle

Hosiery

Little if any reference has been made to appropriate sockware for athletes. Generally, materials consist of either natural fiber (cotton) or synthetic materials (acrylic, nylon, and spandex). The acrylic fiber is superior to cotton in durability, perspiration absorption, washability, and retention of shape. Coolmax by DuPont has even greater wick capabilities than conventional acrylic fibers. Today, such companies as Thor-Lo make sport-specific hosiery, accommodating the specific requirements of walking, running, court sports, and outdoor recreational sports.

Hosiery for running is available in a low-density flat knit acrylic reinforced over the heel and toes. Aerobic socks add Spandex for extra stability and support in the arch during rapid lateral twisting movements. Socks for racquet sports feature high-density padding in the forefoot and heel to absorb foot strike, as well as to protect the toes from sudden changes in movement.

Conclusion

Athletic shoewear no longer serves only to protect the foot during sport but is now considered a highly technical piece of athletic equipment. Shoes are sport-specific, individualized to the athlete's foot morphology and demands. A knowledge of foot and ankle biomechanics, materials, and shoe design features is essential when working with athletes in order to maximize their performance.

Bibliography

1. Bates BT et al: An assessment of subject variability, subject-shoe interaction and the evaluation of running shoes using ground reaction force data, *J Biomech* 16:181, 1983.
2. Bejjani FJ: Occupational biomechanics of athletes and dancers: a comparative approach, *Clin Podiatr Med Surg* 4:671, 1987.
3. Bowers KD, Martin RB: Turf toe: a shoe-surface related football injury, *Med Sci Sports* 8:81, 1976.
4. Brodsky JW et al: Objective evaluation of insert material for diabetic and athletic footwear, *Foot Ankle* 9:111, 1988.
5. Cavanaugh PR: The shoe-ground interface in running, American Association of Orthopedic Surgeons Symposium on Foot and Leg in Running Sports, St. Loius, Mosby–Year Book 1982.
6. Cavanaugh PR: *The running book,* Mountain view, Calif, 1990, Anderson World Pub.
7. Cavanaugh PR, editor: *Biomechanics of distance running,* Champaign, Ill, 1990, Human Kinetics Publishers.
8. Chapman AE et al: Effect of floor conditions upon frictional characteristics of squash court shoes, *J Sports Sci* 9:33, 1991.
9. Cheskin MP et al: *The complete handbook of athletic footwear,* New York, 1987, Fairchild Publication.
10. Clark TE et al: The effect of varied stride rate and length upon shank deceleration during ground contact in running, *Med Sci Sports Exerc* 15:170, 1983.
11. Cook SD, Brinker MR, Poche M: Running shoes: their relationship to running injuries, *Sports Med* 10:1, 1990.
12. Cook SD et al: Biomechanics of running shoe performance, *Clin Sports Med* 4:619, 1985.
13. Dufek JS, Bates BT: Dynamic performance assessment of selected sport shoes on impact forces, *Med Sci Sports Exerc* 23:1062, 1991.
14. Ekstrand J, Nigg BM: Surface-related injuries in soccer, *Sports Med* 8:56, 1989.
14a. Frederick EC: The running shoe: Dilemmas and diemotomies in design. In Segeesser, Pforringer, editors: *The shoe in sport,* London, 1989, Mosby–Year Book (Wolfe).
15. Frederick EC: Biomechanical consequences of sport shoe design. *Exerc Sport Sci Rev* 14:375, 1986.
16. Frederick EC: Kinematically mediated effects of sport shoe design: a review, *J Sports Sci* 4:169, 1986.
17. Frederick EC, editor: *Sport shoes and playing surfaces: biomechanical properties,* Champaigne, Ill, 1984, Human Kinetics Publishers.
18. Jorgensen U: Body load in heel-strike running: the effect of a firm heel counter, *Am J Sports Med* 18:177, 1990.
19. Kalin VX et al: Possible relationships between shoe design and injuries in running, *Sportverletz Sportschaden* 2:80, 1988.
20. Kannus VPA: Evaluation of abnormal biomechanics of the foot and ankle in athletes, *Br J Sports Med* 26:83, 1992.
21. Kaye RA, Shereff MJ: Athletic footwear, modifications, and orthotic devices. In Jahss MH, editor: *Disorders of the foot and ankle,* Philadelpha 1991, WB Saunders
22. Levitz SJ et al: Current footwear technology, *Clin Podiatr Med Surg* 5:737, 1988.
23. Lillich JS, Baxter D: Common forefoot problems in runners, *Foot Ankle* 7:145, 1986.
24. Mann RA: Biomechanics of running. In Ambrosia R, Drez, editors: *Prevention and treatment of running injuries,* Thorofare, NJ, 1989, Slack.
25. McMahon JO: Proper footwear for play and fitting of

painful, deformed feet, American Association of Orthopedic Surgeons Symposium on the Foot and Ankle, St. Louis, Mosby–Year Book 1983.

26. McPoil TG: Footwear, *Phys Ther* 68:1857, 1988.

27. Miller CD et al: The ballet technique shoe: a preliminary study of eleven differently modified ballet technique shoes using force and pressure plates, *Foot Ankle* 11:97, 1990.

28. Monto RR et al: Radiographic abnormalities in the foot and ankle of elite soccer players, poster exhibit, American Academy Orthopedic Surgeons 60th meeting, San Francisco, CA Feb 1993.

29. Nigg BM, editor: Biomechanics of running shoes, Champaign, Ill, 1986, Human Kinetics.

30. Nigg BM, Segesser B: The influence of playing surfaces on the load on the locomotor system and on football and tennis injuries, *Sports Med* 5:375, 1988.

31. Nigg BM, Segesser B: Biomechanical and orthopedic concepts in sport shoe construction, *Med Sci Sports Exercise* 24:595, 1992.

32. Perry J: Gait analysis: normal and pathologic function, Thorofare, NJ, 1992, Slack.

33. Petrov O et al: Footwear and ankle stability in the basketball player, *Clin Podiatr Med Surg* 5:275, 1988.

34. Rheinstein DJ, Morehouse CA, Niebel BW: Effects of traction outsole composition and hardness of basketball shoes and the three types of playing surfaces, *Med Sci Sports Exercise* 10:282, 1979.

35. Segesser B, Pforringer W: *The shoe in sport,* Chicago, 1989, Year Book Medical Publishers.

36. Segesser B et al: Torsion, a new concept in sport shoe construction, *Sportverletz Sportschaden* 3:167, 1989.

37. Smith LS, Bunch R: Athletic footwear, *Clin Podiatr Med Surg* 3:637, 1986.

38. Spring shoe review, *Runner's World* 27:4, 1992.

39. Stacoff A, Kalin X, Stussi E: The effects of shoes on the torsion and rearfoot motion in running, *Med Sci Sports Med* 23:482, 1991.

40. Street GM: Technological advances in cross country ski equipment, *Med Sci Sports Med* 24:1048, 1992.

41. Stussi A: Rapid sideward movements in tennis. In Segesser B, Pforringer W: *The shoe in sport,* Chicago, 1989, Year Book Medical Publishers.

42. Torg JS: Athletic footwear and orthotic appliances, *Clin Sports Med* 1:157, 1982.

43. Torg JS, Quedenfeld T: Effect of shoe type and cleat length on incidence and severity of knee injuries among high school football players, *Res Q* 42:203, 1971.

44. Valiant GA, Cavanaugh PR: A study of landing from a jump: implication for the design of a basketball shoe, *Biomechanics IX,* Champaign, Ill, 1983, Human Kinetics.

45. Williams KR, Cavanagh PR: The mechanics of foot action during the golf swing and implications for shoe design, *Med Sci Sport Exerc* 15:247, 1983.

15

Running Injuries and Treatment: A Dynamic Approach

Kenneth G. Holt

Joseph Hamill

There are few athletes who have not suffered some form of chronic injury from running. Chronic injuries are commonplace and in many cases have led athletes to adopt less punishing forms of exercise. Typically, running injuries are attributed to "overuse." In our opinion the diagnosis "overuse" is inaccurate and misleading. We have all known runners who have run many marathons in a relatively injury-free state. The perennial Boston marathoner Johnny Kelly is an excellent example. On the other hand, many therapists have treated recreational runners (25 miles a week or less) who are chronically injured. If overuse was the sole cause of injury, then the athletes who ran longer distances would inevitably have a greater number of chronic injuries. There is no evidence to support this notion. In fact, there is evidence that runners with low mileage may be injured more than those with high mileage.[15] Why then are some runners more prone to injury than others?

In order to treat a chronic running injury, the therapist must first identify the cause or causes, and treat the cause(s) as well as the symptoms. In several areas of medicine, multiple contributing causes for a disease state have been discovered. Heart disease may be caused by a combination of heavy smoking, poor diet and exercise patterns, and genetic predisposition. One risk factor alone may not cause the disease, but the greater the number of risk factors, the more the person is likely to suffer from the disease. We use this concept to identify the causes of chronic running injuries. It is our opinion that runners who have run long distances for many years in a relatively injury-free state have close to perfect structural biomechanics, along with a minimal number of other risk factors.

As biomechanists and sports physical therapists, our belief and evidence support the notion that the major risk factor for chronic running injuries lies in structural abnormalities. In the following, the important differences between the concepts of *structural abnormality* and *hyperpronation* are clarified. A clear distinction is made between the evaluation and treatment that therapists using a structural abnormality model will employ vs. those using a hyperpronation model. We discuss how even minor structural abnormalities, without hyperpronation, combined with other risk factors may lead to chronic injury. Furthermore, how specific types of abnormality may lead to specific types of injury is discussed. The functional anatomical and biomechanical mechanisms of the most common running injuries are addressed.

As in the diagnosis of chronic running injuries, evaluation and treatment have often been based on the concept of overuse. The theory is, if you overuse something, then use it less, or do not use it at all. Those therapists who have treated avid athletes know that this is an unacceptable treatment for many. Furthermore, given the convenience and physiological benefits of running, and the fact that running is an essential component of many sports, it behooves us to have a more thorough understanding of running injuries so that we can offer more successful and acceptable treatments. The model of injury that we propose leads to specific forms of evaluation and treatment. In the final sections of the chapter those forms are discussed.

Structural Abnormalities vs. Hyperpronation as Cause of Injury

As an alternative to the overuse diagnosis, several therapeutic techniques are based on the hypothesis that hyperpronation results in injuries.[7,12,17] The mechanisms of the relationship between injury and hyperpronation are poorly understood. There is some evidence to support a relationship between hyperpronation and certain types of injury, such as patello-femoral pain syndrome.[18] However, clinical observation reveals a limited correlation between the amount of pronation and the severity or even the occurrence of injury. Some patients have very little hyperpronation, but their injuries respond well to orthotic use. Others have large amounts of pronation and pain that is not helped by orthotic intervention. Research has been equivocal on the benefits of orthoses in both decreasing pain and changing the amount of pronation.[2,4,11]

More recent therapies have stressed the importance of relating the foot structure to the amount of pronation.[3,5,16] From a mechanical standpoint, structural abnormalities may or may not lead to hyperpronation. They may instead, or in addition, lead to inappropriate timing relationships in the actions of joints and muscles, which in turn may lead to torsional stresses on tissues. The model we propose is based on the concept that one must identify the type of structural abnormality and identify its effect on both the amount and timing of pronation in order to understand mechanisms of injury and to successfully treat the injury:

Structural abnormality => Hyperpronation or timing problem => Injury where => indicates causality.

Hyperpronation is seen as one possible effect rather than a cause. For the therapist, the crucial difference between the hyperpronation model and the structural model is that in the latter, one treats the structure and not the hyperpronation per se. Furthermore, if hyperpronation is present, it is a progressive problem in that the occurrence and severity are dependent on the structural abnormality and a number of other factors (such as the amount of exercise) that might influence the dynamic effects on the structures.

Foot Structure Abnormalities

Many foot abnormalities have been associated with athletic injuries to the foot and lower extremity. In this section discussion centers around the structures seen most often clinically. For a more complete discussion of abnormalities, there are a number of texts available.[3,5,16] Emphasis here is placed instead on how the deformity affects the biomechanics, which in turn disrupt the normal functional relationships between joints and muscles.

Varus and *valgus* abnormalities of the foot are clinically defined by the relationships between the structures in nonweight-bearing, with the foot held by the clinician in a subtalar neutral position.[3,5] Hindfoot valgus or varus is assessed by the angle formed by a line that bisects the shank and one that bisects the calcaneus. Forefoot varus and valgus are defined by the angle formed by a line that bisects the calacaneus and one that runs from the first to the fifth metatarsal joint. In the neutral foot, no angle is formed between the hindfoot and shank, and there is a 90-degree angle between the forefoot and hindfoot (Fig. 15-1A). Various combinations of hindfoot and forefoot varus and valgus abnormalities are possible. The most common ones seen clinically are combined forefoot and hindfoot varus (Fig. 15-1B); forefoot varus (Fig. 15-1C); and hindfoot varus (Fig. 15-1D). A forefoot varus deformity that causes the subtalar joint to pronate excessively and the hindfoot to move into a valgus position during weight acceptance is known as a *compensated forefoot varus.* A forefoot varus abnormality that does not cause the foot to move into valgus is called a *noncompensated forefoot varus.* There is a spectrum of states in between these two extremes known as *partially compensated forefoot varus.* Nonweight-bearing valgus deformities are seen much less often in the clinic than varus deformities. Whether this is due to a lack of incidence or because the valgus foot leads to fewer injuries is not known.

A second abnormality often associated with injuries thought to result from poor shock absorption is the *equinus foot,* and particularly the rigid equinus foot. An equinus foot is one in which the forefoot is more distal to the body than the hindfoot when the foot is held at 90 degrees of flexion (Fig. 15-2). The forefoot is plantarflexed relative to the hindfoot.[13] A similar condition in which only the first metatarsal is plantarflexed relative to the hindfoot is the *plantarflexed first ray.* The rigid plantarflexed first ray is particularly important because of increases in the pressures on that structure during weight-bearing activities.

Normal Function of the Lower Extremity in Running

At heel strike the foot is in a slightly supinated and dorsiflexed position. Upon impact, pronation starts to occur. An important point is that the foot is not pronated but pronating. That is, the foot may still be in supination but is in the process of pronating. The necessity of this distinction will become clear when the effects of pronation and supination on the function of other lower extremity structures are discussed. Maximum pronation is reached at about 45% of the total stance time as measured by hindfoot angle (Fig. 15-3).[8] However, when wearing running shoes there is little change (approximately ± 2 degrees) in the pronation angle from about

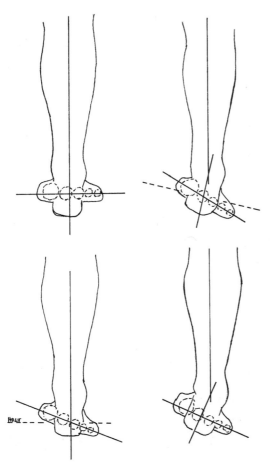

Fig. 15-1 Clinical diagnosis of foot structures in nonweight-bearing. **A,** Neutral foot. **B,** Combined forefoot-hindfoot varus. **C,** Forefoot varus. **D,** Hindfoot varus.

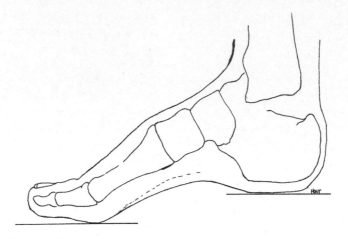

Fig. 15-2 Equinus foot.

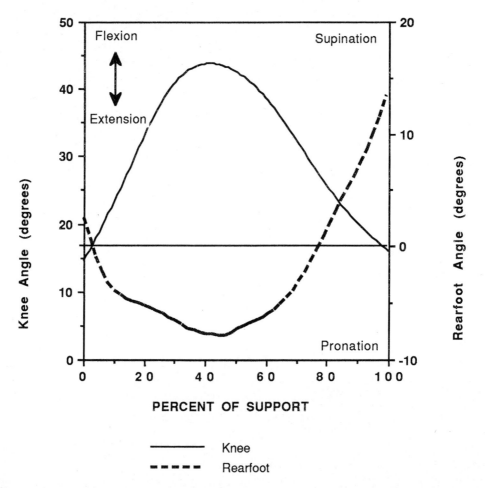

Fig. 15-3 Hindfoot angle and corresponding knee angle as a function of time during the stance phase of running gait.

Rehabilitation of the Athlete's Foot and Ankle

25% to 75% of stance. After 75% stance time there is a significant increase in the rate of resupination. Flexion of the knee joint follows a similar pattern to that of pronation-supination. Maximum knee flexion is reached at about 45% of stance, and the knee immediately begins to extend. The normal complementary relationship between knee flexion and pronating, and knee extension and supinating is crucial for the integrity of the structures that intervene. Subtalar joint pronation causes the tibia to internally rotate, while supination causes external rotation. At the knee joint, flexion allows for the tibia to internally rotate, while extension causes the tibia to externally rotate.[18] It has been hypothesized that a disruption of this normal timing relationship may result in injury.[1] If the act of pronating occurs at the same time as the act of knee extending, an inappropriate torsion around the tibia could occur, resulting in injury to structures of the knee or foot. If those structures are very stable, inappropriate actions at the tibia may even disrupt actions at the hip, pelvis, and back.

Effects on Biomechanics as a Function of Structural Abnormalities

Research on the effects of structural abnormalities on the normal kinetic actions of the foot and lower extremity is extremely limited. In this section the effects of foot structural deformities on normal forces, foot pressures, and kinematic relationships are hypothesized based on biomechanical principles.

Loading and impact of the foot making initial contact with the ground play a vital role in determining the actions of the foot in the stance phase of gait. The foot with a varus deformity of either the forefoot or hindfoot or a combination will hit the ground on its lateral border (Fig. 15-4) compared to a more neutral foot (Fig. 15-5). This means that there

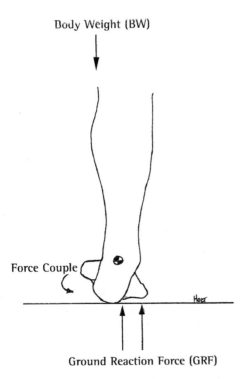

Fig. 15-4 Distribution of forces when the foot hits the ground in a supinated position.

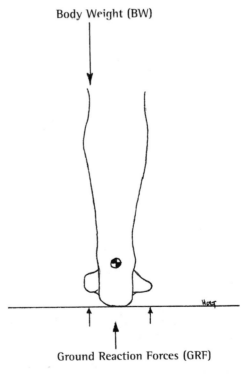

Fig. 15-5 Distribution of forces when the foot hits the ground in a neutral or close to neutral foot position.

is less surface area of contact than if the foot hits in a more neutral position. As a result the force

$$(Mass \times Acceleration)$$

per unit area, or pressure, on a supinated foot is greater. Since the ground reaction force is increased toward the lateral side, there may also be an increase in the distance from the axis of rotation at which the force acts. If the body weight acts on the medial side of the foot (Fig. 15-5), a significant *force couple* will result. Since the actions of the body weight and the ground reaction force act on opposite sides of the ankle axis of rotation, both tend to produce rotation in the same direction. As a consequence of these biomechanical considerations, the moment of the force or torque

$$(Force \times Distance\ from\ rotation\ axis)$$

on the foot is greater than if the foot hits the ground in a more neutral position (compare Figs. 15-4 and 15-5). A second consequence of a varus deformity is the distance the medial foot has to travel before making contact with the ground. In a forefoot deformity, for example, the forefoot may have to travel as much as 20 to 30 degrees before making contact with the ground, compared to 5 degrees in a normal foot.

The greater moment of the force combined with the increased distance the foot has to travel could influence the gait pattern in several ways. One possible scenario is that the varus foot will take longer to reach a fully pronated position on the ground. The act of pronating will continue later into the stance phase than normal, and pronation may continue later into the push-off phase. Thus, when the knee is beginning to extend, the foot may still be in the process of pronating. Resupination will be delayed, and as a consequence the normal timing of foot and knee actions will be disrupted. The second scenario concerns the combined influence of greater torque and increased distance the medial foot has to travel to reach the ground. These factors ensure that the foot has greater velocity and hence momentum

$$(Momentum = Mass \times Velocity)$$

on impact with the ground. One consequence is that specific structures, such as the first metatarsal head, will be subject to greater impact and possible injury. A second consequence is that the foot structures will be subject to greater deformation as the ground decelerates the foot. This may be in the form of greater pronation, greater deformation of the arches, greater deformation of the fat pads, or excessive and high-velocity stretch on muscles that pass from the leg into the foot (e.g., posterior tibialis, anterior tibialis, flexor hallucis longus). Eventually, repeated impacts may cause a breakdown in the medial tissues, perhaps resulting in hyperpronation. In any case the result will be an increase in time for restoration of those structures to their relaxed state. Again, a possible consequence is a change in the timing of foot actions relative to the other lower extremity functions.

Mechanisms of Injury

The most common injuries associated with running, in order of frequency, are knee pain, shin splints, Achilles tendinitis, plantar fasciitis, and stress fractures.[1] In this section the mechanisms of selected injuries are discussed in light of the foregoing biomechanical model and foot types. Injuries to the lower extremity can be viewed as falling into three categories: injuries to intrinsic foot structures, injuries to extrinsic foot structures (the knee, for example), and injuries to intermediate structures. In this latter category, reference is made to structures that originate in the lower leg, cross the ankle, and insert on bones of the feet (Fig. 15-6). This method of categorization is useful because different types of structural deformity tend to cause injuries to structures in one of the categories and are less likely to cause injury in others.

Intrinsic Foot Injuries

Mechanical injuries to the foot include plantar fasciitis, metatarsalgia, sesamoiditis, bunions, and stress fractures. The major structural abnor-

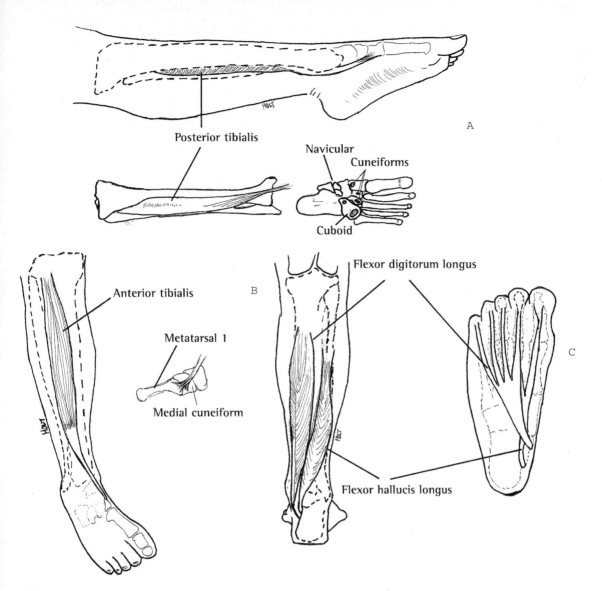

Fig. 15-6 **A,** Origin and insertions of the posterior tibialis muscle. Note the pulley action around the medial malleolus. **B,** Origin and insertion of anterior tibialis muscle. **C,** Origins and insertions of flexor hallucis longus and flexor digitorum longus. All structures are susceptible to abnormally high forces and excessive stretching in feet with varus structural abnormalities.

malities of the foot that are associated with these types of injury are *noncompensated* or *partially compensated forefoot varus deformities*. In both cases the hindfoot cannot fully compensate for the varus deformity by moving into a valgus position. However, the forefoot must necessarily make contact with the ground during the stance phase of gait. Thus, as the forefoot contacts the ground

there is a torsioning of the intrinsic foot structures. The actual mechanism of injury for the most common injury—*plantar fasciitis*—may be the result of two mechanisms during weight acceptance. The first is the increased deformation of the longitudinal arch resulting from the increased torques and momentum when a varus forefoot makes contact with the ground. The high forces generated around the medial forefoot and hindfoot cause the arch to flatten and stretch the plantar fascia more than normal. The second is the "wringing" effect when the forefoot torsions around the hindfoot. The situation is analogous to wringing out a towel. As a towel is wrung out, its length decreases. A similar situation occurs in the foot. As the forefoot approaches the ground, the torsion around the midfoot resulting from the inability of the hindfoot to compensate will effectively shorten the plantar fascia. Unfortunately, the attachments (the calcaneal tuberosity and toes) are not able to respond by coming closer together. Furthermore, the mechanism of higher impact on the medial tissues will ensure that they are inclined to move further apart than in the normal foot as the arch is flattened by the increased load. The fibers of the plantar fascia, being made up of collagen, are incapable of stretching to accommodate these counteractive forces. In fact, as loads become greater, collagen fibers resist deformation to an even greater extent. The net result is that something has to give. The most susceptible link is the origin of the fascia on the calcaneus, although the whole length of the fascia is susceptible to injury.

Plantar fasciitis may also result from late pronation during the push-off phase. As the heel rises, the plantar aponeurosis normally tightens as a function of the "windlass effect." Thus, as the toes dorsiflex, the fascia that inserts on them and wraps around the metatarsals becomes taut. The mechanism is functional in that it helps to make the foot more rigid to assist in push-off. However, if the push-off is from the first metatarsal and first toe, the fascia with insertion on toes two to five is slackened as they move passively into plantarflexion. As a result, the force due to body weight is transmitted only through the fibers that insert on the first toe. Therefore unusually high forces will be incurred on the fascia, and inflammation may occur.

A second injury related to forefoot deformity is the development of *bunions*. Bunions are excessive bone growth (exostosis), development of callus, and thickening of the bursa on the medial side of the first metatarsal head. The deformity is often associated with hallux valgus,[11] but

little has been written about the dynamic etiology of the deformity. No association has been made between the timing of pronation and the development of bunions. However, some runners with forefoot varus deformities present clinically with signs of, and/or complaints of, the development of bunions. As noted earlier, pronation may continue late into the gait cycle for several reasons. The person with a noncompensated varus deformity may be particularly susceptible to this timing issue. As the noncompensated varus forefoot moves into full weight-bearing, it may be slowed by the torsional forces between the forefoot and hindfoot. By the time the forefoot reaches the ground, the heel may already be rising off the ground. Push-off may occur as the weight of the body is being transferred to the first metatarsal head. Heavy callusing of the medial side of the first metatarsal head and the first toe are often seen as a result of the person pushing off these two structures. As a result, the increased stresses placed on the medial head of the first metatarsal and the first toe may produce bone growth (Wolff's law). Thus bunions may be a result of late pronation and push-off from the medial forefoot.

A paradoxical injury related to varus foot abnormalities is *lateral ankle sprain* (inversion sprain). Varus deformities that cause injuries related to hyperpronation and timing dysfunction may also cause sprains. The resolution of these apparently contradictory injuries is in the unstable nature of the varus foot when it hits the ground and the tenuous direction of forces relative to the ankle axis. During running, for example, even small amounts of adduction of the leg at heel strike may result in a force couple that acts in the *opposite* direction to that which normally causes stresses on the medial tissues of the foot and leg (compare Figs. 15-5 and 15-7).

The major point to be made with these examples is that intrinsic foot problems are often associated with noncompensated or partially compensated forefoot varus deformities. If a hyperpronation model is assumed, the therapist will conclude that there is no abnormality, because no calcaneal eversion is observed. The appropriate treatment for such injuries is one that addresses the forefoot deformity. Plantar fasciitis

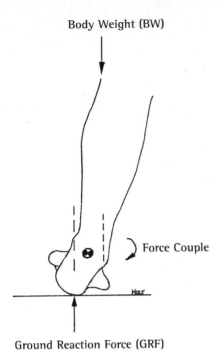

Body Weight (BW)

Force Couple

Ground Reaction Force (GRF)

Fig. 15-7 Distribution of forces when the foot this the ground in supination with adducted lower leg. Note that the force couple is now opposite to that in Fig. 15-5.

due to forefoot varus responds well to the use of an orthosis with a forefoot posting.* Symptomatic treatment meets with limited success. Success with the use of an arch support is also limited because it addresses only one of the problems, the increased deformation due to the increased loading forces. Similarly, surgical intervention on a bunion (bunionectomy) is unlikely to have any long-term benefits for an athlete, since the structure and resulting forces that caused the deformity remain untreated.

Intermediate Structure Injuries

Shin splints is a generic term used to describe tendinitis of the posterior tibialis, anterior tibialis, flexor digitorum longus, and flexor hallucis longus muscles at the site of origin of the muscles on the tibia. A mechanism common to all of these tissues is that they cross the ankle and in-

*Posting refers to the addition of a wedge to an orthosis and is designed to bring the ground up to the foot.

sert on bones on the medial side of the foot. As they cross the ankle joint, the medial structures of the ankle serve as pulleys in transmitting the forces generated by muscle contraction. Severe shin splints may result in a pulling away of bone tissue at the origin, a condition known as stress reaction. Both tendinitis and stress retractions may also occur at the insertion of the muscles on the bones of the foot (see Fig. 15-6).

The mechanism of injury to these tissues may also be the result of structural foot abnormalities, and there may be several mechanisms by which the tissues are injured. Eccentric contraction of several of these muscles is thought to help decelerate the foot to counteract the pronation forces due to ground contact. As noted earlier from a biomechanical perspective, these forces are exceptionally large, or cause exceptional velocity due to the structural deformities. Injury may result from an inability to absorb the high forces and/or to eccentrically contract fast enough to match the higher velocity of pronation.

If the foot is naturally in a varus or supinated position in nonweight-bearing, the natural resting length of the muscles also reflects that position. For example, the posterior tibialis inserts on the bones of the midfoot and is partly responsible for inversion of the foot (see Fig. 15-6A). If the unweighted position of the foot is one of varus, then the resting length of the muscle is relatively short. When the varus foot is pushed into pronation during weight-bearing, there is a passive stretch on the muscle (in this case the posterior tibialis) beyond its resting length. Repeated forced stretch of the muscle beyond its resting length may result in its pulling away from the origin or insertion, thereby resulting in injury.

Achilles tendinitis may result from late pronation or hyperpronation (or excessive supination) during heel-off when there is maximal power production of the muscles responsible for push-off (gastrocnemius, and to a lesser extent the soleus). If the foot is in a pronated position or still pronating, the fibers of the Achilles tendon that insert on the lateral side of the calcaneus will be slack compared to those on the medial side (Fig. 15-8). Most of the contractile force will

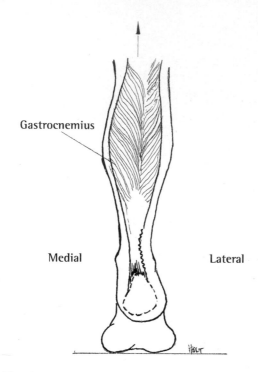

Gastrocnemius

Medial

Lateral

HOLT

Fig. 15-8 Action of gastrocnemius muscle when the foot pushes off with the heel in a valgus position. Injury to the medial fibers of the Achilles tendon may occur.

therefore be transmitted through the medial fibers. The opposite will be true if the foot is in an excessively supinated position at push-off (in a supinated rigid equinus foot, for example). In either case, force is being generated through a diminished number of fibers, with the resultant potential for injury. "Pump bumps" may also result, in which there is an increase in bone growth at the insertion of the fibers that have been subjected to the greatest forces.

Injuries Extrinsic to the Foot

All injuries to the lower extremity and back that are of a nontraumatic nature may *potentially* be caused by structural abnormalities of the foot. Of particular interest are the abnormalities that result in disruption of the normal functional relationships between joints. The disruption of foot pronation/supination and knee flexion/extension is one example that has been discussed. The crucial functional link between the foot and

the rest of the lower extremity is the subtalar joint. The subtalar joint influences tibial rotation, which in turn influences the mechanical functions of other joints. Injuries above the foot that are related to a structural foot abnormality will only occur when that structure influences the action of the subtalar joint. Thus, foot structures that cause either subtalar joint hyperpronation or influence the timing of the pronation will cause injury to more proximal tissues. The foot type that is most likely to produce proximal dysfunction is a *compensated forefoot varus,* in which the forefoot varus is compensated for by excessive subtalar joint pronation. This type of foot has been termed the *destructive foot* because of the many joint and tissue injuries with which it has been associated.[6]

Several injuries to the knee joint may be related to disruption of timing between the knee joint action and foot pronation. *Patello-femoral pain syndrome* refers to pain in and around the patello-femoral joint and has been associated with hyperpronation. The symptoms often respond well to the use of foot orthoses, but the mechanism of injury is not well understood. Knee extension results in a gliding of the patella cranially within the femoral groove. The actual trajectory is rather complex as the various facets come into contact with each other. However, for the purposes of this discussion a thorough description is not necessary. Under normal circumstances the tibia is externally rotating during the last 30 degrees of extension,[18] but if pronation occurs late in the gait cycle the tibia may be internally rotating as the patella glides cranially. From a biomechanical perspective the diagram of forces will be changed such that the angle of force on the patellar ligament is directed more medially. As a result, the effective contraction of the knee extensors (vastus medialis, rectus femoris, and vastus lateralis) will change the direction of patellar tracking compared to when the tibia is closer to the midline (Fig. 15-9). While this change in the direction of pull may be very subtle, the many repetitions characteristic of sports activities can have a devastating effect on the joint.

Chronic *medial and lateral collateral sprains* of the knee may also result from the influence of tibial

Rehabilitation of the Athlete's Foot and Ankle

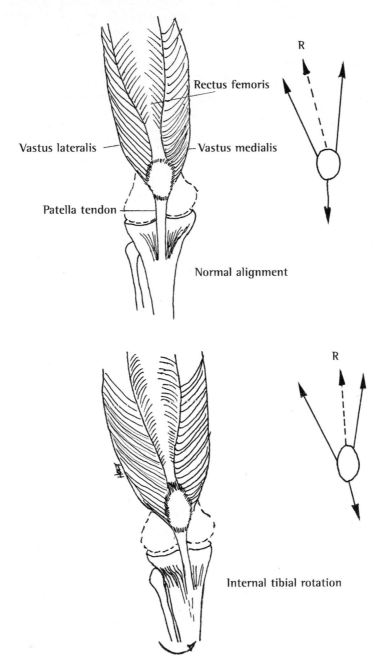

Rectus femoris

Vastus lateralis — **Vastus medialis**

Patella tendon

Normal alignment

R

R

Internal tibial rotation

Fig. 15-9 Effect of internal tibial torsion on action of the quadriceps muscle group. Note changes in the effective direction of the resultant force vector (R) and patella tracking.

rotation on the tibiofemoral joint. In the terminal phases of knee extension, the knee joint is in a close-packed position in which the tibial and femoral joint surfaces are maximally congruent. The ligaments are also thought to be most taut in this position.[18] Internal tibial rotation relative to the femur may serve to increase the tension on the ligaments by virtue of the "wringing" effect between the joint surfaces of the knee. The iliotibial band may be subject to similar forces, resulting in iliotibial band tendinitis at either the hip or the knee.

Effects of Foot Structure on Posture

Standing and locomotory postures may also be influenced by structural abnormalities of the foot. In relaxed stance, the center of mass of the upper body normally passes through both hip joints in the sagittal plane. When a varus or hyperpronated foot is involved, the body weight falls forward of the hip.★ The center of mass is close to the forward edge of the base of support. As a result the person is in very unstable equilibrium. The slightest perturbation may result in a loss of balance. In order to move the center of mass closer to the center of the support base, the individual can use several tactics. In patient populations, two major strategies are often observed: knee hyperextension and a hyperlordotic lower back. Both postures alter the distribution of the forces involved in the back and knee joints and may result in injury when combined with the high forces involved in athletic endeavors.

It is postulated that the old adage 'a chain is only as strong as its weakest link' is true for the joints of the body. Timing and excessive pronation problems may bypass the knee joint completely if it is supported by strong and stable ligaments and muscles. As a result, unusual stresses may occur at the hip joint, the sacroiliac joint, and the spine. While the exact mechanisms of injury to these tissues remain to be elucidated, it is possible that foot dysfunctions could be a cause of such remote injuries as temporomandibular joint dysfunction.

Risk Factors for Injury

We believe that structural abnormalities are the overriding cause of chronic running injuries. However, the severity of the structural abnormality will not determine either the incidence or likelihood of injury. The incidence and severity of an injury will be determined by other risk factors that are present for an individual who has a structural abnormality. These factors include, but

are not limited to, obesity, exercise patterns, prior history of traumatic injury, genetic predisposition, gait patterns, footwear, and nutritional deficits. There is much anecdotal evidence to support the interaction of these factors with structural abnormalities, which may account for some of the puzzling clinical observations.

Loads on the muscles and joints are particularly high in running—up to eight times body weight on impact in the ankle and hip joints. If a large body mass is a result of large bones (and more importantly, joints with a greater surface area) and/or increased muscle mass and strength, the larger impacts may be offset by proportional increases in shock-absorbing capabilities of the larger joints and muscles. Additional loads that do not serve a functional role in absorbing energy and shock will lead to increases in potential for injury. Thus, a person who is carrying the "dead weight" of obesity combined with the unusually high biomechanical torques that result from structural abnormalities is more susceptible to injury.

Similar arguments can be made for exercise patterns. Patients often report that their chronic injury occurred only after gradually increasing their mileage. In increasing daily mileage from 5 to 10 km, a runner is increasing the number of individual footfalls from about 2500 to 5000. A minor structural abnormality, which may produce microtrauma to tissues that can recover at the lower distances, is incapable of doing so when the number of repetitions of the traumatic event is doubled on a daily basis.

A puzzling finding in patients is the report of unilateral pain when examination reveals identical bilateral abnormalities. This finding may be a result of a minor unilateral injury to any joint or tissue at an earlier date. Often the patient has forgotten that the injury occurred, and only remembers it after considerable questioning. In this situation the structural abnormality may be viewed as prolonging or exacerbating the injury because of the unusual mechanical torques associated with the abnormality.

Gait patterns that are freely adopted by an individual and not the result of a structural abnormality may also combine with an abnormality to produce tissue injury. For example, forefoot run-

---

★One can demonstrate this on oneself. In relaxed standing, roll the feet into pronation and supination. The body will rock forward and backward respectively.

Rehabilitation of the Athlete's Foot and Ankle

ners require unusually high eccentric contraction force of the gastrocnemius-soleus group in order to absorb the impact and lower the calcaneus to the ground. If this pattern is combined with a hindfoot valgus resulting from a compensated forefoot, exceptionally high forces might be generated around particular portions of the Achilles tendon (see Fig. 15-8). The forefoot varus alone might be insufficient to produce a problem, but the additional stresses on the Achilles tendon may result in injury.

Shoes that have a low-density midsole may also serve to increase the effects of structural deformities in producing hyperpronation or late pronation. It has been shown that midsole density influences the amount of time a foot is in pronation.[8] As we have argued, late pronation may also be caused by certain structural abnormalities. The combination of the two causes of late pronation may be additive—that is, a person with a forefoot varus abnormality who wears shoes with low-density midsoles will probably pronate later into the gait cycle. The potential for injury may be increased as a result of the two risk factors acting simultaneously.

In the examples presented above, it is clear that the amount of structural deformity is unlikely to be an indicator of the severity of the injury, if an injury occurs at all. However, minor structural deformities may produce significant injury if combined with one or more other risk factors. Clearly, the importance of the history taking becomes highly relevant in this situation.

Evaluation

History

Given the foregoing analysis of the risk factors that contribute to the development of injuries in athletes, it is essential that a thorough and relevant patient history be completed. While the observed structural deformity may be limited, a number of risks may be present that can contribute to the emergence of an injury. Questions to the patient should revolve around the possibility that several risk factors may be present.

The longevity of an injury, response (or lack thereof) to symptomatic treatment, and whether major or minor trauma was involved give the first clues to whether a structural abnormality might be involved. Long-standing injuries that have not responded well to symptomatic treatment and that were the result of minimal or no trauma are a strong indication that structural deformity is present. In a quality assurance study of students who had been prescribed foot orthoses for forefoot varus abnormalities with successful results, 80% reported that they had received previous treatment of symptoms, which had been either totally unsuccessful or had been successful only until they returned to their previous activity.[10]

The patient with a structural abnormality (particularly a forefoot varus deformity) may have experienced injuries to many of the joints of the lower extremity. Unfortunately, patients tend to forget to mention that they have experienced pain or injury to other joints. Their main concern is with what hurts now. Careful questioning about individual joints often reveals a history of injury to several tissues. On physical examination (see next section), tenderness to palpation of several tissues may remain. A history of injury to other tissues of the lower extremity, particularly of a nontraumatic nature, may be indicative of structural abnormalities. Furthermore, multiple chronic symptoms are a good indicator that a compensated forefoot or combined forefoot/hindfoot varus is present. The appropriate questions may lead to the initiation of a differential diagnosis.

Familial inheritance of a specific foot type is not unusual. The patient should be asked about a family history of foot problems, as well as about their own history. Despite a lack of major health screening programs in the United States, patients with foot abnormalities often report that as children they were prescribed "special shoes." Since the effect of structural abnormalities is progressive in terms of the disease process, parents and grandparents of patients often suffer from more advanced pathologies (e.g., bunions, arthritic feet and joints of the lower extremity).

Changes in exercise patterns provide an important clue in the process of evaluating a pos sible structural abnormality. As mentioned previously, increases in mileage produce a multiplicative effect on the number of footfalls. On the other hand, a patient may report that it never felt good to run and that their symptoms are related to walking long distance as a form of exercise. While the forces are lower in walking than running, the person with a structural abnormality is still subject to unusual forces in walking. Questions about changes in shoe type, running surfaces, body weight, and sports participation all give important clues to the risks that might be influential in the development of an injury.

Physical Examination

While an appropriate set of questions in the history taking is crucial to help the therapist understand the potential risks involved for an individual and to initiate a differential diagnosis, a thorough physical examination is also of great importance. The clinical evaluation involves three distinct postures for the patient: weight-bearing, nonweight-bearing, and dynamic activity. Each analysis gives unique information but also allows the therapist to build on and to confirm or reject the hypotheses that have been made from the others.

Weight-Bearing Evaluation

The weight-bearing evaluation is performed with the goal of assessing any postural abnormalities and the position of the feet in stance. A limited amount of information can be obtained in this posture, because most injuries are not incurred in static postures. Foot position in standing gives information on the existence of hyperpronation. Calcaneal eversion and a subtalar joint in rotation imply that there is a hyperpronated foot. The measurement of angles of eversion is of limited use for several reasons. First, the ability to measure angles accurately is limited. Measurement errors using a goniometer may be as large as the angles that are being measured. Second, since any orthotic treatment will be based on the structural abnormality rather than the hyperpronation, angular information is of little practical use. Finally, calcaneal eversion in stance is less than that which occurs dynamically. The forces during locomotory activity ensure that the

angle will increase above that observed in stance. Pes planus (flat foot) and pes cavus (high arch) have also been used extensively as indicators of hyperpronation. However, evidence has shown that the "arch index," a measure of the amount of flat-footedness, is not related to the amount or the timing of pronation[9] and so has limited use in terms of decisions on treatment.

A thorough postural evaluation may give information about the effects of a foot structural deformity or other deformities that might influence the etiology of an injury. For example, although the mechanism is not known, a true leg length discrepancy often results in hyperpronation in the foot of the longer leg. Thus, while the hips may be level, one foot may show a greater amount of pronation than the other. When both feet are held in subtalar neutral, the difference in the levels of the hips is observed. The leg length discrepancy can be confirmed by measurements. Treatment in this situation requires that the provider address both the leg length discrepancy *and* the hyperpronation. The effects of a structural abnormality and hyperpronation can be assessed by having the patient roll in and out of subtalar neutral. If the body moves posteriorly in subtalar neutral, it can be concluded that the foot position may be associated with observed postural abnormalities.

Nonweight-Bearing Evaluation

The nonweightbearing evaluation (NWB) is done with the patient in a prone position with the feet and ankles protruding beyond the end of the table. Mobility of foot structures, tenderness to palpation, and callus patterns are assessed in the NWB position. Hindfoot and forefoot varus and valgus are traditionally measured using goniometry. Again, this method is of limited use because of the large amount of measurement error relative to actual deformity. In addition, there is disagreement about the range of values for the amount of varus or valgus considered to be normal or abnormal.[3,14]

The most common method of assessing foot structures is with the foot held in a subtalar neutral position.[19] In our opinion this also is of limited value. If timing of pronation and hyperpronation are related to the biomechanics of events, as we have described, the variable of interest is not foot structure in subtalar neutral. Rather, the varus or valgus position at which the foot hits the ground is more relevant. This is the biomechanical interface of the foot and the ground that will determine the dynamic forces on the body tissues. In evaluating forefoot and hindfoot abnormalities, therefore, the patient is told to hold the foot in a slight amount of dorsiflexion (perhaps 3 to 5 degrees). This position reflects the angle of the ankle when the foot hits the ground and involves contraction of the ankle dorsiflexors, which are normally contracted just before heel contact. Assessment of the amount of varus or valgus is not "scientific," in that values are categorized as a little (approximately 5 to 10 degrees), a little more (10 to 20 degrees), or a lot (greater than 20 degrees) and are essentially "eyeballed" by the evaluator.

Assessment of the mobility of foot structures is an important part of the NWB evaluation. The major purpose is to determine what accommodations need to be made for immobility in an orthotic device. A rigid plantarflexed first ray is one immobile structure commonly observed. When it hits the ground, large impact forces are generated around the first metatarsal head. An orthotic device that is designed to accommodate some other deformity must also ensure that these high impact forces are attenuated.

Tenderness to palpation helps to establish whether there are areas of the foot and leg that may be sensitive but whose sensitivity is subconscious to the patient. Palpation of the plantar fascia and the medial and lateral borders of the tibia often reveals tenderness of the plantar fascia and origins of the posterior tibialis and anterior tibialis muscles. These tissues may not be perceived as injured by the patient but supply the evaluator with one more piece of evidence supporting a structural abnormality.

Without an actual dynamic analysis, the most important piece of information about the dynamic processes that the foot undergoes is the callus patterns. Callus patterns reflect areas of high pressure. Heavy callusing on the medial side of the first metatarsal head and the first toe are sue indicators that the patient pronates late into the gait cycle and pushes off those structures.

The interested reader is referred to a rich source of information about the meaning of callus patterns with respect to specific foot structures in Root et al.[16]

Dynamic Evaluation

Much has been made in this chapter of the importance of the timing of joint actions in the etiology of injury. Timing relationships between joints are crucial to normal function. They can only be observed in the dynamic situation. Unfortunately, observational gait analysis is highly unreliable. The solution is the use of a video camera with a monitor that allows frame-by-frame advance. The patient performs the activities that produce the pain. For walking and running, the set-up is quite simple. Locomotion on a treadmill is performed at the patient's most comfortable speed (this may be a typical running or walking pace). Filming is performed in the frontal plane from behind and with a close-up view that includes the feet and the knees. Performance is filmed only after the patient has become accustomed to the treadmill. The patient should locomote for at least 15 minutes due to the possibility that compensations may be made to diminish the amount of pain. For example, the foot may be held in an inverted position so that proper timing is maintained, but patients quickly become fatigued and are unable to hold compensatory positions for more than 5 to 10 minutes. The time constraint is particularly important for those patients who report pain only after several minutes of exercise. Thus, after 15 minutes it is safe to assume that the dynamic mechanism of injury may be observed.★

In the analysis of timing dysfunctions, only a limited number of actions must be observed. Freeze-framing at foot strike is important. Observation of the angles at which the hindfoot and forefoot make initial contact and the order of contact allows the therapist to assess the initial conditions for the generation of forces around the foot and ankle. If the medial side of the hindfoot and forefoot are high off the ground, the potential for generation of large forces is great. As the foot moves into weight acceptance, it will

★These are clinical observations.

begin to pronate. Observation of the knee joint action will determine if the appropriate knee flexion is occurring. To observe the action of the knee joint is surprisingly simple in the frontal plane—if the back of the knee is getting larger in the camera view, the knee is extending, and if the knee is getting smaller, the knee is flexing.

Calcaneal eversion (or inversion) at foot flat determines the amount of pronation under dynamic forces. "Normal" feet may seem to show an unexpectedly large amount of pronation if the therapist is experienced only in static analysis. Not too much emphasis should be placed on the amount of calcaneal eversion. More important is the action of the calcaneus during heel-off. At this point, and to toe-off, the foot should be in the process of resupinating. If the same or greater amounts of calcaneal eversion are observed, it may be an indication of late pronation. As the foot rises onto the metatarsal heads, they should all be in contact with the ground. If push-off is clearly occurring at the first metatarsal head and the first toe, it is an indication that the foot is pronating too late into the gait cycle. The combination of continued calcaneal eversion, push-off by the first metatarsal head and first toe, and knee extension is clear evidence of mistiming between the foot and knee.

Treatment

For structurally related injuries, the therapist must treat both the symptoms and the cause. Symptomatic treatment would include all of the clinical therapies normally used for the injury. Treatment of causes has taken two tacks. The first is to attempt to strengthen the muscles that might prevent the foot from hyperpronating. As noted in the previous chapter, pronation and supination are largely passive actions. This is self-evident in the large amount of force that is generated around the subtalar joint axis compared to the relatively small size of muscles (the anterior and posterior tibialis) that potentially control the actions. Although the muscles may be able to control the amount and timing of pronation for short periods, it is unlikely that they

will be able to do so for the time periods and high forces involved in sports activities.

A far more successful treatment method is the use of foot orthoses that compensate for the structural abnormality by bringing the "ground up to the foot." In a group of student athletes (n = 25) who had not responded well to conventional treatments, all reported significant and lasting relief with the use of orthoses.[10] Theoretically, an orthosis that prevents the foot from gaining large amounts of momentum should diminish the possibility of both hyperpronation and inappropriate timing.

Principles of Orthotic Management

An orthosis is not designed to "cure" an injury but to attenuate the excessive forces that are generated as a function of a structural abnormality. Healing of injured tissues requires the therapist to address the symptoms. Orthotic design centers around the concept that one is attenuating biomechanical effects rather than preventing hyperpronation. Thus, the posting of an orthosis is critically dependent on the observed structural abnormality and not simply on hyperpronation. The orthosis will be different when the structural abnormality is treated rather than the hyperpronation. If a forefoot varus is present, that varus must be accommodated for by a forefoot varus posting. In our experience there have been many athletes with forefoot varus abnormalities who have initially rejected the idea of using an orthotic because they "already have one and it doesn't work." Examination of the orthosis shows a molded arch support with no forefoot posting, which clearly does not address the structural problem and its associated biomechanical forces. Unfortunately, there is no way to address a structural abnormality orthotically without posting the structure. Consequently, for individuals with large abnormalities the orthosis may be quite bulky and will only fit into certain types of shoe. We usually recommend that the athlete take the orthosis along when purchasing new shoes (often a half-size bigger).

We also wish to challenge the practice of molding the orthosis with the foot in a subtalar neutral position either in prone or midstance. In this method, the orthotic bed is molded either by a plaster cast or heat-moldable material. The notion is that the molded orthosis fits the contours of the feet, is more comfortable, and tends to hold the foot in subtalar neutral. In the dynamics of gait, however, the foot contours are constantly changing. The subtalar neutral foot occurs for only fractions of a second at two instances during gait: when the foot passes from supination through subtalar neutral to pronation during weight acceptance, and when the foot passes from pronation through neutral to supination during push-off. If a rigid orthosis is used, the foot may be forced into contours that are inappropriate except in those two instances. We prefer to use a material that will be molded by the foot dynamically. There are several durable semirigid running shoe inserts that fit this requirement rather well (e.g., the Stabilizer, Spectrum Sports, Twinsberg, OH). No molding is required in the dynamic method. After a short period of time the bed will mold to the shape of the foot.

The posting of the orthotic bed can be accomplished using composite materials of different densities and thicknesses (Plastazote and Nickelplast, AliMed, Inc, Boston, Mass, are two brand names) that can be glued to the bed and ground to the appropriate shape fairly simply. More important than the materials used is the conceptual basis for posting. An orthotic is posted based on the way the foot hits the ground rather than the clinical diagnosis. For example, in Figure 1D the clinical diagnosis is of a hindfoot varus. However, it is clear that the forefoot will hit the ground in an inverted position. Therefore, equal posting of forefoot and hindfoot would be indicated. This is in contrast to the usual posting methods.[19]

Precise measures of the amount of varus or valgus on which to base posting is scientifically unfounded. In addition, some supination and pronation are normal and essential aspects of foot function. There are widely varying estimates of what constitutes a normal range of motion. In addition, some posting materials will deform more than others under load. Our method of posting is somewhat unscientific: post about what you see on examination of the foot in NWB. This may be a little more than what is actually needed, since the foot still needs to pronate and supinate to serve its shock-absorbing and propulsive functions. However, grinding excess material off the posting is easier than adding it on.

Feedback from the patient after a short period of time (1 to 2 weeks) helps to determine the success of the treatment, as does retesting on the treadmill. If fitted correctly, an orthosis should feel comfortable within a short period of time. There should be no hot spots (areas of high pressure that result in blisters or pain). The athlete will often report that the orthosis "feels right." If the athlete reports discomfort or even that the orthosis feels weird (i.e., too much, not enough), then adjustments should be made. The adjustments should also be made according to simple rules. If there is a hot spot, grind out a small area of the posting beneath it. This will redistribute the forces so that there is a more normal distribution of forces across the foot.

Summary

We have presented a biomechanical model of foot abnormalities as the etiology of specific dysfunctions, with special emphasis on locomotion. The scientific basis of the model is biomechanical, but there is limited scientific experimentation to support it. The evidence supplied is based on the results of limited research but extensive clinical experience and success in the treatment of foot dysfunctions. The approach is different, and the consequent evaluation and treatment procedures are different, from those in other clinical texts. There will, no doubt, be some controversy as a result of these hypotheses. The arguments are moot, however, until scientific data lend support to the claims from either side. We are currently in the process of developing methods to quantify the actions of the forefoot and hindfoot independently during gait and plan to investigate the effects of foot type on biomechanics (forces, pressure distributions, kinematics). We encourage others who would argue these issues to do the same.

Bibliography

1. Bates BT, James SL, Osternig LR: Foot function during the support phase of running, *Running* p 24, Fall 1978.
2. Blake RL, Denton JA: Functional foot orthoses for athletic injuries, *J Am Podiatr Med Assoc* 75:359, 1985.
3. Donatelli R: *The biomechanics of the foot and ankle,* Philadelphia, 1990, FA Davis.
4. Eng JJ, Pierrynowski MR: Effect of foot orthotics on the kinematics of the knee joint, *Proceedings of the 12th International Congress of Biomechanics,* 1989, Los Angeles, CA.
5. Gould JA: *Orthopedic and sports physical therapy,* St Louis, 1990, CV Mosby.
6. Gray GC: When the foot hits the ground everything changes, *Rehabilitation Network,* 1985.
7. Greenfield B: Evaluation of overuse syndromes. In Donatelli R, editor: *The biomechanics of the foot and ankle,* Philadelphia, 1990, FA Davis.
8. Hamill J, Bates B, Holt KG: Timing of lower extremity joint actions during treadmill running, *Med Sci Sports Exerc* 4:807, 1992.
9. Hamill J et al: Relationship of static and dynamic measures of lower extremity, *Clin Biomech* 4:217, 1989.
10. Holt KG: Effects of forefoot orthoses on biomechanical injuries to the foot and lower leg, Quality assurance project, 1987, University of Massachusetts.
11. Lefebvre R, Boucher JP: Effects of foot orthotics upon the ankle and knee mechanical alignment, *Proceedings of the 12th International Congress of Biomechanics,* 1989, Los Angeles, CA.
12. Magee DJ: *Orthopedic physical assessment,* Philadelphia, 1987, WB Saunders.
13. McGlamry DE, Kitting RW: Equinus foot, an analysis of the etiology, pathology, and treatment techniques, *J Am Podiatr Med Assoc* 63:165, 1973.
14. McPoil TG, Brocato RS: The foot and ankle: biomechanical evaluation and treatment. In Gould JA, editor: *Orthopedic and sports physical therapy,* St Louis, 1990, CV Mosby.
15. Pagliano J, Jackson O: The ultimate study of running injuries, *Runners World* 15:42, 1980.
16. Root ML, Orien WP, Weed JH: *Biomechanical evaluation of the foot,* vol 1, Los Angeles, 1971, Clinical Biomechanics.
17. Rothbart BA, Estabrook L: Excessive pronation: a major biomechanical determinant in the development of chondromalacia and pelvic lists, *J Manipulative Physiol Ther* 11:373, 1987.
18. Soderberg GL: *Kinesiology,* Baltimore, 1986, Williams & Wilkins.
19. Wooden MJ: Biomechanical evaluation for functional orthotics. In Donatelli R, editor: *The biomechanics of the foot and ankle,* Philadelphia, 1990, FA Davis.

16

The Foot and Ankle in Football

Thomas J. Herrmann

The range of injuries to the foot and ankle complex in football is considerable. From just "tired dogs" to complex fractures, addressing the complaints of an ever larger and ever more powerful population of football athletes is the routine task of athletic trainers. In order to address most of these complaints in some systematic manner, let's begin with the most distal aspect of the foot and work our way back.

Foot Injuries

Some incredulity is often expressed when a football athlete misses games or ends his career with the complaint of unresolved big toe pain. "Turf toe," however, has become a common and troublesome problem for many athletes. Characterized by pain, swelling, and stiffness at the first metatarsophalangeal (MTP) joint, it means that athletes have great difficulty pushing off from their stance, jumping, cutting sharply, or tolerating having the toe stepped on (a real hazard in football). The etiology of turf toe can be overuse or a traumatic event.[3]

For many football athletes the origin of their great toe complaints lies in a hyperextension injury to the first MTP joint. This hyperextension

may be acute (having the foot fallen on from behind while running, for instance) or chronic (firing out from a three or four point stance). Football athletes are required to generate sprinterlike power from their stance without the benefit of starting blocks; where a sprinter need not hyperextend the great toe, thanks to the angle the blocks provide, a football athlete starts with a relatively flat foot, requiring tremendous ankle dorsiflexion and great toe extension at push-off. The prestretch that this affords the flexor hallucis longus allows the transfer of tremendous energy through the first MTP joint.

The morbid progression of turf toe for many athletes begins with an ache in the first MTP joint, which gradually loses extension. The loss of extension and often painful impingement of the dorsal aspect of the joint with attempted extension now prompts the athlete to externally rotate his foot during high-power maneuvers, thus pushing obliquely through the first MTP joint. Finally, hypertrophic bone along the medial aspect of the joint in response to the stress generates a bunionlike appearance and complaint. The final stage is often a painful hallux rigidus.

Is this progression inescapable? Not always, but to avoid the highly probable morbidity of this injury requires early and aggressive intervention. Baseline X-rays at the time of the injury or at the outset of the complaint are necessary if one is to monitor the progression of the joint pathology. Antiinflammatory measures need to be instituted at the first complaint. Routine icing, oral antiinflammatory medications, phonophoresis or iontophoresis, and joint mobilization are all helpful in combating the progression of joint disease and disability. Trainers and therapists must work aggressively to maintain the plantar/dorsal glide of the MTP joint so that normal joint mechanics can be preserved. A stress-reducing orthosis applied with adhesive tape or in the form of an orthotic is also helpful. Either system must limit the amount of first MTP joint extension to its pain-free range (in some cases as little as 10 degrees). If a valgus deformity is developing or is already present, the orthosis can be modified to bring the toe into line with the long axis of the metatarsal to limit the amount of oblique stress through the joint (see Figs. 22-17 and 22-18). It is also occasionally helpful to support the longitudinal arch and metatarsal arch in order to redistribute the forces through the foot, especially in the case of the athlete who has a pronated foot (Fig. 22-10 and 22-14).

To generalize, it is usually prudent to approach complaints of first MTP joint pain with a double-edged attack; first, reduce the inflammation and stiffness in and around the capsule with aggressive therapy, both pharmacological and physical, and second, reduce the day-to-day stress applied to the joint during activity through the use of some type of orthosis. Working from both directions gives the athlete the best chance of minimizing the often morbid effects that a chronic turf toe has on athletic performance.

Other structures related to the great toe that often present problems for the football athlete are the sesamoid bones of the flexor hallucis muscles and the flexor tendons themselves. Again the problem usually has its roots in chronic hyperextension of the great toe joint and the tremendous forces that are realized at the joint. The insidious implications of a sore great toe along the entire kinetic chain show that there is no such thing as a minor problem with the great toe.

Fractures of the sesmoids, either stress fractures or overt fractures, can be identified clinically through direct tenderness over the sesamoid (usually the medial one) and/or an acute increase in pain with great toe hyperextension and compression of the sesamoid against the first metatarsal.[13] The typical complaint of the athlete is pain with pushing off or with sudden directional changes. The athlete may also relate that the pain can be abated by transferring the weight toward the fifth metatarsal. Documentation of the injury can be made through X-ray and bone scan. When faced with what appears to be a frank fracture, a differentiation should be made between a frank fracture and a congenitally bipartite sesmoid. This can usually be done simply by obtaining comparison views.

The reason for careful differentiation of the diagnosis is so that a prognosis can be delivered with confidence. One can treat a symptomatic congenitally bipartite sesamoid with a tape or manufactured orthosis to relieve pressure and limit great toe extension, much as one would treat an acute tendonitis, with some confidence that the problem will resolve with time. A fracture of the sesamoid may require 6 weeks of casting and nonweight-bearing to finally resolve, followed by a patient and gradual return to sport in order to provide adequate stress accommodation time for the bone to remodel. Even with weeks or months of gradually increasing stress exposure, the athlete may find the use of an orthosis necessary and continue to experience discomfort at full activity levels.

The excision of a symptomatic sesamoid, or the bone grafting of a nonunion, in an athlete is sometimes problematic. Intratendon scarring can develop and can often represent a source of complaints equal to the sesamoid. If a surgical course is taken, however, aggressive therapy to restore tendon elasticity and foot/ankle strength and power must follow, and the return to activity is painfully slow for the athlete. Nevertheless, this approach usually presents the athlete who is experiencing unrelenting symptoms with the best opportunity to return to sport with minimal complaints.

Forefoot pain at the distal aspects of the metatarsals is not uncommon, especially if the football athlete plays on artificial turf. The possible injuries in this region of the foot range from metatarsalgia to metatarsal stress fracture to neu-

Rehabilitation of the Athlete's Foot and Ankle

roma. Any or all of these problems respond well if the trainer or physician intervenes early in the event.

When an athlete complains of forefoot pain, one of the first items that requires assessment is the integrity of the metatarsal arch. The normal anatomy of the forefoot includes a small arch across the metatarsals so that the first and fifth come into contact with the ground first and the midmetatarsals then settle to the ground.[7] One must suspect that this arch has been compromised when an athlete develops a callus under the second, third, and/or fourth metatarsal heads. The presence of this callus suggests that the midmetatarsals are now the primary weight-bearing metatarsals. Athletes with cavus feet or a pronounced Morton's toe are especially susceptible to this type of weight-bearing pattern.[11]

Metatarsalgia with no definite X-ray or bone scan findings is common among athletes. Stress fractures of the second and third metatarsal are also found quite often. Finally, a neuroma must be suspected if the athlete complains of forefoot pain that includes numbness between the toes. All of these problems respond well to pressure relief orthotics, usually of a soft material such as felt or a viscopolymer.

The trainer has two available routes in developing a forefoot pressure relief pad. One is to pad the entire forefoot and leave a gap in the pad under the tender metatarsal. This is effective if the integrity of the metatarsal arch is intact; if the arch has been compromised, then the gap simply permits the bone to fall further. The other is to create a teardrop-shaped pad and place its wide end just behind the midmetatarsal heads (see Fig. 22-14). This acts as a post for the midmetatarsals, causing the weight to be pushed toward the first and fifth metatarsals. This is effective when callus formation suggests a loss of metatarsal arch integrity or when the complaints of pain include the shaft of the metatarsal as well as the head. The teardrop-shaped pad also seems to be effective in relieving the pain produced by a neuroma by creating a little more space between the bones and by diverting force away from the middle of the foot.

Treating a *Morton's type neuroma* in the athlete can be a difficult problem. In the football ath-

lete in particular, the problem of sheer size and weight becomes a factor. It is generally difficult to develop a soft system that can stand up to the pressure that even a small football athlete generates. A felt padding system that works usually needs to be recreated on a weekly basis. A more rigid, and thus more durable, system compromises the shock-attenuating qualities that most athletes prize in their footwear and can lead to more problems than it solves. But while the mechanical problems of pressure relief are being addressed, the therapeutic problems of reducing the neuroma and its symptoms also need to be addressed.

It is typical to treat Morton's type neuromas with ultrasound therapy and oral antiinflammatory medications in conjunction with pressure relief orthotics. When using ultrasound, care must be exercised to minimize bone penetration since the metatarsals are very prominent and superficial. For this reason, a pulsed 3-MHz signal is desirable along with a small sound head, 1 or 3 cm if available.[12] Occasionally the use of a corticosteroid injection is warranted in the persistently or acutely painful neuroma. This, followed by therapeutic modalities and padding, is often very effective.

The final attack on a Morton's neuroma is to excise it surgically. This must be approached with caution in the athlete. Postsurgical scarring can sometimes present as persistent a problem as the neuroma, and failure to pay careful attention to the strengthening of the intrinsic muscles of the foot often leads the athlete to doubt the value of the surgery. While surgical attention to the neuroma is sometimes the only option to relieve the athlete's complaints, the physician, therapist, and trainer must develop a well-orchestrated recovery plan that minimizes scarring and restores strength, power, and proprioception along the entire kinetic chain in order for the athlete to realize the full benefit.

If low back pain is the plague of the American worker, heel pain is the plague of the athlete. Call it what you will, *"plantar fasciitis,"* "painful heel syndrome," "heel spurs," or whatever else fits the descriptive requirements, but complaints of pain at the origin of the plantar fascia are some of the most difficult to address in the athlete. The confounding factors with the football athlete are again the sheer size of the athlete and the power that the athlete can generate.

For our purposes, let's reduce the description of plantar heel pain to "painful heel syndrome" (PHS).[1] For most athletes, the historical description of the problem includes painful walking when first arising in the morning or after prolonged sitting. The pain usually subsides somewhat after a few minutes of walking. Pain with repeated loading of the foot, especially in high-power moments, becomes progressively worse, and the athlete will relate that firing out of a three or four point stance is becoming impossible. Finally, even standing for any period causes significant pain.

The root of PHS lies in the chronic tightness or inflexibility of the entire plantarflexing mechanism. For our purposes, this includes the gastroc-soleus complex, the long and short toe flexors, and the plantar fascia. Failure to address the need for flexibility in all of these structures will only partially remedy the excessive traction problem that gives rise to the problem.[1]

The mechanical processes of the windlass mechanism of the foot have been well described[4,7] (Fig. 16-1). Briefly, the insertion of the plantar fascia at the base of the proximal phalanges causes the plantar fascia to supinate and slightly externally rotate the calcaneus as the toes are extended at the initiation of the push-off phase of walking or running. This in turn assists in the elevation and supination of the midfoot, providing a stiff foot for the efficient transfer of force. The origin of the plantar fascia at the medial calcaneal tubercle is a focal point of tension in this mechanism, with forces acting on either side of it at the ankle and the MTP joints.[1,9]

It doesn't take a lot of imagination to picture how pathomechanics or injury to the structures on either side of the origin of the plantar fascia can lead to problems. A tight gastroc-soleus complex causes the ankle to lose dorsiflexion. The lack of dorsiflexion at the ankle causes a compensatory increase in dorsiflexion of the toes in order to preserve the duration and power production of the gait cycle. An increase in toe dorsiflexion causes an increase in traction at the origin of the plantar fascia by increasing the distance between origin and insertion.[9] This increase in traction leads to microtrauma and its sequellae.

A valgus heel, pronated foot, or combination of both often reflect uncompensated hindfoot or forefoot pathomechanics that put excessive traction at the origin of the plantar fascia through failure of the normal windlass pattern. As the foot remains pronated in the push-off phase of gait, the midfoot fails to elevate. This presents a twofold problem: the traction component of the plantar fascia increases due to the increasing distance between origin and insertion, and the softness of the foot causes an increase in muscular work due to inefficient transfer of force. In this case, the athlete has a compounded problem of increased tension and mechanical inefficiency.[9] Again this leads to microtrauma, inflammation, and chronic pain.

The resolution of PHS in athletes is often more an exercise in patience than a marvelous medical/therapeutic achievement. The ultimate resolution of the problem lies in reduction of the traction forces at the origin of the plantar fascia. This is obviously accomplished through stretching and mechanical adjustments in foot pathomechanics if required.[5] The pharmacological approach has a role in the acutely sore athlete. The application of therapeutic modalities should fol-

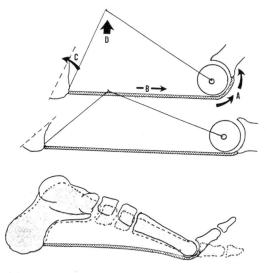

Fig. 16-1 The windlass mechanism. (From Cailliett R: *Foot and ankle pain,* ed 2, Philadelphia, 1968, FA Davis.)

Rehabilitation of the Athlete's Foot and Ankle

low some rational progression or regression pattern based on the desired effect. Not so obvious, however, is the need to gradually expose the fascial tissue to stress so that it can remodel at a rate that is equal to the stress loads. This is where the patience comes in.

If the athlete is in acute pain, there may be some benefit in the use of a corticosteroid injection to control the inflammation. If this approach is taken, the athlete must endure a strictly enforced 7- to 10-day period of complete rest because of the steroid's tissue-weakening effect.[1] During this rest period, however, the athlete may begin a period of ultrasound treatments and gentle stretching of the fascia. What appears to be most effective is using ultrasound at the medial calcaneal tubercle with the fascia on stretch. The sound can be fairly aggressive at first, a 1-MHz frequency for penetration, pulsed 50% in the 1.2 to 1.4 W/cm^2 range. This seems to have the desired tissue-softening and inflammation control effects. As the athlete begins to become active, it is necessary to change the ultrasound to a 3-MHz frequency to avoid high bone penetration and to change the pulse rate to 20% or even 10%. This enhances the mechanical effect of the sound on soft tissue while minimizing its effect on the bone.[12]

The use of orthotics is sometimes helpful, but it may be best to begin with a simple longitudinal arch or Low-Dye arch tape to take some of the load off the plantar fascia (see Figs. 22-10, 22-11, 22-12, and 22-13). If this is successful, then the addition of a soft arch support for activity will probably work as the pain becomes less acute. It is usually not necessary to generate a pressure relief post for a heel spur unless the spur is palpable and painful.[1]

Stretching and gradual stressing are the key ingredients to the program. A position that puts the entire plantar mechanism on stretch is essential. A modified wall lean stretch with the toes extended will accomplish the task. The athlete stretches in this position at a level just below pain for at least 2 minutes 3 or 4 times a day. Along with the stretching, the athlete begins a walking program designed to gradually introduce stress. The athlete walks a distance short of one that causes pain, whatever that distance is. The athlete must then walk that distance daily and add no more than 10% a week to that distance to allow for tissue accommodation. Running can be introduced in the same manner, establishing the pain-free distance and adding no more than 10% a week.[1] Most athletes find this pace excruciating, but it helps to ensure that the fascia is not being overtaxed. If at any point in the activity program the athlete experiences pain, the athlete must return to the previous activity level and remain there another week; then move up again. Guarding against exacerbation of symptoms is our first goal; eliminating complaints is our final goal.

A *painful midfoot* in the football athlete represents a myriad possibilities. In a sport where it is likely that the foot will be stepped on repeatedly, contusions to the dorsum of the foot are common. While usually not debilitating, they are painful and may require some accommodation of the footwear to relieve the pressure of the laces. A pressure-induced or contact tendinitis of the toe extensors is a real risk. For that reason, icing and pressure relief should be a matter of course until the complaints are resolved.

More of a problem is a sprain or fracture in the midfoot. Often following a forced plantarflexion injury or forced dorsiflexion injury, an intratarsal sprain or fracture can be a source of pain and dysfunction for months. It is possible that a midfoot injury will evolve into a season-long challenge. The top of the midfoot nightmare list is a Lisfranc fracture or fracture/dislocation. The disruption of the tarsometatarsal joints creates a mechanically unsound midfoot. In effect, the midfoot collapses during the stance portion of the gait and never recovers.[6]

A sprain of the midfoot that permits an abnormal amount of micromotion of the intratarsal and tarsometatarsal joints may not be classified as a true midfoot instability, but these sprains represent a painful problem and a difficult problem to manage.[6] Again, usually following an injury in the extremes of plantarflexion or dorsiflexion or a direct blow, the athlete will find weight transfer from the hindfoot to the forefoot very painful. The athlete may try to externally rotate the foot during push-off to divert force to other structures or hold the foot supinated to splint the midfoot. Neither of these compensatory patterns is desirable for both anatomical and mechanical reasons.

The athlete with a midfoot sprain will often complain of pain in the longitudinal arch or pain along the extensor tendons on the dorsum of the foot. Stressing the midfoot during the exam and finding point tenderness along the tarsal joints should lead the examiner to suspect a midfoot injury as opposed to a sprain of the plantar ligament or dorsal tendinitis, especially if the injury history includes a mechanism of extreme forced motion in plantarflexion or dorsiflexion.

With a midfoot sprain, a longitudinal arch support system is required to relieve the stress. This can be accomplished with tape or with a soft orthosis. The simple X-type longitudinal arch tape is usually a good start. In the larger athlete or the athlete who already has a pronated foot, the more aggressive Low-Dye tape is sometimes necessary (see Figs. 22-10, 22-11, 22-12, and 22-13). The tape, combined with heel cord stretching to ease the stress of dorsiflexion, therapeutic modalities for pain and swelling control, and strengthening of the intrinsic foot muscles, usually permits the athlete with a midfoot sprain to return to participation comfortably once the acute episode has passed.

A midfoot injury that is not very common but that is difficult to manage is a *navicular stress fracture*. The presentation of this injury is not dissimilar from that of a midfoot sprain or fracture. There will be point tenderness over the navicular, however, which is typically not present with other midfoot injuries. Bone scan documentation is necessary.

The athlete who is returning from a navicular stress fracture must do so with caution. An arch support system with an aggressive, but not rigid, longitudinal arch post is required. A medial heel post may also be of some help in limiting the amount of pronation of the foot during the stance phase of the gait. This should eliminate some of the stress realized by the navicular during activity. Gradual exposure to the stress of sport over a period of weeks is also recommended. Again, accommodation to stress rarely happens at a rate greater than 10% per week.

Resolution of the injury and restoration of function may well take months.[8]

On the lateral aspect of the midfoot, the proximal end of the fifth metatarsal has presented itself as a source of concern, especially in large, high-power athletes. Repetitive stress, acute inversion events, or high-velocity rotational forces applied through the foot can produce *fractures at the proximal fifth metatarsal*.[3] This type of fracture presents a wide variety of problems.

The fracture described as a Jones fracture is a fracture at the proximal metaphyseal-diaphyseal junction. An argument can be made that this fracture is often the sequella of a stress fracture that the athlete has been ignoring, but a Jones fracture can also occur during an inversion-internal rotation injury, especially if force is applied focally at the distal end of the fifth metatarsal (slipping off an opponent's foot, for instance). In any event, the athlete will complain of pain along the lateral aspect of the foot and will usually relate a history that includes a "pop" or "snap" during the accident.

Avulsion of the peroneus brevis tendon and fracture of the fifth metatarsal styloid at its insertion on the proximal fifth metatarsal is another possibility and occurs after an acute inversion event. Arguably, the proprioceptive response of the peroneal muscles as the ankle is acutely inverted is to fire aggressively to try and protect the joint. If the inversion force is high enough, the force overcomes the structural strength of the tendon-bone junction, and the peroneus brevis tendon pulls loose, bringing its bony attachment with it.[13]

Again, a range of possibilities exists in terms of treatment. Casting is obvious, but in the case of the athlete the possibility of internal fixation of the avulsion or the Jones fracture must be considered. While a fibrous union of an avulsion may provide adequate healing for the average person, this sometimes represents a considerable source of irritation for the high-power athlete. Internal fixation of these fractures also helps reduce the risk of delayed union or nonunion and may permit the athlete to participate in early rehabilitation to minimize the loss of motion and strength.

Rehabilitation of the Athlete's Foot and Ankle

When supporting an injury along the fifth metatarsal, the trainer must be conscious of the need to support the bone along its entire length. When taping an ankle or foot routinely, the trainer should cover the proximal fifth completely or stay posterior to it completely in order to avoid undo pressure at the fifth metatarsal's proximal articulation. When the lateral foot requires support, however, the tape should extend all the way to the distal aspect of the metatarsal in order to restrict the spread of the forefoot. If the trainer fails to consider this, the distal edge of the tape represents a focal point of pressure along the shaft of the bone, causing pain and occasionally additional risk to the bone itself.

Working to unload the fifth metatarsal to protect a stress fracture or a healed or healing Jones fracture requires a whole foot approach. It is necessary to support the longitudinal arches of the foot and to continue the support out to the distal ends of the metatarsals. Then a gap must be created under the fifth metatarsal head so that it doesn't realize as much ground force. By doing so, the proximal articulation and the shaft of the bone are supported, but shearing and oblique forces are not transferred back up through the bone.

Ankle Injuries

Probably the most commonly injured joint in sport is the ankle.[3] Mild twists and turns of the ankle are experiences shared by nearly every athlete. The nature of these twists and turns, however, differs from sport to sport. In football, in addition to the common inversion injury, there are a host of high-torsion injuries that represent considerable challenge in treatment and restoration of function. This discussion will begin with the most common and then proceed to the difficult variations on the theme. The vast majority of ankle injuries in football fall into the inversion or inversion with plantarflexion category. This mechanism produces injury to the anterior-lateral and lateral ligament complex of the ankle and also exposes the proximal fifth metatarsal to

risk (as discussed earlier). The anatomical alignment of the anterior talofibular ligament establishes its long axis as the primary restraint to inversion if the ankle is plantarflexed. The calcaneofibular ligament has the most advantageous angle to resist inversion when the ankle is in neutral. There has been some discussion stating that the lateral ankle ligaments tear in a priority depending on whether the ankle is in neutral, plantarflexed, or dorsiflexed.[2,3,13]

An *ankle sprain* that produces instability on acute exam requires support and protection in some sort of device that puts the ankle in neutral. This seems logical enough since the neutral position approximates the normal anatomical length of the healing ligament. In order to take advantage of the ankle's favorable response to early treatment, however, it is beneficial to use a removable protective orthosis, such as a walking boot or posterior splint, as opposed to a cast.[13] The use of a removable device, however, requires that the athlete be trusted to cooperate thoroughly with the program. Casting can always be held in reserve for the athlete who fails to follow the directions of the physician or the trainer.

Following even a severe ankle sprain, the ankle joint responds favorably to early motion and strengthening. This effort for early functional training has little deleterious effect on the healing process or residual instability. It is important, however, to make sure that the rehabilitation effort is carefully planned to protect the injury. Early motion should be limited to dorsiflexion, plantarflexion to pain tolerance, and no inversion or eversion.[3]

Movement in straight plantarflexion or dorsiflexion, without forced plantarflexion, encourages appropriate scar formation in the ruptured ligaments while limiting the formation of random, extraneous scar, which will only have to be broken later to restore normal motions. It has been stated that only scarring along the mechanical axis of the ligament contributes to the ligament's integrity without compromising the motion of the joint that the ligament supports.[13] For this reason a number of therapeutic modalities as well as range of motion exercises should be employed early in the recovery process.

The use of cold and cryokinetics is of particular value in treating ankle sprains.[3,13] The reflex vasoresponses initiated by the combination of cold and movement help activate the lymphatic and venous return system, which leads to evacuation of the swelling. The anesthetic effect of the cold allows the motion to be less painful, and the deep vasodilation near the joint helps accelerate the healing response.[13] The combination of cold whirlpool (50° to 55°F) followed immediately by elevation (greater than 45 degrees) and active motion in plantarflexion-dorsiflexion works quite well.

The use of muscle or electrical stimulation is useful in the control of pain and in early muscle reeducation. Acutely, the use of stimulation for pain control is best accomplished by placing the pads along the joint lines so that the capsule can be reached and desensitized. A high-frequency and a medium pulse width will accomplish this best. As the acute pain subsides, the pads of the muscle stimulus can be moved to the peroneal and posterior tibial muscles. Since the proprioceptive signals to these muscles are severely compromised in a severe ankle sprain, use of the stimulus to reeducate the muscles is indicated. Muscle reeducation is best accomplished with a medium frequency and a wide pulse width.[12] It is also helpful to require the athlete to fire the stimulated muscles voluntarily in concert with the stimulus, isometrically early in the recovery phase and concentrically in the later stages of recovery.

In the case of a severe ankle sprain, a period of 2 to 3 weeks should pass before any inversion or plantarflexion into a painful range should be introduced. This allows adequate time for the ligaments to stick together but does not permit extraordinary scarring. Allowing that soft tissue healing takes approximately 6 weeks, the trainer or therapist should be patient in getting inversion and not be too concerned if a few degrees is lost in the process. The therapist or trainer should be concerned if there is a loss of dorsiflexion, however. This will compromise the athlete's ability to protect the ankle and puts the Achilles tendon and the plantar fascia at risk for overuse and strain. A detailed description of an ankle rehabilitation protocol will follow.

Injuries that appear to be ankle sprains at the outset but that can present a considerable challenge to the football athlete and to the trainer or therapist have usually involved rotational forces in conjunction with the more routine mechanisms. A plantarflexion-inversion-rotation injury adds considerable shearing force. The athlete may also have experienced a posterior process fracture, a medial malleolar fracture, or a Maisonneuve type fracture up the leg. One can witness this in the football running back who plants to make a cut and inverts his ankle while turning on the leg.[2]

Eversion type injuries of the ankle, while possibly more common in soccer than in football, are difficult in and of themselves without the compounding variables of rotation. Slow to resolve at best, an eversion injury not only puts the medial ankle ligaments at risk but often compromises the ankle syndesmosis.[13] If such an injury is coupled with dorsiflexion and/or external rotation, the athlete may be faced with a bimalleolar or trimalleolar fracture that totally disrupts the ankle mortise. In football, these are generally contact-initiated injuries incurred while tackling or blocking and having a force applied to the distal or lateral leg.

Hyperdorsiflexion or hyperplantarflexion injuries can wreak havoc on the ankle syndesmosis. A rupture of the tibiofibular ligament and the interosseous membrane compromises the stability of the ankle mortise and often leaves the athlete with a chronically painful ankle. In a sport like football, where the shearing and rotational forces are very high, the athlete may find it difficult to stop, cut, or even tolerate the day-to-day pounding of practice. These sprains often require a specially designed tape job in an attempt to bind the tibia and fibula together and limit plantarflexion and dorsiflexion (Figs. 22-7, 22-8, and 22-9). An increase in the shock-attenuating quality of the athlete's shoes is also in order.

Fractures of the talar or calcaneal processes can occur during an inversion event and can often be missed during the acute assessment. A high suspicion of posterior process fracture should exist if the athlete has sustained a severe inversion injury or a forced hyperplantarflexion injury where the posterior talus is forced up into the ankle

Rehabilitation of the Athlete's Foot and Ankle

mortise. The athlete will complain of posterior lateral tenderness and pain with active great toe flexion or passive great toe extension (since the posterior process of the talus forms the tunnel for the flexor hallucis longus tendon).[2]

Lateral talar process fractures can occur after a dorsiflexion-inversion event. The physical exam is similar to a typical severe ankle sprain, with marked swelling and lateral joint line pain. For this reason, the trainer or physician should be acutely aware of the injury mechanism and rule out this injury acutely. The morbidity of this fracture is high if untreated because it often affects the congruity of the subtalar joint and leads to chronic pain and disability.[2]

Fracture of the anterior process of the calcaneous is yet another obscure possibility after a severe inversion-plantarflexion event or inversion-plantarflexion compression (inverting the ankle and getting it stepped on, for example). Exquisite tenderness anterior and distal to the lateral malleolus, just posterior to the calcaneocuboid joint, should be a warning that this fracture exists. Other complaints consistent with a typical severe ankle sprain will be present, so discrete palpation of specific structures is required.[2]

All of these articular process fractures require early recognition and generally conservative management with periods of immobilization and nonweight-bearing. Large displaced fragments may require surgical reduction. Nonunited fragments after conservative treatment may require excision secondary to chronic pain, but this should be delayed for months, sometimes up to a year, to provide every opportunity to resolve.[2]

Finally, when considering ankle injuries and some of the morbid sequellae that may occur, the trainer has to consider the possibility of intraarticular lesions. A chronically sprained ankle or a single severe event may produce enough compression or shear to cause an osteochondral lesion of the talus.[2,8] This should be a major concern when the athlete complains of "catching" in the joint. Dealing with this type of problem in any athletic population is difficult, but when adding the size and power of the typical football athlete, it is permissible to be guarded in the prognosis. Even after surgical debridment and drilling, prolonged nonweight-bearing and limited weight-bearing, and gradual and closely protected return to activity, it is not uncommon for the athlete to continue to experience pain, swelling, and occasional popping in the joint.

There are two reasons this discussion is important when dealing with football athletes. First is the obvious one; many football athletes are very large, and high compression and shear forces are practically inescapable during ankle sprain mechanisms. Second, the nature of the sport introduces high torsional moments, twisting and cutting at high speeds, with occasional simultaneous collisions. This sets up tremendously high forces applied to discrete anatomical structures in patterns those structures are ill designed to accept. The trainer and physician must be suspicious of obscure or occult fractures in and around the ankle joint any time a football athlete—or any athlete who participates in a high-velocity, horizontally oriented sport—sustains an inversion injury, especially one that includes a rotational or compressive component.

Dealing with a football athlete who has a foot or ankle injury is a mixture of blessings and curses. The blessings are that most football athletes have learned to accept some level of pain because of the nature of the sport and that most of the forces are torsional or horizontal in nature and respond to external support systems reasonably well. The curses are that the athletes are usually large and powerful, so the forces one is working to control are amazingly high and the forces introduced through collision with the opponent are completely unpredictable.

For these reasons, being willing to adapt and adjust on an incident-by-incident basis, and sometimes on a day-to-day basis, is necessary. It is also necessary to be very sensitive to the atypical complaint and the unusual injury mechanism, because these are the circumstances that produce the often missed, and often morbid, injuries.

Bibliography

1. Amis JA: Painful heel syndrome, *University of Cincinnati Sports Care Newsletter* 1(3): July 1987.
2. Amis JA, Gangl PM: When inversion injury is more than a "sprained ankle," *J Musculoskeletal Med* 4(9):68, 1987.
3. Arnheim D: *Modern principles of athletic training,* ed 7, St Louis, 1989, Mosby.

4. Cailliett R: *Foot and ankle pain,* ed 2, Philadelphia, 1968, FA Davis.
5. Chandler TJ, Kibler WB: A biomechanical approach to the prevention and treatment of plantar fasciitis, *Sports Med* 15(5):344, 1993.
6. Curtis M, Myerson, M, Szura B: Tarsometatarsal joint injuries in the athlete, *Am J Sports Med* 21(4):497, 1993.
7. Hicks JH: The three weightbearing mechanisms of the foot. In Evans FG, editor: *Biomechanical studies of the musculoskeletal system,* Springfield, Ill, 1972, Charles C Thomas.
8. Khan KM et al: Outcome of conservative and surgical management of navicular stress fracture in athletes, *Am J Sports Med* 20(6):657 1992.
9. Kibler WB, Goldberg C, Chandler TJ: Functional biomechanical deficits in running athletes with plantar fasciitis, *Am J Sports Med* 19(1):66 1991.
10. Kimura IF et al: Effects of the Airstirrup in controlling ankle inversion stress, *J Orthop Sports Phys Ther* 9(5):190 1987.
11. Nachbauer W, Nigg BM: Effects of arch height of the foot on ground reaction forces in running, *Med Sci Sports Exerc* 24(11):1264, 1992.
12. Nelson RM, Currier DP: *Clinical electrotherapy,* East Norwalk, Conn, 1987, Appleton-Century-Crofts.
13. Roy S, Irvin R: *Sports medicine: prevention, evaluation, management and rehabilitation,* Englewood Cliffs, NJ, 1983, Prentice-Hall.

17

The Foot and Ankle in Basketball

Thomas J. Herrmann

Basketball and other sports, such as volleyball, that have a significant vertical component present an interesting set of demands for the foot and ankle complex. Not only do these sports require quick directional changes and sudden acceleration and deceleration in a horizontal plane but also sudden acceleration and deceleration in a vertical plane. This repeated jumping and landing is usually coupled with a turn, twist, or anticipated directional change as the foot or feet are returning to the floor. In short, the athlete's expectation of the foot and ankle is that they will accept considerable force and redirect that force instantly along different lines in two planes of motion.

By far the most often occurring injury to the ankle in these vertical sports is the *inversion-plantarflexion ankle sprain*.[2] Commonly the aftereffect of landing on another athlete's foot, this injury usually leaves the jumping athlete unable to continue, at least temporarily, due to pain. While many athletes in primarily horizontal sports may be able to "walk off" a Grade I ankle sprain and return with a good tape job, it is the unusual jumping athlete that will return and play effectively after even a mild ankle sprain.

Basically, during an inversion-plantarflexion event, the anterior lateral ligament structure of the ankle is placed in a direct line with force being applied. As the talus inverts, the anterior talofibular ligament is put on stretch and eventually fails. (If extrapolation of data from knee ligament studies is valid, whether the ligament sustains a midsubstance rupture or an avulsion seems to depend on the rate at which the force is applied.) As the talus continues to invert and plantarflex, the calcaneofibular ligament, posterior talofibular ligament, and occasionally the ankle syndesmosis fail.[2]

Exposure to high-force/high-velocity events in plantarflexion-inversion is common in basketball. The incidence of mild to moderate, as opposed to severe, injuries can be attributed to many positive characteristics of athletes, including a high degree of strength, coordination, and proprioception. Basically, athletes have a well-developed ability to protect themselves, which helps to limit but does not eliminate the risk.

The troublesome variations on the inversion theme that appear in jumping sports are inversion injuries in neutral. This mechanism not only puts the lateral side of the joint at risk but the medial side and the syndesmosis as well. In what is referred to as an inversion–axial load mechanism, the inverted talus is forced up against the medial malleolus and can act as a wedge in the ankle mortise. This mechanism can produce concomitant injuries ranging from medial capsular impingement to bimalleolar fractures to osteochondral injuries.[13] The trainer and physician must be very sensitive to medial ankle complaints after an inversion event when examining a jumping athlete.

In my experience inversion–axial load mechanisms have produced some unusual injuries in jumping athletes:

A male intercollegiate basketball player sustained a Grade III injury and missed the remaining 7 weeks of the basketball season. Despite aggressive therapy and rehabilitation, he continued to complain of sharp anterior-medial ankle pain. Multiple imaging techniques (this was before the advent of magnetic resonance imaging technology) did not reveal any bony problems. Postseason arthroscopy revealed a scarred and hypertrophic anterior medial capsule.

A female high school basketball player missed 5 weeks after a Grade I inversion–axial load event. Her chief complaint was pain at the medial malleolus. Bone scan revealed a line of increased uptake obliquely from mid to proximal malleolous. This was interpreted as a *medial malleolar stress fracture*.

A male intercollegiate gymnast landed on an inverted ankle during a dismount from the rings. The high force of the landing caused a bimalleolar fracture and disruption of the syndesmosis. While this was not a difficult injury to recognize at the time of the incident, the athlete never returned to his performance level prior to the injury. Surgical reduction of the fractures and restoration of joint congruence was very good and therapy was extensive, but he continued to have chronic stiffness and pain in the extremes of motion required when performing and in high-impact events like tumbling and dismounts.

Although these brief injury scenarios digress a little from the idea of basketball injuries, they share a common factor: their etiology includes a significant vertical component. This vertical component adds an interesting and sometimes troubling wrinkle to the typical ankle sprain. It requires special attention in the rehabilitation process as the athlete develops protective mechanisms for use after a return to activity, which will be discussed later.

Other troubling consequences of high-force inversion and especially inversion-plantarflexion injuries are the occasional neurological insults they cause. The anatomical position of the superficial branch of the peroneal nerve and the sural nerve put them at considerable risk in severe inversion-type injuries. If the translation of the foot is great enough, the nerves can realize a traction force high enough to cause injury. It is important to recognize problems along the distribution of these nerves early in the treatment program so that an accurate assessment and prognosis can be made. Any athlete suffering from an ankle sprain who complains of numbness over the dorsal and lateral aspect of the foot must be carefully examined for *injury to the superficial peroneal nerve.* The lateral aspect of the foot and the fifth toe are innervated by the sural nerve, so numbness there must give rise to suspicion of sural nerve injury. Numbness in the web space between the first and second toe and/or motor deficits in the short toe extensors suggest an injury to the deep peroneal nerve.[1,3]

The integrity of these nerve distributions must be documented acutely and routinely checked as the athlete recovers. As the sprain heals, it is possible for the scarred ligament and capsular tissue to entrap one the branches of the nerve and cause problems that do not manifest themselves until weeks after the initial injury.[1]

If a nerve injury is suspected and documented, it can have a braking effect on the treatment protocol. Pain control and protection of the nerve(s) become a priority. Limiting motion that produces traction on the nerve is necessary. Electrical stimulation around the injury site with an interferential current may assist with pain control, and pulsed ultrasound may limit scarring around the nerve.[10] The athlete must be prepared for a slow recovery, however.

Reflex sympathetic dystrophy (RSD) is an uncommon but difficult problem to manage should it develop. Almost always following extremity trauma, it leaves the athlete experiencing exquisite pain, which is not always discrete to the injury. The trainer or physician must be sensitive to complaints of pain that seems disproportionate to the level of injury or that is described as burning or shooting. Characteristics of RSD include temperature changes, global swelling, hypersensitivity, and erythema as well as the pain complaints. Early clinical suspicion of RSD should be high even without hard diagnostic evidence, since diagnostic evidence via bone scan may take weeks or months to develop.[3,7]

If RSD is suspected or diagnosed, immediate measures to control the swelling should be initiated. Sensory desensitization, gentle compression, and range of motion within pain tolerance are key. It is sometimes necessary to pursue aggressive pain control measures such as nerve blocks for patient comfort and to facilitate therapy.[7] The athlete who develops RSD after an ankle sprain should be prepared for a long and arduous recovery over a period of months and be aware of the possibility of recurrence even after mild subsequent injury.

Achilles tendinitis secondary to an ankle sprain is not too uncommon an occurrence when working with jumping athletes. The most likely etiology is a loss of dorsiflexion on the injured side, which may lead to higher moments of force at the Achilles tendon. Another contributing factor may be that pushing the athlete to an early return while the ankle is still painful causes gait changes and muscle guarding, which lead to higher forces at the Achilles tendon and rapid overuse symptoms. Whatever the cause, a painful Achilles in the jumping athlete represents a considerable challenge and, left unresolved, can have devastating consequences.

Any athlete with mildly painful or Grade I Achilles tendinitis should be provided with a supportive orthosis for activity. This may be as simple as a ¼- to ½-inch heel lift or a tape application where the heel is slung in elastic tape to limit dorsiflexion and assist in push-off.[2] Grade II tendinitis, with swelling and range of motion limitations, requires the usual support regimen as well as limitations on activities more strict than "pain as guide." It is often necessary to restrict jumping and sprinting activities as well as repetitive drills for the basketball athlete in order to minimize the instantaneous loading of the inflamed Achilles.

Grade III Achilles tendinitis, with crepitus, severe motion restriction, and painful daily activity, is a condition that should preclude the jumping athlete from participation.[11] It is nearly impossible to protect this athlete adequately with tape, brace, or pad from the potentially disastrous event of an Achilles tendon rupture. It may be necessary for the athlete to spend some time nonweight-bearing or at least in a plantarflexed walking orthosis in order to protect the tendon while it is acutely inflamed. A gradual restoration of the normal length, elasticity, and strength of the tendon is vital. Maintenance of the athlete's general level of conditioning should also be a high priority through the use of swimming and other aquatic exercise programs, stationary cycling if tolerated, and weight training.[12] The return to jumping activities may be weeks or months away based on the response of the athlete to treatment and rehabilitation.

Other problems that frequently arise when working with basketball athletes are problems of the forefoot. Sudden directional changes, pivoting, and twisting put tremendous pressure on the metatarsals and metatarsophalangeal (MTP) joints. Calluses, blisters, and various forms of metatarsalgia are common.

Calluses may seem harmless, and some athletes mark their development with a sort of pride as evidence of how hard they are working. The buildup of calloused skin, can present a problem, however, if left unattended. Thickened callus at the first and fifth MTP joints is common and typical of normal force distributions. When this buildup is extensive, however, the dead skin may become mobile on the live skin below, causing friction between the layers. This friction leads to *blister formation* between the live skin and the callus, which is painful and often disabling to the athlete. Many of these blisters become bloody or infected and difficult to manage. Complete removal of the callus exposes so much tender new skin that the athlete usually cannot bear to play. Failure to remove any of the callus and simply addressing the blister does not remove the irritant. The most effective approach is usually to pare down the callus to a level where it is almost translucent, then drain the underlying blister using sterile technique. A sterile dressing must then follow and should be applied with some pressure to inhibit any refill of the blister. A donut pad for pressure relief should be applied during activity to reduce the force at the blister.[2] As the tenderness subsides, the callus should be spared routinely, but one should exercise considerable patience when approaching the new skin below. Exposing this new skin too soon will cause the athlete considerable discomfort and is likely to prohibit activity. One should only totally remove the callus and expose the new skin fully if the blister below the callus is infected or continues to refill with pussy or bloody fluid.

Callus under the midmetatarsals should alert the trainer to a failing or failed metatarsal arch. These athletes may also have a Morton's foot, hammer toes, a cavus foot, and/or all of the above. The chief complaint of the basketball athlete with this type of callus formation is pain at the heads of the midmetatarsals and occasionally dorsal foot pain. Considering the amount of time the basketball athlete spends on the forefoot, forefoot discomfort can become quite distracting and eventually debilitating.

Most pain at the second, third, and fourth metatarsal can be relieved by placing a teardrop-shaped metatarsal post just proximal to the heads of the bones. This acts to distribute the force away from the middle of the forefoot and to allow the first and fifth to bear the brunt of the force at footfall. A pad under the entire forefoot will not redistribute forces but will cushion the forefoot when general metatarsalgia is the athlete's primary complaint. It is important to note that failure to address metatarsal pain early may lead to less manageable problems, such as metatarsal stress fractures, fractures, or neuroma.

Arch and heel pain in the jumping athlete is not uncommon and can have various etiologies. More often than not, it is repetitive jumping that underlies the problem. The constant loading and unloading of the plantar fascia and plantar ligaments at high velocity can lead to sprains of the longitudinal arch structures, strains of the long toe flexors, especially the flexor hallucis longus, painful heel syndrome, or midfoot pain.[12]

One of the simplest ways to thwart the insidious attack of the sport on the arches and foot and their supporting structures is to carefully watch for signs of degraded footwear. Much of the risk from vertical forces can be managed well with a maintenance or increase in the shock-attenuating characteristics of the shoes.[8] For the high-performance high school or college athlete, it is unlikely that one pair, or even two pairs, of shoes will survive the season. Even the best athletic footwear loses its shock-attenuating and foot-controlling qualities long before it loses its looks. The gradual loss of shoe quality is sometimes best assessed by the athlete. Have the athlete put on an identical pair of new shoes and move about. If the shoe is appreciably softer to the feel and firmer with directional changes, then the old shoes are clearly on their way out.

The practice of many basketball players of holding a "good" pair of shoes in reserve for the games and wearing a practice pair at other times also contributes to leg and foot wear and tear. Athletes practice longer and more frequently than they play games. Why hold a good pair of shoes in reserve for the less demanding activity and suffer through the tougher activity in old, hard, worn shoes? It makes more sense for an athlete to wear a single pair of shoes until it is time to retire them to the back of the closet and replace them with a new pair. With this system, the athlete may go through three or four pairs of shoes in one basketball season. (I have worked with college basketball players who have gone through as many as seven pair of shoes in one season, though this was rare.)

Fifth metatarsal fractures of various descriptions are common in a population of jumping athletes. Turning or pivoting at high velocity during basketball creates considerable torsional forces through the midfoot and puts the fifth metatarsal at considerable risk. A midshaft fifth metatarsal fracture often follows an incident during which the athlete is turning and is stepped on by another player. As the athlete pushes off, the opponent's foot acts as a lever across the midfoot or fixes the forefoot to the floor as the athlete moves the hindfoot away. Either of these can

Rehabilitation of the Athlete's Foot and Ankle

cause a fracture through the shaft of the metatarsals and seems to put the fifth at particular risk.

Jones fractures in basketball athletes, or any vertically oriented athlete, present a difficult scenario. Given the propensity for delayed union or nonunion of these fractures in the general public, a high-performance basketball athlete should be made well aware of that probability. For many sports medicine orthopedists, internal fixation of the Jones fracture is the treatment of choice so that the athlete's ankle motion and lower leg strength can be maintained while limiting micromotion at the fracture site. While it is unlikely that an athlete can participate in sport early after internal fixation, at least they can participate in early rehabilitation.

Lisfranc sprains and fractures present great difficulty for the jumping athlete. Even a small amount of abnormal motion through the tarsometatarsal joints can cause disability and preclude jumping or high-force directional changes. Protection of the midfoot with tape or a pad offers some relief, but the athlete should be prepared for a slow return to full activity. It is sometimes necessary for the athlete to undergo surgical stabilization of the affected joint in order to obtain acceptable pain relief and function.[4,5]

Rehabilitation of the foot and ankle complex in the jumping athlete presents some interesting challenges. Of course the primary concern of the athlete is the return of jumping power and height. The primary concern of the trainer or therapist, however, should be the return of basic strength and neuromotor control. The power will return, but in the absence of proprioception and intrinsic foot control, the power is wasted.

In the acute phase, cryokinetic techniques have a dramatic effect on swelling and pain.[12] By applying cold, with immersion baths, ice packs, or cold-compression devices, in conjunction with or immediately followed by active motion and muscle action, the vascular and vasomotor responses are accentuated. With elevation, gravity also lends a helping hand in the movement of the swelling. This activation of the venous and lymphatic pumping action is vital to the evacuation of swelling, and the evacuation of swelling is vital to pain control and muscle function.

One must resist the temptation to move too quickly to restore what the athlete believes are the essential components of lower leg strength, the gastroc-soleus complex, at the expense of basic strengthening of the intrinsic and extrinsic foot muscles. Early in the rehabilitation process, great attention must be paid to strengthening of the short and long flexors and extensors of the toes. Toe pumps, towel gathering exercises, and marble pick-up exercises are very valuable. Isometric exercises for the primary ankle movers can be begun immediately to help offset the loss of neuromotor control and to minimize the loss of strength (though some strength loss is inevitable).

Early progressive resistance routines after an ankle or foot injury to a jumping athlete must still focus on restoring control and power in the evertors and invertors. The function of the peroneal muscles in protecting the ankle is well documented, and the function of the posterior tibialis in supporting the midfoot and providing propulsion is also well known.[6] Their role is even more important when the primary risk to the ankle comes through a vertical plane, where the decelerative forces are higher and the reaction times are shorter. Concentrating on these muscles early in the process of rehabilitation helps assure that they are up to the demands created when the most powerful movers of the ankle come up to speed.

Retraining the gastroc-soleus complex and the anterior tibialis for the production of power, especially jumping power, sometimes requires some unusual activities. While toe and heel raises and aggressive progressive resistance activities will provide strength and girth, the production of jumping power and repetitive power requires a short response time and high muscle fiber recruitment. Failing to develop, or redevelop, these performance characteristics will cause the athlete to feel "slow off the floor," a considerable problem for the basketball athlete (or any jumper). Most of these performance qualities of the lower leg can be well addressed through the use of plyometric activities.

The essence of plyometric activities is to create some sort of external load, have that load applied to the muscle at velocity, and then respond to that load in the opposite direction. Basically, the muscle is required to accept force and then generate force in response.[2] While there is some risk inherent in this type of training, there are considerable benefits to be gained as long as the risks are introduced progressively and controlled.

For the jumping athlete recovering from a foot or ankle injury, plyometric activities can be broken down into rehabilitation activities and performance activities. The rehabilitation activities are done in controlled environments, at low velocities and in definite patterns. The performance activities are done in environments that are less controlled but not totally free, at higher velocities and in patterns that can be changed or that are undetermined. The trainer or therapist can mark out a pattern on the floor and have the athlete hop or jump to specific marks in a set pattern. This pattern may include X's, Z's, straight lines forward or backward, and squares. If the marks are numbered or colored, the trainer or therapist can advance the athlete into a more aggressive pattern by simply calling out the number or color of the mark to which to move.

The upper end of the plyometric training program in a rehabilitation setting is to add small barriers to the movement routine. These can vary in height from a few inches up to a foot or more. The athlete then has to clear the barriers through the same patterns that were established earlier in the program. The benefit to this variation is that the athlete must accentuate the vertical component of the movement and must rebound in a vertical plane instantly to clear the next barrier. This helps the athlete restablish the "speed off the floor" that many jumpers find essential. It also has considerable confidence-building effects, for it is often quite suprising to find the anxiety that a 3-inch barrier causes the athlete who is recovering from an ankle or foot injury.

Needless to say, all of these upper end activities are performed with considerable protection. A solid ankle or foot tape job (sometimes both), or a brace, and shoes that are in competition condition are essential to minimize the risk while maximizing the activity. This stage of the rehabilitation and training process also provides the trainer with the opportunity to try out a number of options for the creation of an external support system in a controlled environment. This gives the athlete confidence in the system prior to the return to participation and leaves the athlete with one less thing to worry about.

In summary, landing from a jump is a challenge, in terms of both the skeletal and musculoskeletal forces involved and the neuromotor responses required. Add to this the in-air collision in basketball, which changes posture and position, the proximity of the feet of opponents and teammates, and the fact that in almost all instances, the athlete is concentrating on something other than landing, and it is clearly fortunate that more ankle and foot injuries do not occur.

High-velocity directional changes in two planes of motion exert tremendous torsional forces through the midfoot and metatarsals. In these events, the skeletal system cannot take full advantage of its inherent strength along the long axis but must accept and generate forces through oblique planes. This places high focal forces on the fifth metatarsal, the navicular, and the tarsometatarsal joints. Exposure to the risk of overuse injuries and stress fractures in these areas is high, and this requires considerable awareness on the part of the trainer or physician.

Finally, the loss of proprioception is considerable and rapid after an ankle or foot injury. Failure to address this loss early and thoroughly will ensure a disappointing return to participation for the athlete. Building a rehabilitation program that provides good neuromotor functioning early will make the restoration of power easier and the recovery of the athlete ultimately quicker and more complete.

Bibliography

1. Amis JA, Gangl PM: When inversion injury is more than a "sprained ankle," *J Musculoskeletal Med* 4(9):68, 1987.
2. Arnheim D: *Modern principles of athletic training,* ed 7, St Louis, 1989, Mosby.
3. Cailliett R: *Foot and ankle pain,* ed 2, Philadelphia, 1968, FA Davis.
4. Curtis M, Myerson, M, Szura B: Tarsometatarsal joint injuries in the athlete, *Am J Sports Med* 21(4):497, 1993.
5. Faciszewski T, Burks RT, Manaster BJ: Subtle injuries to the Lisfranc joint, *J Bone Joint Surg* 72A:1519, 1990.

6. Hartley A: *Practical joint assessment,* St Louis, 1990, Mosby.

7. McNerney JE: Reflex sympathetic dystrophy, traumatic and post-operative presentation and management in the lower extremity, *Clin Podiatr Med Surg* 8(2):1991.

8. Milgrom C, Finestone A, Shlamkovitch N: Prevention of overuse injuries of the foot by improved shoe shock attenuation: a randomized prospective study, *Clin Orthop* 1992.

9. Nachbauer W, Nigg BM: Effects of arch height of the foot on ground reaction forces in running, *Med Sci Sports Exerc* 24(11):1992.

10. Nelson RM, Currier DP: *Clinical electrotherapy,* East Norwalk, Conn, 1987, Appleton-Century-Crofts.

11. Rovere G et al: Retrospective comparison of taping and ankle stabilizers in preventing ankle injuries, *Am J Sports Med* 16:1988.

12. Roy S, Irvin R: Sports medicine: prevention, evaluation, management and rehabilitation, Englewood Cliffs, NJ, 1983, Prentice-Hall.

13. Taga I et al: Articular lesions in ankles with lateral ligament injury, *Am J Sports Med* 21(1):1993.

14. Torg J: Ankle and foot problems in the athlete, *Clin Sports Med* 1:1982.

18

Rehabilitation of Baseball Injuries

Richard V. Abdo

The games of baseball and softball are characterized by periods of relative inactivity interspersed with sudden and explosive action. Initiation of a sprint to steal a base or retrieve a ball can create rapid and appreciable forces on soft tissue structures, leading to acute injury. Poor weather conditions or an improperly groomed field with divots increases the risk of acute injury to the foot and ankle. When collisions in the base paths as well as hitters and fielders being struck by the baseball are added to this spectrum, it becomes easy to understand that the majority of injuries to the foot and ankle are acute conditions rather than conditions caused by overuse.

In contrast, pitchers and catchers will have more injuries to soft tissue caused by chronic overuse. The repetitive action of a pitcher's windup and delivery can expose both the pivot and lead foot to tendinopathies and to impingement of the ankle and first metatarsophalangeal (MTP) joint. The catcher has probably the most physically demanding position in baseball. This position requires the repetitive alternation between a squatting and vertical position as well as explosive thrusts to make throws to second base and sprints to back up first base on ground balls. Impingement syndrome or inflammatory conditions of the posterior ankle or heel may result.

Base sliding is the single activity that places a player most at risk for an injury, particularly of the foot and ankle. Although an injury can be sustained by the player covering the base, the player performing the slide is more frequently injured. The mechanics of sliding have been previously analyzed.[11] The four phases of sliding are sprint, attainment of sliding position, airborne, and landing. Injuries most frequently occur during the landing phase when the body is absorbing the impact from the ground and the base. The most popular and probably the safest slide is feet first in a semisitting position with the extended leg making initial contact with the base and the bottom leg bent beneath the player. It is important to maintain the top leg about 6 inches off the ground. If the cleats catch the ground or the foot strikes the base improperly, an injury involving plantarflexion or external rotation of the ankle may occur. This may result in an ankle sprain, fracture, syndesmotic disruption, or an injury to the os trigonum. In performing the hook slide, a player slides to the side of a base to avoid a tag and attempts to hook the base with the toes and forefoot of the lead leg. Mechanically, this is a poor slide that carries an increased risk of a lower extremity fracture. The head-first slide is potentially dangerous because it exposes the player to upper extremity, head, and neck injuries.

Prevention of base-sliding injuries would greatly improve the safety of the game. Many of the injuries could be avoided by instruction to improve sliding technique, better conditioning of the player, avoidance of alcohol use during recreational games, and changes in the league rules to make sliding illegal. However, these measures are either impractical or require an active role by the participants and therefore are subject to less than ideal compliance. Many foot- and ankle-related injuries incurred on the base paths are caused by the rapid deceleration and torque that are experienced by the player when stationary bases are encountered. Break-away bases have been found to appreciably decrease the rate of injury from base sliding. A 98% reduction of injuries has been achieved by installing break-away bases in fields used by recreational softball leagues.[18] More recently, an 80% reduction in sliding-related injuries has been noted in the high-performance college and professional baseball population because of the use of break-away bases.[17] It is highly recommended that break-away bases be used as the single most important preventive measure in decreasing softball and baseball injuries, particularly those injuries related to the foot and ankle.

This chapter reviews the common goals and basic methods of rehabilitation that are generic to most foot and ankle injuries sustained while playing baseball. The injury-specific concepts of evaluation, treatment, rehabilitation, and prevention are presented for acute injuries, including ankle sprains and fractures, posterior ankle impingement, peroneal tendon dislocation-subluxation, and contusions. The review of chronic injuries includes Achilles tendinitis, retrocalcaneal bursitis, and hallux synovitis-rigidus.

Goals of Rehabilitation

It is critical to recognize that rehabilitation of an injury begins at the time of the injury rather than at a specified interval after the injury or after tissues have healed. It is helpful to conceptualize the goals of rehabilitation as occurring in three phases: early, intermediate, and late.[2] In the early phase, the goals of rehabilitation are to diminish the inflammatory response and pain to permit more rapid return of pain-free motion and flexibility. This will have far-reaching benefits in the later phases of rehabilitation by minimizing adhesions and contractures, thereby permitting efficient return of muscle function. The intermediate phase involves restoration of the strength and endurance of specific muscles. The late phase of rehabilitation concentrates on the functional return to sport-specific activities as well as the enhancement of cardiovascular endurance. The attainment of these goals is accomplished by specific rehabilitative methods.

Several important rehabilitation modalities that can be applied to the treatment of injuries to the foot and ankle include heat, cold, electricity, mechanical manipulation, and therapeutic exercise.[3] Heat may be applied superficially (by whirlpool, contrast baths, hot packs, or hydrocollator baths) or through the deep thermal effects of ultrasound therapy. Cryotherapy may be applied through the use of ice bags, ice massage, ice baths, gel packs, and coolant sprays. Electrical therapy can be used in various forms, including transcutaneous electrical nerve stimulation, electrical muscle stimulation, and iontophoresis. Mechanical manipulation includes massage, traction, and compression. Therapeutic exercise can involve various types of strength training (e.g., isometric, isotonic, isokinetic), stretching for motion and flexibility, and cardiorespiratory endurance activities, such as swimming or use of a cross-country ski machine (Fig. 18-1) for aerobic conditioning.

Ankle Sprains

Injury to the lateral ligamentous structures of the ankle commonly occurs from an inversion and plantarflexion force. In baseball, this injury typically occurs during base sliding when the foot strikes the stationary bag. An ankle sprain may also occur when a fielder steps on an area of uneven ground, such as the junction between the base path and infield grass on a well-groomed diamond. Because the anterior talofibular liga-

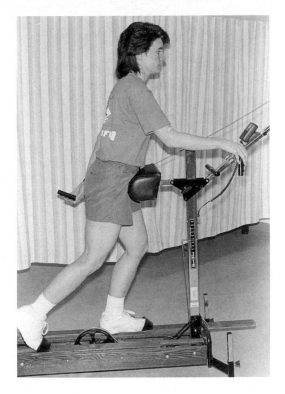

Fig. 18-1 A cross-country ski machine provides cross-training for aerobic conditioning.

ment is more taut in plantarflexion and the calcaneofibular ligament is more taut in neutral position, the position of the foot at the time the force is applied will determine the degree and nature of the injury. The anterior talofibular ligament is the most commonly injured ligament. The posterior talofibular ligament is rarely affected.

Diagnosis

The diagnosis of an ankle sprain is made by a history of a twisting injury to the ankle combined with lateral pain and swelling of the ankle. The severity of the injury depends on the structures torn and the consequent degree and extent of pain, swelling, and tenderness. A Grade I sprain is a partial tear of the anterior talofibular ligament. Swelling and tenderness are isolated to the anterolateral aspect of the ankle just anterior to the fibula and over the sinus tarsi. The anterior drawer sign will be negative.

Roentgenography reveals no increased talar tilt with application of inversion stress. Grade II sprains involve a complete tear of the anterior talofibular ligament with the calcaneofibular ligament remaining intact. Swelling and tenderness may be more appreciable. The anterior drawer sign will now be positive such that anterior displacement of the heel will create forward subluxation of the talus. A dimple sign overlying the site of injury to the ligament at the anterolateral corner of the ankle joint is created by the negative pressure between the joint and skin as the talus moves forward.[5] Roentgenography with application of inversion stress continues to reveal normal findings with an intact calcaneofibular ligament. Grade III sprains involve complete rupture of the anterior talofibular and calcaneofibular ligaments. Swelling and tenderness are extensive; the anterior drawer sign is distinctly positive. Talar tilt is positive, with inversion stress both clinically and radiographically. It is important to use radiographs to compare the talar tilt of the injured side with that of the uninjured side. Most authors believe that a difference of 10 degrees or more is significant and indicates extensive instability of the lateral ligament.[19]

It is critical that the routine ankle sprain be differentiated from the more uncommon syndesmosis or "high" ankle sprain. Relatively little information exists in the literature regarding syndesmosis sprains that are not accompanied by a fracture.[7,9,13] An external rotation force to the ankle will create a medial ankle injury (rupture of the deltoid ligament or fracture of the medial malleolus) and tearing of the ligaments of the distal tibiofibular syndesmosis. This injury almost always occurs during base sliding, when the cleats catch on the ground or when the foot strikes the base and is forced into external rotation. It may also occur as a fielder sprints to tag a base and hits the base awkwardly, causing dorsiflexion, eversion, and external rotation. The swelling and tenderness more preferentially will be located proximal to the ankle joint over the syndesmosis. On examination, external rotation of the foot while stabilizing the leg will create pain at the syndesmosis. The squeeze test will also be positive.[16] Pain at the syndesmosis with compression of the fibula to the tibia at the level of the middle calf suggests a diagnosis of syndesmosis sprain. These acute injuries have been classified as a sprain without diastasis (Type I), latent diastasis (Type II), or frank diastasis (Type III).[13] In Type I, no diastasis exists between the fibula and tibia on external rotation-abduction stress radiography. With the latent type, diastasis between the tibia and fibula occurs on stress radiography, but the syndesmosis remains reduced on unstressed radiography. Type III reveals diastasis of the syndesmosis on radiography even without stress. It is important to obtain full-length tibia–fibula X-rays to determine whether a proximal fibula fracture is present. The syndesmosis sprain typically produces longer disability than does the more routine ankle sprain.[16]

Treatment

The first phase of rehabilitation is to diminish the inflammatory response and pain. This is accomplished by protection, rest, ice, compression, and elevation (PRICE). An air stirrup provides functional protection by preventing inversion and eversion while permitting plantarflexion and dorsiflexion. Initially, crutches are usually needed for comfort, but progressive weight-bearing to tolerance is encouraged. Cryotherapy is applied in the form of ice packs, ice massage, or cold water immersion, providing analgesia, diminished muscle spasm, and decreased permeability of vessels and edema by vasoconstriction. Application of cold substances should be performed several times a day, limited to 20 to 30 minutes at each application to avoid frostbite. Cold water immersion, although more effective around the bony and contoured ankle, has the disadvantage of requiring a dependent position, which would act to increase swelling. Cryotherapy should be avoided in patients with underlying vascular disease or in patients with sensitivity to cold. Compression is typically accomplished by the use of an elastic wrap starting distally and wrapping proximally. When swelling is severe, commercially available compression pumps may be more effective during the initial several days of acute swelling. Elevation above the level of the heart with pillows is important

to decrease swelling. If the patient finds it difficult to maintain the extremity on the pillows during sleep, placement of a suitcase or another large object beneath the mattress at the foot of the bed may be helpful to achieve elevation. The inflammatory response may also be diminished during the first week after injury by the use of nonsteroidal antiinflammatory medication.

The second phase of rehabilitation to restore motion, strength, and endurance commences with reduction in swelling and improvement of the athlete's comfort with regard to motion and progressive weight-bearing. The initial efforts at regaining motion should be through open chain exercises in which the extremity is free in space rather than fixed, such as with the foot planted on the ground. Passive and active assisted exercises are performed to eliminate adhesions that will have formed about the ankle and subtalar joints. These exercises should be performed with the athlete relaxed and without causing pain. The Achilles tendon should be stretched. Mobilization of the intrinsic muscles of the foot can be accomplished by toe curl exercises. The patient is instructed to use his or her toes to wrinkle a towel placed on the floor. Eventually, weights can be added to the opposite end of the towel to increase resistance. Isotonic resistive exercises are typically accomplished by the use of surgical (rubber) tubing for plantarflexion, dorsiflexion, inversion, and eversion. Emphasis is placed on the return of eversion strength. The peroneal muscles are strengthened to the maximum degree when the ankle is in a position of plantarflexion. This objective is most simply accomplished by having the patient lie on the side with the medial aspect of the involved ankle resting on the arm of a couch with a 2- or 3-pound weight about the forefoot.[14] With the foot in plantarflexion, eversion of the ankle is performed. The weight is increased by 2 pounds when the patient can perform 3 sets of 10 repetitions of the exercise twice a day. A total of 15 to 20 pounds is the goal.

The final phase of rehabilitation for an ankle sprain is the functional return to baseball by the use of agility exercises for balance and proprioception. Conditioning is initiated with bicycling, swimming, and aquatic running. With improvement in comfort and strength of the ankle, the exercise of running in a straight line on even ground is added to the program. During this phase, progression to closed chain exercises (foot planted on the ground) includes heel raises as well as a balance board (Fig. 18-2) to regain proprioception. Agility drills are then advanced to the performance of hopping maneuvers, back peddling, running in figure eights and zigzags, and carioca running (sidestepping, alternating one foot over the other). In baseball players, plyometric exercises are important to regain the power necessary for the explosive maneuvers needed in the base paths and the field. The principle of plyometric exercise is that eccentric prestretching of muscles creates tension and ultimately increased power during a concentric contraction.[1] As training progresses, the rate of this

reflex eccentric prestretch followed by concentric contraction will increase, as will neuromuscular efficiency. Examples of plyometric exercises include power jumps or leaps and the throwing of a weighted object. These exercises should not be performed more than 2 to 3 times a week.

Controversy exists regarding the need for surgery for Grade III ligamentous injuries to the ankle.[7] Some physicians believe that the relatively low number of patients in whom functional instability develops after a severe ankle sprain does not justify surgical repair in all patients. Other professionals recommend operative repair of acute Grade III ligament injuries to the ankle in the young high-performance athlete.

Type I syndesmosis sprains are treated symptomatically and according to the same principles as a standard ankle sprain. Type II syndesmosis sprains require cast immobilization and nonweight-bearing for 4 weeks, followed by 2 weeks of partial weight-bearing. Type III syndesmosis sprains require surgical reduction and stabilization with a syndesmosis screw. If plastic deformation of the fibula prevents satisfactory reduction of the syndesmosis, a proximal fibular osteotomy is performed to bring the distal tibiofibular joint into proper position.[13] It is important for the athlete to realize that even a Type I syndesmosis sprain may take nearly twice as long for recovery as a Grade III standard ankle sprain.[16]

Prevention

Because many ankle injuries occur during base sliding, one of the most important preventive measures would be to substitute break-away bases for standard stationary bases. Wellgroomed playing surfaces will help to eliminate the twisting injuries that occur on uneven ground or in divots. A regular program to maintain strength and flexibility is important. Proper footwear and protection of the ankle can be accomplished through the use of taping, ankle stabilizers, or functional orthotics. Biomechanical problems, such as a varus heel, should be identified and addressed through the use of modifications to the shoe or orthotic devices.

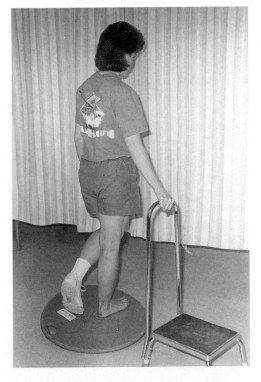

Fig. 18-2 The Biomechanical Ankle Platform System (BAPS) board (Camp International, Jackson, Mich) provides proprioceptive training for ankle sprain rehabilitation.

Ankle Fractures

Similar to ankle sprains, ankle fractures tend to occur on the base paths and are caused by the athlete's cleat catching the ground or by excessive abnormal force when the foot collides with the base. Many ankle fractures are caused by an inversion plantarflexion force, but pronation and external rotation may also be the mechanism of injury.

Diagnosis

Patients with ankle fractures typically present with severe pain and swelling beyond what would be anticipated with an ankle sprain. Swelling and tenderness will be more preferentially located over the site of fracture rather than at soft tissue and ligamentous structures. Crepitance or frank deformity and instability through the fracture site(s) may be present. Nearly all fractures of the ankle involve the lateral malleolus. Medial swelling and tenderness signify a rupture of the deltoid ligament or medial malleolus (bimalleolar) fracture. A more severe injury may be accompanied by a posterior malleolus (trimalleolar) fracture. Tenderness at the level of the proximal fibula should alert the physician to a Maisonneuve's injury. This injury is created by an external rotation abduction force that ruptures the deltoid ligament, ankle capsule, syndesmotic ligaments, and interosseous membrane, with the force finally exiting at the lateral proximal leg with a fracture of the fibular neck. Radiography of the ankle in this injury will show no fracture but may demonstrate widening of the syndesmosis and medial clear space.

Treatment

The athlete should be initially immobilized in a splint, with application of ice and elevation of the extremity above the level of the heart. Radiography is necessary to delineate the exact nature of the injury and the degree of fracture displacement. A nondisplaced fracture, particularly an isolated lateral malleolus, is treated by 6 weeks of cast immobilization, nonweight-bearing for the initial 3 to 4 weeks, and then by partial weight-bearing. After cast immobilization, the ankle will need to be protected for an additional 4 to 6 weeks, typically with an ankle stirrup. During this time, the focus of rehabilitation is on restoring joint mobility of the ankle as well as the hindfoot. This goal can be accomplished through a series of mobilization techniques to achieve satisfactory glide between the tibia and talus as well as the talus and calcaneus. Stretching can be accomplished through proprioceptive neuromuscular facilitation, particularly for the Achilles tendon.[1] In performing the hold-relax technique, the trainer places the ankle in an initial stretch position of dorsiflexion, after which the athlete isometrically resists the force, holding for a count of 10. This is followed by placement of the ankle in a new stretch position beyond the original position. Isokinetic exercises on one of the commercial machines (e.g., Cybex Systems, Cybex, Ronkonkoma, NY; LIDO Systems, Loredan Biomedical Co., Davis, Calif; Biodex, Biodex Medical Systems, Shirley, NY) is important to regain muscle strength and endurance (Fig. 18-3). Even during the period of cast immobilization, conditioning can be accomplished by aquatic training and bicycling. The commencement of running and agility drills requires satisfactory healing of bone.

Prevention

Prevention of ankle fractures in baseball is similar to that of ankle sprains: the use of break-away bases, well-groomed playing fields, and, to prevent the recurrence of fractures, proper ankle rehabilitation and protection of the ankle for several months after the return to competition.

Posterior Ankle Impingement

In baseball, posterior ankle impingement injury may occur acutely with forced plantarflexion of the ankle, most commonly the result of a hook slide into a base. On a chronic basis, the catcher is at risk for development of posterior talar impingement because the ankle is kept in repetitive plantarflexion during maneuvers in the

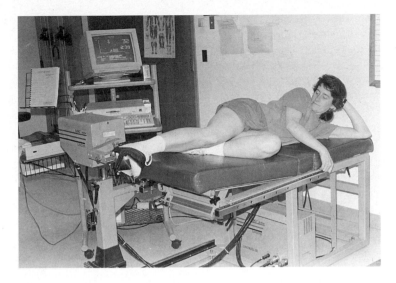

Fig. 18-3 Isokinetic exercises are performed for muscle strength and endurance.

stance position behind the plate. This is sometimes referred to as os trigonum syndrome when radiography demonstrates a bony ossicle off the posterolateral tubercle of the talus. Whether from thickened inflamed capsule and synovium or a bony ossicle, extremes of plantarflexion will cause compression between the tibia and calcaneus.[15]

Diagnosis

The athlete will complain of posterolateral ankle pain located anterior to the Achilles tendon and retrocalcaneal space. Tenderness will occur with deep palpation over the posterolateral structures of the ankle. This injury can usually be differentiated from that in the more laterally placed peroneal tendons. Flexor hallucis longus tendinitis can be differentiated from this condition by the location of symptoms posteromedially and the lack of exacerbation of symptoms by forced plantarflexion. In cases that are difficult to localize or diagnose, a bone scan may be helpful.

Treatment

Relative rest by avoiding the inciting activities or position is important for resolution of posterior talar impingement. During the initial phase, gentle dorsiflexion stretching exercises are important to minimize posterior ankle and subtalar joint capsular adhesions. Application of ice and the use of nonsteroidal antiinflammatory medication is recommended. The athlete should avoid shoes with increased heel height. If these treatment measures fail, a local injection of cortisone can be considered. Surgery through a posterolateral approach for debridement and excision of an os trigonum is infrequently needed for the patient whose condition is refractory to conservative management.

Prevention

Instruction on proper sliding technique, avoidance of the hook slide, and the use of break-away bases would help to prevent the acute injuries that initiate posterior talar impingement syndrome.

Peroneal Tendon Dislocation/Subluxation

The peroneal tendons are restrained behind the fibula in their fibroosseous tunnel by the superior peroneal retinaculum (SPR) and a fibrocartilaginous rim extending along the posterolateral lip of the lateral malleolus. Dislocation or subluxation typically occurs when a force creates dorsiflexion of the ankle and valgus of the heel accompanied by reflex contraction of the peroneal muscles. This forces the peroneus longus and brevis tendons laterally and anteriorly, rupturing the soft tissue restraints or avulsing a fragment of bone from the lateral malleolus. In baseball, this injury may occur when the athlete plants the foot with an unexpected lack of support beneath the heel. A fielder may land on the forefoot with the heel sinking into a divot, or a baserunner may land on a base with the forefoot only, while the heel drops to the ground.

Management will depend on the type of injury sustained (Fig. 18-4).[8,12] With a Grade I injury, the SPR and periosteum are torn from the lateral malleolus. The tendons may be stable when reduced. With a Grade II injury, the fibrocartilaginous rim is ruptured. In a Grade III injury, a cortical rim avulsion occurs. The tendons are usually unstable when reduced in Grade II and III injuries.

Diagnosis

A history of an injury with a mechanism of ankle dorsiflexion and heel valgus accompanied by posterolateral ankle pain, swelling, and ecchymosis will raise the suspicion of dislocation of the peroneal tendons. The athlete will often hear a snap at the time of injury and be unable to ambulate. If still dislocated at the time of evaluation, the tendons will be palpated in their abnormal position. Radiography is important to check for the presence of an avulsion fracture. This is a pathognomonic sign that is best visualized on the mortise view. The athlete with chronic dislocation of the peroneal tendon will complain of a sensation of the ankle giving way or popping, and apprehension or frank dislocation of the tendons may occur with resisted eversion.

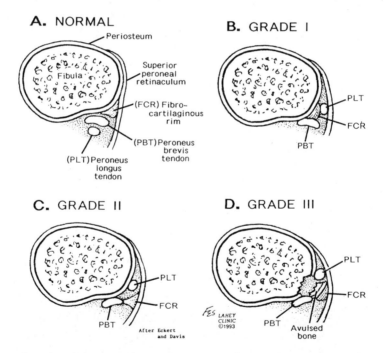

Fig. 18-4 Peroneal tendon dislocation. **A,** Normal anatomy. **B,** Grade I: rupture of superior peroneal retinaculum and periosteum. **C,** Grade II: rupture of fibrocartilaginous rim. **D,** Grade III: avulsion of cortical rim from posterolateral aspect of lateral malleolus. (Adapted from Mann RA, Coughlin MJ, editors: *Surgery of the foot and ankle*, ed 6, vol 1, St Louis, 1993, Mosby–Year Book, p. 1170; with permission; conceptualized using the grading system found in Eckert WR, Davis EA Jr: Acute rupture of the peroneal retinaculum, *J Bone Joint Surg* 58(A):670, 1976; with permission; reprinted with permission of the Lahey Clinic, Burlington, Mass.)

Rehabilitation of the Athlete's Foot and Ankle

Treatment

For an acute peroneal tendon dislocation, if the tendons are not already located behind the fibula, a reduction is attempted by recreation of the original force followed by gentle pressure over the tendons with plantarflexion and inversion of the foot. If the tendons are stable (Grade I), the athlete is placed in a short leg cast with enough plantarflexion to maintain reduction and is kept nonweight-bearing for 6 weeks. Surgery is required for the acute injury with unstable tendons or an avulsion fracture or for a chronic condition. Surgery for an acute injury involves repair of the ruptured soft tissue and plication of the SPR (Grades I and II), or internal fixation (Grade III). For the athlete with chronic dislocation of the peroneal tendon, a variety of described procedures exist that involve repair or reconstruction of the SPR, rerouting of the tendon, or deepening of the posterior fibular groove. Operation is typically followed by 4 weeks of nonweight-bearing in a short leg cast. Rehabilitation is similar to that of ankle fractures, with increased emphasis on flexibility and strength of the peroneal muscle. Conditioning in the pool or on the bike is performed during the early stages of phase II of rehabilitation, when the concentration is on return of strength and endurance of the ankle. Flexibility and strength of the hip and knee are also emphasized to avoid biomechanical deficiencies during gait that may abnormally stress the lateral leg musculature. Electrical muscle stimulation may be helpful to promote initial retraining of peroneal muscle contraction and to diminish edema after exercise by enhancement of local circulation.[10] As with ankle sprains, work with a balance board will help to regain proprioception. The athlete returns to functional activities, running, and agility drills (phase III of rehabilitation) with diminution of swelling and discomfort. Peroneal strength (ankle eversion) should be approximately 90% of the normal side. During this phase, taping of the ankle with a J-shaped pad over the peroneal tendons can act as a useful external restraint.

Prevention

Well-groomed playing fields and proper techniques of base running will decrease the incidence of dislocation or subluxation of the peroneal tendon.

Contusions and Subungual Hematomas

In baseball, contusions and subungual hematomas occur when the foot or ankle area is struck by a baseball. This most commonly happens to the batter when a ball is hit directly down to the feet. The catcher can also be hit by a foul ball, but the leg guard equipment provides some protection.

Diagnosis

A contusion after direct trauma will be manifested by localized swelling, ecchymosis, and tenderness. Involvement of a cutaneous nerve will cause altered sensation and possibly paresthesias in the appropriate distribution. A subungual hematoma is a collection of blood beneath the toenail, usually involving the hallux. It can be intensely painful because of the pressure of the contained blood by the nail plate. Radiography should be obtained to confirm the absence of a fracture.

Treatment

The principles of PRICE, as initially outlined for ankle sprains, are applicable to the initial treatment for the pain and swelling of a contusion. A vapocoolant spray may be applied to the skin to provide initial relief of pain on the playing field until more standard cryotherapy is used. For contusions of the foot and subungual hematomas, use of a stiff-soled shoe provides protection. After several days, with cessation of acute bleeding and soft tissue reaction, healing of a contusion is aided by local massage and ultrasound to enhance circulation and diminish adhesions and induration of soft tissue.[10] Voluntary splinting by the athlete is discouraged, and the use of gentle passive and active assisted range of motion exercises is encouraged.

Decompression of a subungual hematoma is accomplished by boring a small hole through the nail plate. This is most easily accomplished with a sterile needle or the end of a paper clip heated over a flame. The nail plate is left in place and taped, if loose. Eventually, the toenail typically falls off and is replaced by a new one. If radiography reveals a fracture of the distal phalanx, the injury should be considered open, and a dose of intravenous antibiotics followed by 1 week of oral antibiotics should be provided.

Prevention

It is difficult to prevent these injuries because they are a natural consequence of the game. A recent injury can be protected by a steel toe plate, but this may interfere with the athlete's agility and proprioception.

Achilles Tendinitis and Retrocalcaneal Bursitis

The Achilles tendon and posterior heel region are subjected to concentrated and repetitive stress during virtually all sport activities. Consequently, these areas are prone to the inflammation and degeneration associated with overuse. Increased torque in the biomechanically deficient foot, such as the stiff pes cavus or flexible pes planus, may predispose the athlete to these conditions. In baseball, the catcher is particularly at risk for the development of posterior heel complaints. Classically, the term Achilles tendinitis is reserved for the inflammatory process that occurs approximately 4 to 5 cm proximal to the Achilles tendon insertion. The retrocalcaneal bursa is located between the Achilles tendon at its insertion and the superior prominence of the calcaneus. Inflammation of this structure is called retrocalcaneal bursitis. Secondary degeneration and calcification of the Achilles tendon insertion may be present. Athletes with cavus feet and varus heels have limited ankle dorsiflexion and are more prone to the development of retrocalcaneal bursitis.

Diagnosis

Achilles tendinitis presents with nodular thickening and tenderness 4 to 5 cm proximal to the insertion. Pain is typically worse in the morning, at the beginning of activity, and after exer-

cise. Retrocalcaneal bursitis will have a pain pattern similar to Achilles tendinitis. Tenderness is located just proximal and anterior to the Achilles tendon insertion. Local swelling may progress to diffuse thickening of soft tissue as the condition becomes chronic. Radiography may reveal a spur or calcification at the Achilles tendon insertion. Dorsiflexion of the ankle is often limited in both Achilles tendinitis and retrocalcaneal bursitis. These conditions are often associated with excessive pronation or a high-arched foot, which can lead to abnormal torque on the Achilles tendon.

Treatment

Nonoperative treatment for both conditions is similar. The acute inflammatory symptoms are diminished by rest, antiinflammatory medication, and application of ice. Contrast baths are useful to enhance local circulation and healing of tissues[3] and usually consist of two whirlpools: a hot bath, lasting 3 to 4 minutes, and a cold bath, lasting 1 to 2 minutes. A heel lift or an orthotic device to correct a biomechanical abnormality may be useful. An Achilles tendon stretching program is important. If symptoms are initially appreciable or refractory to the treatment efforts mentioned previously, a short period of immobilization (up to 4 weeks) may help. Although an injection of cortisone into the retrocalcaneal space can be beneficial in resistant cases of retrocalcaneal bursitis, it is generally not recommended for Achilles tendinitis. Phonophoresis (ultrasound with hydrocortisone cream) can diminish local inflammation and promote tissue healing.[10] Ultrasound is not recommended for use over areas of poor vascularity, decreased sensation, or open physes.

Surgical treatment is considered when the athlete's condition has not improved within a minimum of 3 to 4 months of conservative therapy. Results of surgery for retrocalcaneal bursitis are better when performed within 1 year of the onset of symptoms.[4] Surgery involves debridement of the retrocalcaneal bursa and any insertional bony abnormalities of the Achilles tendon. Ostectomy of the superior angle of the calcaneus is performed. For Achilles tendinitis, debridement of the inflamed sheath is followed by

Rehabilitation of the Athlete's Foot and Ankle

palpation and inspection of the tendon proper through a small longitudinal incision parallel with the fibers.[21] Mucinoid degeneration within the tendon is excised. After operation, the ankle is immobilized in neutral position with a short leg cast for 2 weeks. After immobilization, flexibility and strength are regained by passive and active assisted motion exercises and progressive resistance exercises. A heel lift is used for 6 to 8 weeks. Return to functional activities may take 2 to 3 months.

Prevention

It is important to recognize any biomechanical abnormality in the athlete and to correct or compensate for these by modifications to the shoe or with orthotics. A regular program of stretching, particularly of the Achilles tendon, is completed before and after sport activities. A slant board should be readily available for this purpose. Avoidance of training errors, such as too rapid an increase of workout intensity or duration, will further help prevent Achilles tendinitis and retrocalcaneal bursitis.

Hallux Synovitis/Rigidus

Inflammation of the first MTP joint can occur from repeated hyperextension of the hallux. This condition creates dorsal compression and stretching of the plantar plate and collateral ligaments. In baseball, the pitcher subjects the hallux of the pivot foot to repetitive microtrauma (Fig. 18-5). During delivery, the great toe lies over the edge of the rubber. The pivot foot rotates nearly 90 degrees at push-off, causing compression and torque at the first MTP joint. Some have coined the term *pitcher's toe* for this condition.[20] In essence, this is a chronic form of acute turf toe. Entrapment of the medial hallucal nerve (Joplin's nerve) at the fascia of the abductor hallucis muscle may also cause pain in the great toe in the baseball pitcher.[6]

Diagnosis

The athlete will complain of pain at the first MTP joint. Dorsal tenderness and edema will be

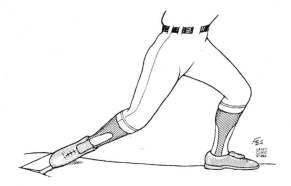

Fig. 18-5 The hallux of the pivot foot of a baseball pitcher is exposed to repetitive compression and torque during delivery. (Reprinted with permission of the Lahey Clinic, Burlington, Mass.)

present. Synovial thickening and dorsal osteophytes may be palpable in the more advanced cases. Initially, limitation of dorsiflexion may be mild; however, the condition can progress to hallux rigidus with more marked restriction of motion. Localized pain and tenderness at the plantar medial aspect of the first MTP joint raises the suspicion of medial hallucal nerve entrapment. Results of radiography will be negative if the condition is early and mild. In more advanced cases, radiography may reveal dorsal osteophytes, joint-space narrowing, and subchondral sclerosis. It is helpful to compare these findings to those from radiography of the contralateral first MTP joint.

Treatment

The initial thrust of treatment is to decrease the acute inflammatory reaction by rest, nonsteroidal antiinflammatory medication, and application of ice. Alternative conditioning that does not stress the great toe includes bicycling and swimming or running in water. Passive and active assisted range of motion exercises are performed within tolerance and with emphasis on dorsiflexion. As symptoms subside and the athlete returns to activity, the hallux is protected from excessive dorsiflexion by taping made in a figure-eight loop around the proximal phalanx and attached to the plantar surface of the foot. This treatment may be supplemented by buddy taping the hallux to the second toe. The sole of the athletic shoe should be stiff. A steel plate or shank can be added to the sole of the shoe. However, an excessively stiff-soled shoe may interfere with the motion and delivery of the high-performance pitcher.

Prevention

Prophylactic taping of the hallux and modifications to the shoe to stiffen the sole will decrease the repetitive stress placed on the great toe. In addition, exercises to increase dorsiflexion should be instituted in the athlete identified as having limited motion of the first MTP joint.

Summary

Foot and ankle injuries sustained during the games of baseball and softball do not occur as frequently as with other sports, such as basketball, football, and running. Nonetheless, the physician and athletic trainer who evaluate and treat baseball-related injuries need to be familiar with the typical foot and ankle conditions that can occur. Most injuries of the foot and ankle are acute injuries and occur during the landing phase of base sliding: ankle sprains and fractures, posterior talar impingement, peroneal tendon dislocation-subluxation. The most useful preventive measure in decreasing baseball and softball injuries would be to substitute break-away bases for stationary bases.[17,18] Contusions are a natural consequence of the game when a ball strikes the foot and ankle region. The most common chronic conditions resulting from baseball are posterior heel inflammation (Achilles tendinitis, retrocalcaneal bursitis) and hallux synovitis.

The rehabilitation of a foot and ankle condition commences with the occurrence of the injury and progresses through three phases until the athlete returns to the sport.[2] The goals of the early phase of rehabilitation are to diminish the inflammatory response and pain by protection and rest of the injured area, cryotherapy, compression, and elevation. The goals of the early phase and the transition from the early to the in-termediate phase of rehabilitation may be better achieved with the use of phonophoresis and electrical stimulation.[10] These modalities enhance local circulation, decrease muscle spasm and edema, and promote tissue healing. The intermediate phase of rehabilitation restores strength and endurance of local muscles through isometric, isotonic, and isokinetic exercises.[3] The proximal musculature of the hip and knee should not be ignored during this phase. A stretching program for the return of motion and flexibility is important. The late phase of rehabilitation is heralded by functional activities and agility training. Progression through the final stages of rehabilitation and the athlete's return to baseball will be more efficient when cross-training (e.g., bicycling, running in water) is performed during the earlier phases of rehabilitation.

Acknowledgement

A special thanks goes to the Lahey Clinic Photography, Medical, Art, and Editorial departments and also to Sandra Falzarano for their help in preparation of this manuscript.

Bibliography

1. American Academy of Orthopaedic Surgeons: Chapter 45. In *Athletic training and sports medicine,* ed 2, Rosemont Ill, 1991, AAOS.
2. American Academy of Orthopaedic Surgeons: Chapter 49. In *Athletic training and sports medicine,* ed 2, Park Ridge, Ill, 1991, AAOS.
3. American Academy of Orthopaedic Surgeons: Chapter 50. In *Athletic training and sports medicine,* ed 2, Park Ridge, Ill, 1991, AAOS.
4. Angermann P: Chronic retrocalcaneal bursitis treated by resection of the calcaneus, *Foot Ankle* 10:285, 1990.
5. Aradi AJ, Wong J, Walsh M: The dimple sign of a ruptured lateral ligament of the ankle: brief report, *J Bone Joint Surg* 70(B):327, 1988.
6. Baxter DE: Functional nerve disorders in the athlete's foot, ankle, and leg. In Heckman JD, editor: *American Academy of Orthopaedic Surgeons instructional course lectures,* vol 42, Park Ridge, Ill, 1993, AAOS.
7. Boruta PM et al: Acute lateral ankle ligament injuries: a literature review, *Foot Ankle* 11:107, 1990.
8. Brage ME, Hansen ST Jr: Traumatic subluxation/dislocation of the peroneal tendons, *Foot Ankle* 13:423, 1992.

Rehabilitation of the Athlete's Foot and Ankle

9. Clanton TO, Schon LC: Athletic injuries to the soft tissues of the foot and ankle. In Mann RA, Coughlin MJ, editors: *Surgery of the foot and ankle,* ed 6, St Louis, 1993, Mosby.

10. Cooper M: Use of modalities in rehabilitation. In Andrews JR, Harrelson GL, editors: *Physical rehabilitation of the injured athlete,* Philadelphia, 1991, WB Saunders.

11. Corzatt RD et al: The biomechanics of head-first versus feet-first sliding, *Am J Sports Med* 12:229, 1984.

12. Eckert WR, Davis EA Jr: Acute rupture of the peroneal retinaculum, *J Bone Joint Surg* 58(A):670, 1976.

13. Edwards GS Jr, DeLee JC: Ankle diastasis without fracture, *Foot Ankle* 4:305, 1984.

14. Hamilton WG: Foot and ankle injuries in dancers. In Mann RA, Coughlin MJ, editors: *Surgery of the Foot and Ankle,* ed 6, St Louis, 1993, Mosby.

15. Hardaker WT Jr, Margello S, Goldner JL: Foot and ankle injuries in theatrical dancers, *Foot Ankle* 6:59, 1985.

16. Hopkinson WJ et al: Syndesmosis sprains of the ankle, *Foot Ankle* 10:325, 1990.

17. Janda DH et al: Sliding injuries in college and professional baseball: a prospective study comparing standard and break-away bases, *Clin J Sports Med* 3:78, 1993.

18. Janda DH et al: A three-phase analysis of the prevention of recreational softball injuries, *Am J Sports Med* 18:632, 1990.

19. Leach RE, Schepsis AA: Ligamentous injuries. In Yablon IG, Segal D, Leach RE, editors: *Ankle injuries,* New York: 1983, Churchill Livingstone.

20. Pappas AM: Personal communication, May 1993.

21. Schepsis AA, Leach RE: Surgical management of Achilles tendinitis, *Am J Sports Med* 15:308, 1987.

19

Foot and Ankle Injuries in Soccer

Janet C. Limke

Soccer is the most popular sport in the world. In the past two decades soccer interest and participation have surged in the United States, making soccer the third most popular youth sport. According to the Soccer Industry Council of America, there were an estimated 14 million participants in 1992 (Table 19-1).

The male/female ratio was 3:2. Looking at 10-year trends (Table 19-2), youth participation in soccer doubled between 1982 and 1992. The greatest increase occurred among female players at both youth and college levels (with nearly triple the number of high school female players and more than quadruple the number of female collegiate teams). Comparing this to other sports at the high school level shows that soccer participation has dramatically increased while baseball and basketball have modestly declined (Table 19-3).

With this rise in soccer participation, there are increasing challenges for health professionals, coaches, and trainers to deal effectively with soccer-related injuries. This chapter deals with common foot and ankle injuries in soccer in a framework that emphasizes causes and prevention. This is not meant to be a thorough reference to foot and ankle injuries occurring in soccer. Other chapters in this text and current orthopedic and sports medicine texts may be used when further information is needed.

The portions of this chapter devoted to soccer injury epidemiology, injury prevention, and soccer-specific rehabilitation should not be overlooked. They contain vital information for trainers, therapists, and health professionals who work with soccer players. Much of this information is based on prospective studies of both amateur and professional youth and adult soccer. The research provides the basis for treatment and training strategies that may lessen lower extremity injury and its recurrence.

Table 19-1 Demographics of Soccer Participation (U.S.) 1992

	No. of Participants	Percent
Total	14,567,000	100
Male	8,955,000	61
Female	5,612,000	39
Under age 18	11,099,000	76
Under age 12	5,934,000	41

Adapted from Soccer Industry Council of America: *Soccer in the USA,* 1992, SICA.

Table 19-2   Ten-Year Trends

U.S. Soccer Youth	1981-1982	1991-1992	% Change
Affiliate registrants	1,072,706	2,156,235	+101
High school participants (male)	161,167	236,082	+ 46
High school participants (female)	51,869	135,302	+161
NCAA teams (male)	521	581	+ 12
NCAA teams (female)	77	348	+352

Adapted from Soccer Industry Council of America: *Soccer in the USA,* 1992, SICA.

Table 19-3   Ten-Year Trends: High School Soccer vs. Other High School Sports

	1981 Participants	1991 Participants	% Change
Soccer	190,495	350,102	+83.79
Baseball	422,310	419,015	−0.79
Basketball	977,270	903,446	−7.56

Adapted from Soccer Industry Council of America: *Soccer in the USA,* 1992, SICA.

Epidemiology

Most of the data on soccer injuries come from Europe, in particular Sweden and Denmark. Only a few well-designed prospective studies have been published. The injury rates reported vary from 3.7 per 1000 hours of total play (including practice and competition) for male youth during 1 year to 16 per 1000 hours of competition in a senior age group. It is difficult to compare the studies because of differences in the definition of injury, practice vs. game time, competitiveness, and age and sex of players. However, several conclusions are apparent:

1. Studies of youth soccer in both Europe and the United States reveal that nearly twice as many girl athletes sustain injuries as boys. When maturity is reached, the injury rates are nearly equal. Researchers are uncertain about the reason for this sex difference.
2. Adolescents suffer less frequent and less serious injuries than adults.
3. There are greater numbers of injuries during games than during practice.
4. Lower extremity injuries account for 70% to 88% of all injuries in soccer.
5. About 90% of lower extremity injuries consist of sprains, strains, and contusions.[12,26]

Further breakdown of lower extremity injuries reveals that thigh strains are the most common, followed by nearly equal numbers of injuries to the ankle and knee. Foot and ankle injuries make up approximately 24% of all soccer injuries. In terms of overall injury rate, soccer has been determined to be approximately equal to basketball and safer than football.[26]

Biomechanics

Before addressing injuries to the foot and ankle in soccer, consider the biomechanics of soccer play. First one must appreciate the forces distributed through the lower extremity during kicking. High forces are transmitted throughout the entire lower extremity and spine in a closed chain reaction, with relatively little force actually translated to ball motion. Three types of kick are described, as follows:

Rehabilitation of the Athlete's Foot and Ankle

1. The *straight-ahead kick* involves powerful use of hip flexors, knee extensors, and ankle dorsiflexors. It is used for volleys and long passing shots and lacks some of the control of the inside kick.

2. The *inside (power) kick* requires strong hip flexors, adductors, knee extensors, ankle dorsiflexors, and ankle invertors to drive the ball. For both the straight-ahead and the inside kicks, 800 to 2000 pounds of varus torque are generated before and after ball contact. Smooth follow-through is very important to dissipate energy. There is great vulnerability to the player when follow-through is blocked.

3. The *outside kick* is less powerful and is executed with great finesse. Hip external rotators, vastus lateralis, tensor fascia lata, peronei, and extensor digitorum communis are activated in concert to control the ball with this kick.[26]

Factors Involved in Soccer Injury

The intrinsic and extrinsic factors listed in Table 19-4 account for most of the identifiable causes of soccer injury. By first understanding the factors that lead to increased injuries, one can then postulate prevention strategies.

First, consider the intrinsic factors. Given what has already been noted about the high incidence of thigh strains, it is not surprising that soccer players have been found to be *inflexible* in the thigh adductors and quadriceps.[4]

Ekstrand and Gillquist have published a series of well-designed prospective analyses of soccer injury.[4] In one controlled study of Division 4 Swedish soccer players, they looked at the effects of a prophylactic stretching program on injury incidence over a period of 6 months. They controlled for several important variables, including optimal equipment, correction of training errors, and ankle taping. They reported an impressive reduction of 75% in injury incidence in those who participated in the prophylactic program as compared to the control group. This study shows

Table 19-4 Factors Contributing to Soccer Injuries

Intrinsic	Extrinsic
Inflexibility	Frequency/duration/ intensity of play
Muscle imbalance	Person-to-person contact
Inadequate aerobic/ anaerobic capacity	Contact with ground Contact with objects
Poor nutrition	Coach/referee lenience
Dehydration	Inadequate equipment
Pes/planus/cavus deformity	Improper footwear
Improper technique	Surface characteristics

how a clear analysis of epidemiologic factors in injury can lead to practical interventions that may result in a dramatic reduction of injuries.[26]

Muscle imbalances are frequently found in soccer players who suffer recurrent injuries. Adequate strengthening of ankle evertors must follow a lateral ankle sprain so as to rebalance forces around the ankle and prevent instability.

One study looked at the muscular balance around the knee joint during the kicking motion of soccer players and nonsoccer players. It was found that antagonist muscle (hamstring) contractions were greater in the soccer players than the nonsoccer players. Soccer players kicked the ball farther and with greater control. This was thought to be due to the eccentric (lengthening) contraction of the antagonist in synergy with the concentric agonist (quadriceps) muscle contraction. Thus it is recommended that soccer training include eccentric hamstring strengthening along with concentric quadriceps strengthening for optimal performance. Good proximal control is key to maintaining distal function and alignment.[21]

The optimal physiological profile of the soccer player has been studied by comparing *aerobic* and *anaerobic capacity* in amateur and professional soccer players. Despite the fact that many consider soccer a primarily aerobic sport, with players running 6 to 8 miles per game, Faina et al found that soccer players have only average aerobic fitness compared to other athletes.[21] The distinguishing feature between amateurs and professionals was found in anaerobic, not aerobic, fitness. The professional soccer players were found to have greater "explosive muscle power" than the amateurs. Thus the researchers recommend that training should emphasize progressively more intense and repeated loads with fast muscular activation. They further state that long-duration, low-intensity drills should be avoided.

Adequate *nutrition* and *hydration* are essential for players. Tournament games may be back to back or on successive days, leaving no time for muscle repair processes to occur or for replenishment of muscle glycogen. There is evidence that high carbohydrate intake may help replete muscle glycogen stores and ensure adequate fuel for training and competition. Thus, nutritional counseling is recommended.[10] The Federation Internationale de Football Association (FIFA) has enforced restrictive policies that limit times for hydration of players during international competition. Dehydration and electrolyte imbalance, particularly when exacerbated by high ambient temperatures, lead to problems of declining performance. This in turn can lead to difficulty maintaining muscular control during the most intense portions of the game. Pregame overhydration and, when possible, using breaks in play for hydration are ways to minimize this problem.

Pes planus and *cavus deformities* of the foot, when left uncorrected or unsupported, may lead to a variety of disorders affecting the closed chain of the lower extremity and back. These problems will be addressed later in relation to tendinitis and other overuse injuries.

Extrinsic factors that predispose to overuse injury include the *frequency, duration,* and *intensity* demands of soccer practice and competition. Intensity of participation has increased in recent years such that a youth soccer player may compete in two outdoor seasons per year with an optional indoor season. "Select" teams, which may begin at age 10, may play 30 to 40 weeks per year with 2 to 3 practices per week and 1 to 4 games per week. There are no rules limiting the number of games, practices, or length of the sea-son. Cumulative trauma injuries had occurred in 20% of the youth soccer players in Kibler's study.[9]

Stresses along any portion of the chain can result in *improper technique,* with compensatory strategies that overstress other parts of the linkage. For example, chronic adductor strain may lead to hesitation due to pain with inadequate follow-through during kicking. Poor follow-through may cause the forces generated by the kick to be focused on another portion of the linkage (e.g., the knee or ankle). When evaluating such a player with medial knee pain, an astute clinician or trainer may also discover tightness and discomfort at the adductor longus insertion onto the pubis. For another example, when looking for factors contributing to pain at the lateral aspect of the ankle, as in peroneal tendinitis, one may find a tight iliotibial band and weak hip external rotators. Relative weakness at the hip may contribute to improper technique and greater stress further down the chain of the lower extremity (Fig. 19-1).

Kibler reported the causative factors of injury during four consecutive years (1987 to 1990) of a large soccer tournament of male and female youth. Extrinsic causative factors were led by *person-to-person contact* (43%). *Contact with the ground,* as in kicking the ground instead of the ball, or falling, and *contact with other objects,* such as goalposts, sideline equipment, and spectators, together accounted for an additional 24% of the injuries. Thus, using shin protectors, padding goalposts, and clearing a larger radius around the playing field, are all potential ways to decrease injuries.[9]

In order to ensure safety during games, *coaches* and *referees* should encourage good sportsmanship and consistently call penalties for inappropriate actions such as jersey pulling and deliberate "take downs." Equipment should be checked for optimal condition.[9]

Soccer players prefer tightly fitting, lightweight *footwear*. The design allows for maximum "feel" of the ball during kicking but provides minimal protection. The best soccer shoes are made of soft, flexible leather with the shoe upper slightly overlapping the insole. This relationship of the upper to the insole is unlike that in

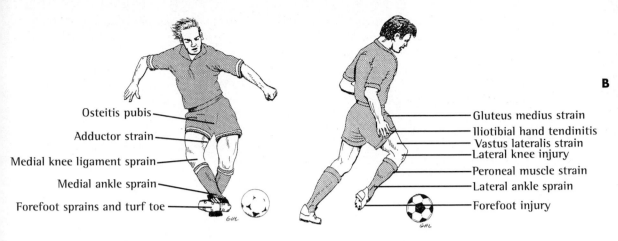

Fig. 19-1 **A**, Force distribution during the inside kick can lead to problems anywhere along the chain of the lower extremity. **B**, Examples of problems associated with forces transmitted through the lower extremity during the outside kick.

Labels (left figure, A):
Osteitis pubis
Adductor strain
Medial knee ligament sprain
Medial ankle sprain
Forefoot sprains and turf toe

Labels (right figure, B):
Gluteus medius strain
Iliotibial hand tendinitis
Vastus lateralis strain
Lateral knee injury
Peroneal muscle strain
Lateral ankle sprain
Forefoot injury

other sport shoes. It gives better contact with the ball during kicking but contributes to overuse problems such as turf toe, described later.

The study of different *surfaces* and the frictional characteristics of the sole vs. the ground is an area in need of research. Too little traction impedes running progress and causes slippage and falls. Too much traction may increase knee injuries and lower extremity fractures as excessive torque is applied to the foot that is firmly fixed to the ground. On hard ground and Astroturf, a multistudded or turf toe shoe seems to provide a reasonable amount of friction, good weight distribution, and comfort. In contrast, fewer studs allow better traction on soft ground. Screw-in stud systems have been developed out of rubber, leather, nylon, or polyurethane to allow interchanges for different ground conditions. FIFA permits no more than 6 screw-in studs of 10-mm (⅜-inch) diameter.[3] (See Fig. 19-2 for examples of various sole configurations.)

Soccer players less than 12 years of age do best with multistudded or turf shoes. Even distribution of force is particularly important for young players, who have not yet had fusion at calcaneal growth centers. A child running on few studs may aggravate the heel pain seen with Sever's disease, as described later.[21]

A strong heel counter for hindfoot control and torsional rigidity are important stabilizing fea-

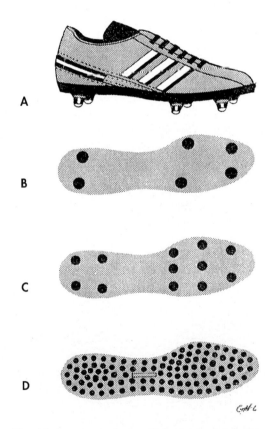

Fig. 19-2 Soccer shoes with various sole configurations. **A,B,** Screw-in 6-stud system. **C**, Multistudded system. **D,** Turf shoe.

tures of any sport shoe. Torsional rigidity is resistance to excessive forefoot pronation. In soccer, some stability and foot protection are ultimately compromised in order to get a lightweight, flexible shoe that allows the most "feel" and contact with the ball during kicking.[3]

Foot Injuries

Sprains

Acute foot injuries, including sprains, contusions, and fractures, are more frequent in soccer than in other running sports. Both the kicking action required and the frequency of being stepped on by opponents make these injuries common.

Contusions occur most often. X-rays including posteroanterior, lateral, and oblique views are done to rule out fracture. Contusions respond well to ice, elevation, compression, and protective padding over tender areas until healing is complete.

Sprains most frequently affect the dorsum of the foot. Most forefoot sprains occur while the foot is plantarflexed. This puts tension over the dorsal structures. When a soccer player unintentionally kicks the ground or a ball that is being blocked, severe torque is exerted on these already taut dorsal structures. The intrinsic muscles and plantar fascia partially protect the undersurface of the foot from sprains.[26]

With the inside kick, the medial ligaments of the forefoot [medial midtarsal joints over the first and second metatarsophalangeal (MTP) joints] are most at risk. With the outside kick, the lateral ligaments (subtalar and lateral midtarsal joints) are most vulnerable. The straight-ahead kick can affect any of the above.

Diagnosis of acute sprains should be made at the time of injury in order to institute treatment immediately and prevent complications arising from progressive edema. The foot is painful during weight-bearing and tender over the affected ligaments. X-rays are used to rule out a concomitant avulsion fracture. Treatment includes a compressive dressing, ice, elevation, and limited weight-bearing until gait is pain-free. Next, jog-

ging is started and gradually increased. Cutting maneuvers are added before the player can progress to kicking the ball. Firm insoles such as orthotics made of Orthoplast should be utilized to dampen the torque transmission through the forefoot during cutting and kicking maneuvers.[26]

Forceful hyperextension strain to the first MTP joint is known as *turf toe*. The unyielding characteristics of synthetic turf combined with the pliable lightweight shoes worn by soccer players are both to blame for this condition. The treatment is the same as for other sprains. Prevention of reinjury can be achieved with the use of a stiff-soled shoe or a semirigid orthotic that extends beyond the first MTP joint.[7]

The same mechanism of injury that causes sprains can result in avulsion fractures and/or joint dislocations and fractures. The importance of adequate follow-through in order to dissipate the high forces involved in kicking was mentioned previously. When follow-through is blocked by an object such as the ground or an opponent, extreme torque is exerted on the blocked portion of the extremity. Avulsion fractures that are commonly encountered involve the following ligaments: (1) the sustentaculum tali at both its anterior and posterior border, (2) the talonavicular ligament to the navicular, and (3) the peroneus brevis muscle to the fifth metatarsal. Exquisite tenderness over the avulsed site is noted, and radiographs will confirm the diagnosis.[26]

Sustentaculum fractures involving the anterior process will heal without a weight-bearing restriction. Posterior sustentaculum fractures involve a weight-bearing area and are best treated with 6 to 8 weeks of nonweight-bearing progressing to full weight-bearing over 3 months. Surgical excision may be needed to excise the fragment if a painful nonunion occurs. Navicular avulsion requires a shorter period (approximately 2 weeks) of nonweight-bearing restriction.[26]

Lastly, avulsion of the peroneus brevis tendon deserves special attention due to the importance of distinguishing it from a Jones fracture. Avulsion fractures occur acutely and are due to forceful inversion of the foot. These heal well with a short leg cast and partial weight-bearing as tolerated. Fracture of the shaft of the fifth metatarsal, or Jones fracture, occurs within 1.5 cm of the tuberosity in a poorly vascularized area. This fracture is due to cumulative trauma, typically presenting as insidious lateral foot pain followed by an acute injury for which the athlete seeks medical attention. An acute Jones fracture may heal with 2 to 3 months of nonweight-bearing, although subacute or chronic fractures may not. Nonunion occurs when there is sclerosis within the fracture site after medial displacement of the distal segment. These require surgical repair with either curettage and bone grafting or intramedullary screw fixation.[8,23]

Stress Fractures

Bone is continually being remodeled in response to stresses. When an athlete has a sudden change in activity, as at the beginning of the season, there is a greater chance of overuse injuries, including stress fractures. Stress fractures are most common in the tibia and fibula and may present as pain or aching in the lower leg or ankle. In the foot, the second metatarsal is most frequently affected. It is wedged into the transverse tarsal arch and is directly in line with force transmission during the push-off phase of gait.

Tenderness in a well-circumscribed area may be the only finding on physical examination, although focal swelling might be palpable. Plain X-rays will usually be negative for at least the first 3 weeks after onset of symptoms. Bone scan is more sensitive and is the first test ordered by some sports physicians when a stress fracture is suspected. Garrick and Webb recommend that an athlete be pain-free for 10 consecutive days before increasing activity.[7] Pain is the guide for each consecutive increase in training, and careful titration of activities is the key to successful treatment.

Plantar Fasciitis

The plantar fascia is the tough fibrous sheet extending from the anterior border of the calcaneus to the base of the metatarsals and supporting the longitudinal arch of the foot. Both flat feet with excessive pronation and high-arched rigid feet may predispose to plantar fasciitis.[11]

Symptoms of pain are most pronounced when first arising in the morning or at the onset of activity. As the condition progresses, the pain may persist and limit athletic competition. Tenderness is noted at the proximal insertion of the plantar fascia. X-rays may reveal calcaneal heel spurs, which are a local reaction to inflammation. Excision of these does not address the biomechanical problem and so is not usually recommended.[7,13]

Local treatment consists of friction massage and ultrasound to the medial arch of the foot and progressive resistive exercises to strengthen intrinsic foot muscle strength. Toe flexor exercises may be performed by placing a towel on the floor and a book on the end of the towel. The toes then grab the towel to pull the book along the floor. Progressively heavier books are used to achieve strengthening. Street shoe and soccer shoe modifications are crucial for successful treatment. The ideal shoe has a stiff, rocker-bottom sole and a longitudinal arch support. This will decrease MTP joint dorsiflexion during gait and limit pronation, together decreasing the stresses over the plantar fascia.[13]

Sesamoiditis

Sesamoid problems at the great toe are a diagnostic and therapeutic challenge. Medial and lateral sesamoid bones lie within the flexor hallucis brevis tendon. It has been estimated that forces equal to three times body weight are transmitted through the sesamoid bones during the push-off phase of gait. Numerous pathological processes may affect the sesamoids, including stress fracture, inflammation, osteoarthritis, osteochondritis, and bursitis. Sesamoiditis may represent inflammation of a variety of structures, including the flexor hallucis longus tendon as it passes between the sesamoids, and the sesamoid bursa. The player may find it painful to land from a jump and to accelerate forward from a stopped position.[8,15]

Tenderness is present at the sesamoids on the base of the great toe, and passive dorsiflexion of the great toe causes pain. X-rays are used to rule out a fracture, which may be confusing in the 10% to 33% of people with bipartite sesamoids.[15] In fact, Monto et al found that bipartite sesamoids were among the radiographic abnormalities found to be of higher incidence in elite soccer players.[12]

The key to successful management is limiting weight-bearing through the sesamoids. Again, a firm sole with a rocker bottom is helpful by allowing the foot to roll through the push-off phase of gait.[13] In addition, routing out the sole beneath the great toe and replacing this with soft foam helps to inhibit contraction of the flexor hallucis brevis muscle since there is nothing substantial left for the toe to push against.[20] Icing, nonsteroidal antiinflammatory drugs (NSAIDs), and modified activity are other usual adjuncts of conservative management. Excision of a sesamoid bone is considered a last resort after months of "aggressive" nonsurgical management, since biomechanical imbalances can occur that result in a poor functional outcome.[7]

Cornal/Calluses/Blisters

Tight soccer shoes contribute to what are perhaps the player's most common physical annoyances: corns, calluses, and blisters. *Corns* are hyperkeratotic lesions in response to pressure either from the inside out (exostoses) or from the outside in (ill-fitting footwear). Filing the corn down, wearing U-shaped pads, and adjusting footwear to redistribute pressures constitutes effective treatment in most cases. Surgical excision of osteophytes may be needed if conservative management has failed to control symptoms.[7,26]

Calluses form most over the highest weight-bearing areas, especially at the base of the first and second metatarsals. Two and a half times body weight is transmitted through the ball of the foot with each step. While leaping for the ball, as in heading, the force of impact can nearly triple. Placing an arch support and metatarsal pads inside the soccer shoe will redistribute forces and decrease the discomfort from painful calluses located at the base of the metatarsals.[7]

Blisters are caused by frictional forces within the skin. Sheer injury occurs as the surface of the skin momentarily sticks to that which overlies it (e.g., the shoe). Large blisters should be sterilely drained and covered by Second Skin or even adhesive tape. If tape is used, it should be coated on the outside by a silicone spray to act as an interface between the sock and the skin, thus limiting frictional forces within the skin's layers. Small blisters or preblisters may be treated with the protective Second Skin alone or other similar interface.[7,26]

Subungual Hematoma

Subungual hematoma occurs more commonly in soccer than in any other sport. The soles of the soccer shoes are either flush with or recessed from the upper leather portion to allow better foot contact with the ball. During kicking, the longest toe is jammed up against the tightly fitting toe box. An opponent stepping on the shoe also causes these injuries. Severe pain may be relieved by drilling holes in the center of the nail to drain the hematoma. Complete or partial nail avulsions should be taped back in place to protect the nailbed.[3,26]

Ankle Injuries

Acute tendinitis around the ankle in soccer is due to both external mechanical trauma and the intrinsic factor of repetitive activation of the muscle. External trauma may be due to contact with the ball, the ground, other players, goalposts, equipment in the sidelines, or tight footwear. As stated, average distances run during a game range between 6 and 8 miles, with midfielders running most and defenders least. The game is intermittent; it requires bursts of energy, with frequent starting, stopping, jumping, and acceleration. When requirements of aerobic capacity are exceeded, control becomes difficult to maintain. The player is unable to maintain proper form. Poor technique combined with increased intensity, duration, and frequency of play contribute to a variety of injuries, including tendinitis and tenosynovitis. Often more than one tendon is involved. At the anterior aspect of the ankle, the anterior tibialis tendon and sheath is vulnerable. Both direct trauma from the ball during the straight-ahead or inside kick, and microstresses along the musculotendinous unit during kicking action add up to cause this overuse injury. Similarly, the inside kick may initiate me-

Rehabilitation of the Athlete's Foot and Ankle

dial ankle tenosynovitis, which may involve the tibialis posterior tendon, flexor digitorum profundus, and/or the flexor hallucis longus tendons. Lateral ankle tendinitis is seen with irritation of the peroneal tendons. Subluxation of the tendons anteriorly over the lateral malleolus should be noted, if present. This can contribute to lateral instability. Posterior ankle pain is seen in processes affecting the Achilles tendon and its insertion[26] (Fig. 19-3).

Signs and symptoms include pain, tenderness, crepitus, swelling, and erythema along the course of the involved tendon. If tenderness is noted at the insertion of the bone, partial avulsion should be considered. If tenderness is prominent near the musculotendinous insertion, a partial rupture may be present. Plain X-rays occasionally reveal bony avulsion or chronic calcific tendinitis. They are not needed routinely except to rule out suspected fractures. Magnetic resonance imaging has become increasingly useful in those with chronic symptoms or slow response to treatment, to determine the extent of intratendinous damage. This can directly aid in treatment decisions. Thus, a simple Achilles tendinitis may be treated with a course of rest, NSAIDs, and a heel lift, whereas an impending rupture of the Achilles tendon requires more aggressive treatment. The choices include casting with a nonweight-bearing restriction for several weeks and gradual return to activity *or* surgical repair.

Physical therapy treatment of acute tendinitis may include massage and electrical stimulation to help pump edema out of the surrounding tissues, followed by gentle stretching. A progressive resistive eccentric and concentric strengthening program is initiated once the pain associated with stretching has subsided. In chronic tendinitis, heat in the form of ultrasound and friction massage may help break up adhesions that have formed. The goal is to restore normal pain-free motion against resistance.[7]

It is important to provide a substitute activity for the soccer player to maintain general fitness while running and jumping activities are curtailed. Swimming or bicycling with low resistance results in minimal loading of the tendons and helps maintain endurance during the recovery phase. Bicycling, as described by Garrick and Webb, is a partial weight-bearing activity and involves very little ankle motion in the midrange.[7] Thus it is an excellent adjunct to continuing endurance training in soccer players with ankle injuries.

Factors contributing to tendinitis should be identified. In the case of the soccer player, excessive pronation is common, particularly with sidekicking and turning maneuvers. Orthotic arch supports and ankle supports may help maintain alignment and lessen the effect of torque on the ankle at the time of impact with ball or ground or after a lateral passing shot. Pronation is implicated as a cause of posterior tibial tendinitis due to the excessive stretch on the tendon in this position. Tight heel cords or hamstring tendons, increased Q angle, and weak or strained hip external rotators may be associated with excessive pronation.[13]

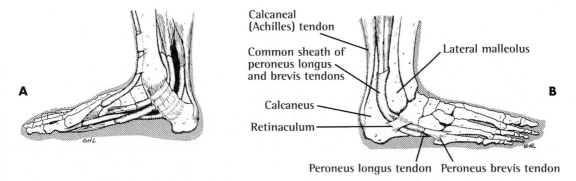

Fig. 19-3 **A,** Anterior and medial tendons of the ankle. **B,** Lateral tendons of the ankle: peroneus longus and brevis.

A rigid or *high-arched foot* does not absorb shock well and thus may predispose to overuse syndromes such as tendinitis. The athlete must adhere to proper technique or risk a variety of injuries along the linked chain of the lower extremity. Adequate warm-ups, flexibility exercises, and gradual increase in intensity of play are recommended adamantly by researchers who have studied the epidemiology of soccer injury.[4,5]

Sever's Disease

Sever's disease, or traction apophysitis of the heel, is a harmless condition occurring in children during growth of the calcaneal apophysis. It is analogous to Osgood-Schlatter's disease at the tibial tubercle. The child, usually aged 8 to 13, will have heel pain and a slight limp while running. Tenderness is noted at the posterior aspect of the calcaneal tubercle. Soccer shoes with too few studs inadequately distribute forces along the heel. Tight Achilles tendons may also exacerbate the problem. Modifying the child's activity temporarily, changing footwear, and gentle heel cord stretching will lead to resolution of pain in a short time in most cases.[21]

Fractures of the Ankle Joint

Ankle fractures in soccer frequently involve severe torque as a player's body weight is exerted over the foot that is fixed to the ground. It is beyond the scope of this chapter to discuss the classification and treatment of ankle fractures. Unstable or displaced fractures should be treated with open reduction and internal fixation. Achieving as close to perfect anatomical alignment as possible is important to lessen the development of degenerative arthritis.[26]

As the number of children involved in athletic competition rises, so does the incidence of growth plate injuries attributable to sports. Fractures in children who play soccer, as in other sports, occur at their weakest link, the growth plate, or physis. The skeletally immature child with open growth plates rarely sustains severe ligamentous injury since the ligaments at that stage are stronger than bone. The periosteum of a child or adolescent is stronger, thicker, and has greater osteogenic potential than that of an adult. This results in fewer open fractures, greater stability after reduction, and more callus formation. As the adolescent reaches age 15 to 16, the growth plates close and the pattern of injury becomes similar to that found in the adult athlete.[17,25]

Ankle Sprains

Ankle sprains account for 17% to 36% of all injuries in soccer.[6,19] This is not surprising considering the frequent jumping, turning, and kicking from all sides. As in the general population, inversion injury is most common. The medial aspect of the ankle is supported by the strong deltoid ligaments, which are rarely sprained. The lateral side has three major ligaments (common), listed in the order of injury frequency: (1) the anterior talofibular ligament (ATL), (2) the calcaneofibular ligament (CFL), and (3) the posterior talofibular ligament. The player is frequently landing from midair with the ankle in plantarflexion (Fig. 19-4). When the ankle is in plantarflexion, the ATL becomes aligned in the vertical position, where it provides the greatest stabilizing force. In this position it is also most vulnerable when inversion occurs. With the ankle in neutral, the ATL is aligned horizontal to the ground and is less likely to be sprained, while the CFL, which crosses the ankle mortise vertically, is more vulnerable to injury.[1,2,20]

It is important to realize that the degree of ankle swelling on physical examination has no correlation to the severity of the injury but only to early efforts to control edema. Edema, if not aggressively treated, will cause restriction in range of motion and interfere with recovery. Palpable tenderness is present over the involved ligaments. Anterior subluxation of the talus when the tibia is stabilized and the heel is moved forward occurs with disruption of the ATL. This constitutes a positive anterior drawer sign. Excessive talar tilt with inversion stress may be seen in rupture to the CFL. Stability testing using the talar tilt and anterior drawer signs, if positive, indicates a more severe sprain. Such testing can be difficult to perform in the acute stages when there is a painful, swollen ankle. Also, early stress radiographs may be falsely negative. They may

Rehabilitation of the Athlete's Foot and Ankle

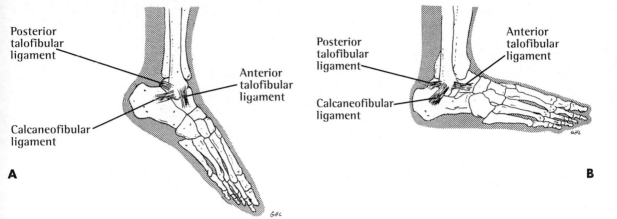

Fig. 19-4 **A,** The anterior talofibular ligament is aligned vertically when the ankle is plantarflexed. **B,** In neutral ankle position, the calcaneofibular ligament is vertical and most vulnerable to injury.

be better performed after swelling has subsided and if recovery is delayed. X-rays in the acute phase are used to rule out occult fractures and should include anteroposterior, lateral, and mortise views.[1,2,7]

Ankle sprains are graded from I to III based on the degree of ankle instability. Grade I is a partial tear of a ligament, Grade II is a more severe tear of one or more ligaments, while Grade III constitutes complete disruption of one or several ligaments and is the least common.[20]

The eponym PRICE (Protection, Rest, Ice, Compression, and Elevation) covers the most important principles of acute ankle sprain management. Grades I to III can all be managed nonoperatively, although early surgical intervention in Grade III injuries may speed recovery in the young athletic population and prevent chronic instability. Physical therapy should begin early and may include electrical stimulation, icing, massage, Ace bandage wrapping, and isometric strengthening. Since new collagen bundles form parallel to lines of stress, it is believed that gentle stretching and progressive resistive exercises should begin as soon as pain control permits. This also helps prevent contracture formation. The ultimate goals of an ankle rehabilitation program are to restore full range of motion, strength, and proprioceptive function and to provide graduated sport-specific exercise training.[1,7] An ankle rehabilitation protocol such as that out-

lined by Garrick is useful in guiding decisions regarding return to activity and play (Fig. 19-5).

For soccer, ankle sprains are often undertreated. This leads to recurrent sprains and chronic ankle instability. In Ekstrand and Tropp's study of the incidence of ankle sprains in four male senior soccer divisions, those who had had a previous problem with the ankle had a 50% chance of resprain, whereas those with no injury in the past had only a 10% chance of ankle sprain.[6] Efforts to prevent ankle sprains with ankle stabilizers and prophylactic taping should at least be utilized for those with previous ankle sprains. These efforts have been successful in significantly reducing morbidity in several studies of soccer and football players.[6,18] Taping is more costly due to the time required for application and materials and may be less effective in limiting motion. Lace-up ankle supports can be frequently tightened by the athlete, affording more consistent support throughout a game or practice.[18]

Strengthening should include both eccentric and concentric exercises and be performed in diagonal as well as horizontal and vertical planes. Use of an elastic band of various tensions allows a trainer or therapist to gradually increase the work load to the affected areas. Once open chain exercises such as these have progressed without difficulty, one can proceed with closed chain activities. Proprioceptive retraining with the use of a

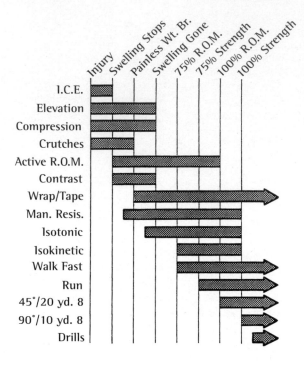

Fig. 19-5 Ankle rehabilitation. (Adapted from Garrick JG: A practical approach to rehabilitation of the ankle, *Am J Sports Med* 9:67, 1981; with permission.)

balance board is recommended. The balance board is an excellent challenge to develop well-controlled motions in all planes while in the loaded position. Walking, jogging, running, and finally, soccer drills are added. Soccer drills should include progressively more intense bouts of play, including cutting, jumping, sprinting, and stopping maneuvers. Aerobic and anaerobic capacity of the athlete is needed to adequately respond to the demands of competition.[20,21]

Meniscoid Lesions

A small subset of soccer players who have recurrent ankle sprains, persistent swelling, and a sensation of catching have been found to have meniscoid lesions on arthroscopy of the ankle. In each of several cases described by McCarroll et al, conservative management failed, no instability of the ankle was noted under anesthesia, and a fibrous white band of tissue was found between the fibula and talus.[16] Those authors postulate that the band represents redundant synovium that formed during the inflammatory stage of a previous sprain; while Drez believes it is residual torn ligament that becomes entrapped be-

tween the lateral malleolus and the talus.[16a] Regardless of its origin, arthroscopic examination and resection has been found to be an effective treatment.[16]

Soccer Player's Ankle

Soccer player's ankle, or footballer's ankle as it is called outside the United States, initially presents as pain over the anterior aspect of the ankle joint when kicking the ball hard or having the kick blocked by an opponent. During extreme plantarflexion, the anterior portion of the ankle joint is placed under tension. Forceful impact with the ball may cause ligamentous injury similar to dorsal foot strain. Repetitive trauma in this area leads to calcifications in the soft tissues and bony spurring from the anterior aspect of the talus and navicular bones (Fig. 19-6). Extreme dorsiflexion of the ankle may also aggravate the condition by causing anterior impingement between the talus and midtarsal bones.[14,26]

The posterior tubercle of the talus can also become impinged between the tibia and calcaneus during extreme plantarflexion of the ankle.

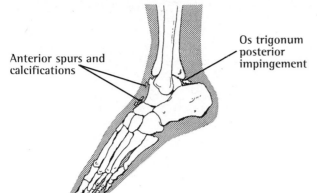

Fig. 19-6 Soccer player's ankle, diagrammatic representation. Repetitive trauma at the anterior ankle leads to calcifications in the soft tissues and bony spurring. At the posterior ankle, the os trigonum is shown as it is impinged between the tibia and calcaneus during plantarflexion.

Anterior spurs and calcifications

Os trigonum posterior impingement

Symptoms of pain and swelling may thus occur in the posterior ankle as well. With repetitive trauma, the posterior tubercle may break off and resemble an os trigonum. The os trigonum is found in 5% of the general population but has a higher incidence (up to 16%) in soccer players.[14,26]

Dramatic statistics come from a study by Massada.[14] He looked for X-ray abnormalities consistent with anterior or posterior impingement in professional soccer players. The X-ray abnormalities of repetitive dorsal strain injury overlap with anterior impingement (dorsal spurring and soft tissue calcifications). He found changes in more than half of the ankles, with very few (less than 7%) reporting symptoms. Those most likely to have symptoms had osteophytic projections in the affected area, similar to those seen in soccer player's ankle.

Conservative management includes NSAIDs, a heel lift to prevent the anterior impingement, orthotics, and limitation of pain-provoking activities such as forceful kicking and running uphill. Surgery may be necessary to excise osteophytes that remain symptomatic.[14,26]

emphasis on kicking and running causes proportionately greater stresses on the foot and ankle. Understanding the biomechanics of kicking and the factors predisposing to injury provides a basis from which to approach the rehabilitation of the soccer player. The most holistic approach includes evaluation of the entire closed linkage of the lower extremity, shoewear, playing surfaces, equipment, and training strategies.

Ultimate return to play follows stepwise increases in activity guided by frequent assessments. One can learn much about soccer injury and prevention by studying the literature in Europe where soccer has been the most popular team sport for decades.

With the recent increase in indoor soccer and longer seasons of play, the game's physical demands have changed. Future research should look prospectively at the epidemiology of injury in the face of these trends. Outcomes of such studies may then lead to specific recommendations to coaches and trainers that will enable players to minimize injury while continuing to strive for excellence.

Conclusion

As soccer's popularity continues to rise, health professionals, trainers, and coaches will be challenged not merely to treat injuries but to maximize the player's performance. Soccer's

Acknowledgment

I would like to acknowledge my father, George H. Limke, for his contribution of time and talent for the medical illustrations in this chapter.

Bibliography

1. Arendt E: Inversion injuries to the ankle, *Surg Rounds Orthop* June:15, 1989.
2. Balduini FC, Tetzlaff J: Historical perspectives on injuries of the ligaments of the ankle, *Clin Sports Med* 1:3, 1982.
3. Cheskin MP: *The complete handbook of athletic footwear,* New York, 1987, Fairchild Publications.
4. Ekstrand J, Gillquist J: The frequency of muscle tightness and injuries in soccer players, *Am J Sports Med* 10:75, 1982.
5. Ekstrand J, Gillquist J: Soccer injuries and their mechanisms: prospective study, *Med Sci Sports Exerc* 15:267, 1983.
6. Ekstrand J, Tropp H: The incidence of ankle sprains in soccer, *Foot Ankle* 11:41, 1990.
7. Garrick JG, Webb DR: *Sports injuries: diagnosis and management,* Philadelphia, 1990, WB Saunders.
8. Keene JS, Lange RH: Diagnostic dilemmas in foot and ankle injuries, *JAMA* 256:247, 1986.
9. Kibler WB: Injuries in adolescent and preadolescent soccer players, *Med Sci Sports Exerc* 25:1330, 1993
10. Kirkendall DT: Nutrition in soccer performance, *Sci Football* 4:32, 1991.
11. Kwong PJ et al: Plantar fasciitis mechanics and pathomechanics of treatment, *Clin Sports Med* 7:119, 1988.
12. Lohnes JA, Garrett W: The epidemiology of soccer injuries, Annual Meeting of ACSM, Orlando, FL, 1991.
13. Marshall P: The rehabilitation of overuse foot injuries in athletes and dancers, *Clin Sports Med* 7:175, 1988.
14. Massada JL: Ankle overuse injuries in soccer players, *J Sports Med Phys Fitness* 31:447, 1991.
15. McBryde AM Jr, Anderson RB: Sesamoid foot problems in the athlete, *Clin Sports Med* 7:51, 1988.
16. McCarroll JR et al: Meniscoid lesions of the ankle in soccer players, *Am J Sports Med* 15:255, 1987.
16a. Andrews JR, Drez DJ, McGinty JB: Symposium: Arthroscopy of joints other than the knee. *Contemp Orthop* 9(4):71, 1984.
17. McManama GB Jr: Ankle injuries in the young athlete, *Clin Sports Med* 7:547, 1988.
18. Miller EA, Hersenroeder AC: Prophylactic ankle bracing, *Pediatr Clin North Am* 37:1175, 1990.
19. Nielsen AB, Yde J: Epidemiology and traumatology of injuries in soccer, *Am J Sports Med* 17:803, 1989.
20. Norris RN: Some common foot and ankle injuries in dancers. In Solomon R, Minton SC, Solomon J, editors: *Preventing dance injuries: an interdisciplinary perspective,* Reston, Va, 1990, American Alliance for Health, Physical Education, Recreation and Dance.
21. Reilly T et al, editors: *1st World Congress of Science and Football, Liverpool, April, 1987,* Suffolk, England, 1988, St Edmundsburg Press.
22. Schmidt-Olsen S et al: Injuries among young soccer players, *Am J Sports Med* 19:273, 1991.
23. Torg JS: Fractures of the base of the fifth metatarsal distal to the tuberosity, *Orthopedics* 13:731, 1990.
24. Wiktorsson-Mölller M et al: Effects of warming up, massage, and stretching on range of motion and muscle: Strength of the lower extremity. *Am J Sports Med* 11:249, 1983.
25. Wong JC, Gregg JR: Knee, ankle and foot problems in the preadolescent and adolescent athlete, *Clin Podiatr Med Surg* 3:731, 1986.
26. Xethalis JL, Boiardo RA: Soccer injuries. In Nicholas J, editor: *The lower extremity in sports medicine,* vol II, St Louis, 1989, CV Mosby.

20

Rehabilitation of Volleyball Injuries

Keith S. Feder

Volleyball is a sport in which the participant must combine vertical and horizontal motion. The athlete must utilize lateral, backward, forward, and rotational motion complemented with jumps. The physical properties of the playing surface can significantly accentuate these demands. With the growth of beach volleyball as well as court (indoor) volleyball, there are injuries that are distinct to each and common to both.

Over the past several years, injury to players on the U.S. Volleyball Association (USVBA) National Team (Fig. 20-1) and participants in the Association of Volleyball Professionals (AVP) Beach Tour were tracked. Foot and ankle injuries to the USVBA indoor players comprised 19.82% of the total, with ankle injuries (10.81%) slightly greater than foot injuries (9.01%). Ankle injuries ranked third, behind those to the shoulder and the knee. On the beach, the incidence of foot and ankle injuries ranked fourth, behind those to the lumbar spine, shoulder, and knee. On the indoor surface, the number of foot injuries was greater than the number of ankle injuries.

Injuries can be divided into two categories: overuse and traumatic. Common overuse injuries in the sport of volleyball occur at the anterior tibial and posterior tibial muscles and the Achilles tendon (Achilles tendinitis). Plantar fascitis, metatarsal stress fracture, and tarsal-navicular stress fracture also occur at a fairly high rate. Traumatic injuries include ankle sprain, avulsion fracture to the base of the fifth metatarsal, Jones fracture to the proximal shaft of the fifth metatarsal, Achilles tendon rupture, hyperextension of the first metatarsophalangeal (MTP) joints with secondary hallux rigidus, and hyperflexion of the MTP joints with secondary instability and capsulitis.

Ankle Injuries

Lateral ligament injuries to the ankle are the most common injuries. Inversion stress can result from landing on another player's foot, sudden directional change, an inadequately rehabilitated previous injury, and from improper conditioning. The most common biomechanical mechanism of injury is the combination of inversion and rotation on a plantarflexed foot. This injury occurs more often indoors because of the increased coefficient of friction between the floor and the athlete's shoe. Furthermore, with indoor volleyball there are more players on the court (six vs. two), and side-to-side blocking

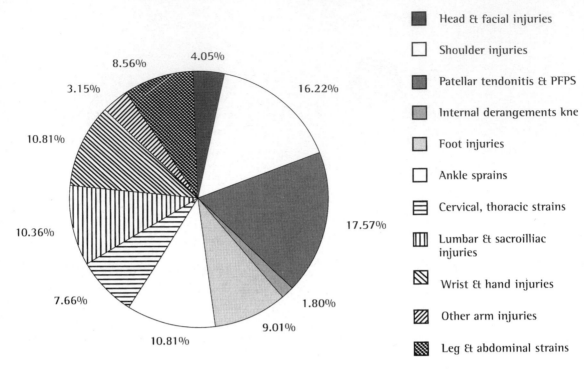

Fig. 20-1 Injuries to volleyball players by regional anatomic location. (USVBA/AVP)

techniques are utilized, which increase the risk of injury. Among the beach player population, the combination of a more forgiving surface (sand) and the increased proprioception and tendon strength in a shoeless foot decreases the incidence of lateral ligamentous injury.

Ankle sprains are classified as Grade I, II, or III. A Grade I sprain is defined as a minor tear or stretch of the ligament fibers. This injury is characterized by mild pain and little or no swelling, ecchymosis, or point tenderness. No instability is present on stress tests. A Grade II sprain is characterized by an incomplete ligament tear with moderate pain and point tenderness. Moderate swelling and hemorrhage are present as well as slight to moderate instability. A Grade III sprain consists of a complete ligament rupture, global swelling and hemorrhage, marked tenderness, significant instability, and abnormal motion.

Initial conservative treatment of all ankle sprains is that for all soft tissue injury: PRICEMM, or *Protection* of the injured area (im-

mobilization), *Rest* or activity modification (cross-training), *Ice, Compression* (elastic or hydraulic), *Elevation, Medication* (nonsteroidal antiinflammatory drugs), and *Modalities,* such as interferential, galvanic, and ultrasound (phonophorisis). Electrical stimulation can be used to both increase muscle pumping action and decrease local inflammation (Fig. 20-2). This is achieved by varying the current type and waveform employed by the modality during the course of treatment.

Cast immobilization is reserved for either Grade II injuries with moderate instability or Grade III sprains where severe instability is often present. The initial immobilization is for 2 weeks in a neutral, dorsiflexed position. The ankle is then reexamined and immobilized further if significant joint laxity remains.

The rehabilitation program is similar for all grades of ankle sprain, beginning with range of motion exercises. These exercises include plantarflexion/dorsiflexion, inversion/eversion, and "alphabet writing." The program begins with

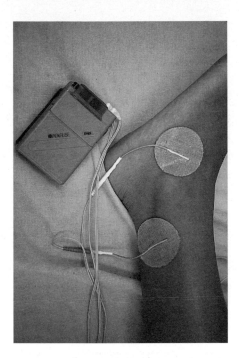

Fig. 20-2 *Muscle Stimulation.* Neuromuscular stimulation has been shown to be effective when used to increase local blood circulation and the movement of body fluids. Whenever possible, the limb should be elevated while ice and electrical stimulation are being applied.

manual resistance exercises with a therapist and progresses to elastic band resistance exercises. Double- and single-leg heel raises and BAPS board follow when tolerated, progressing to jump rope and sport-specific activity, such as digging drills and jumping drills.

Avulsion Fractures

Avulsion fractures of the base of the fifth metatarsal involve an avulsion of the peroneus brevis. Stewart[9] classifies these into fractures of the junction of the shaft and the base (IA), and comminuted fractures of the styloid with articular involvement (IB). The injury is the result of forced inversion and plantarflexion from a position of eversion and dorsiflexion. This can happen when awkwardly landing following a block or spike or

when landing on another player's foot. This is initially conservatively treated in the same fashion as Grade I and II ankle sprains. A figure eight elastic bandage is employed for support. Rarely, a short leg walking cast is necessary.

A Jones fracture was defined by Jones in 1902 as a diaphyseal fracture occurring ¾ inch distal to the tip of the styloid of the fifth metatarsal. The mechanism differs significantly from that of an avulsion fracture in that athletes that have sustained it describe an elevated heel and maximum load over the lateral aspect of the foot.[3,6,9] However, the Jones fracture in a majority of cases is a stress fracture and not an acute fracture resulting from a single traumatic event.

Initial treatment should consist of nonweight-bearing cast immobilization for a minimum of 4 to 8 weeks or until clinical healing occurs. If symptoms were present prior to fracture, or in cases where nonunion is documented, open reduction internal fixation (ORIF) with bone grafts must be considered. In studies by both Delee et al[3] and Kavanaugh et al[6] involving highly competitive athletes, primary ORIF was carried out with 100% healing in 8 to 12 weeks postoperatively.

Achilles Tendon Injuries

The Achilles tendon initiates the jumping motion. With the volleyball athlete, Achilles tendinitis occurs more frequently in the indoor player. Poor flexibility, poor conditioning, a hard surface, and the repetitive jumping that occurs indoors are all predisposing factors to this condition.

In general, Achilles tendon rupture is more common in athletes over 30 years old. The patient will describe a sudden "pop" sensation over the back of the leg. The injury will more often occur with the initiation of a jump (while blocking), as opposed to a sudden directional motion change (which occurs while digging). Chronic injury, chronic inflammation (long-standing tendinitis), previous corticosteroid injection, and poor flexibility are contributing factors. The diagnosis is made with a positive Thompson test and/or a palpable tendon defect. The Thompson test may not be positive with an intact plantaris. If there is a diagnostic dilemma, magnetic resonance imaging may be helpful.

Conservative treatment, rest, casting, and rehabilitation can be considered in the recreational and older athlete, as well as in the patient with a partial tear. However, studies have shown a higher rate of rerupture with nonoperative treatment.[4]

Operative treatment is strongly considered in the younger athlete, the elite athlete, and in those patients with a tear at the calcaneal insertion. Postoperative treatment is becoming more aggressive, with full weight-bearing in a short leg walking cast at 2 weeks. Cast changes are recommended at 2-week intervals with a gradual increase in dorsiflexion. At 8 weeks, the patient is taken out of the cast and placed into a shoe with a tapered heel lift. The heel lift is gradually decreased over the next 8 to 12 weeks. An aggressive physical rehabilitation exercise program is initiated with an expectation that the athlete will return to competitive volleyball 9 to 12 months from the time of operative intervention.

The remaining injuries—plantar fascitis, sesamoiditis, arch sprains, MTP joint hyperextension, and MTP joint hyperflexion—occur both indoors and on the sand. Plantar fascitis, sesamoiditis, arch sprain, and hyperextension injuries to the toe are more common indoors because of the unresilient nature of the playing surface. Hyperflexion injuries of the toes are rare indoors but common in beach volleyball.

Plantar fascitis, sesamoiditis, and arch sprains are all injuries to the plantar aspect of the foot

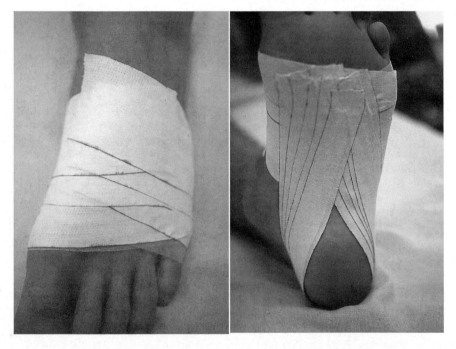

Fig. 20-3 *Arch Taping.* Arch taping supports the longitudinal arch and stabilizes the forefoot. The following steps may be followed; the athlete lying face down on the table with the foot extended out over the table:
1. Place anchor strips around the ball of the foot.
2. Start the next strip at the base of the great toe; take tape around the heel, crossing to the arch, and then return to the starting point.
3. Start the next strip at the base of the second toe and repeat, covering the arch 3 to 4 times, depending on the size of the foot.
4. Close tape with anchors around the ball of the foot.

Rehabilitation of the Athlete's Foot and Ankle

occurring secondary to the repetitive trauma of jumping. This repetitive trauma occurs as a result of both the takeoff and landing actions of jumping. Initial treatment is PRICEMM. Indoors, the injury can be treated with the appropriate pad, heel wedge, and/or orthotic (semiflexible medial longitudinal arch support). The only way to treat these injuries in a beach volleyball player is to employ an appropriate supportive taping technique (Fig. 20-3). Prevention of these injuries begins with an appropriate stretching regimen, off-season conditioning, and correct jumping technique.

Hyperextension injuries of the great toe (turf toe) and lesser toes are seen both indoors and outdoors. Initial treatment is PRICEMM. Taping techniques used to prevent hyperextension can ameliorate the problem (Fig. 20-4). Ongoing hyperextension trauma can lead to hallux

rigidus.[2,8] Predisposing factors for hallux rigidus of the great toe have been reported to include an abnormally long first metatarsal[1,8] and pronation of the forefoot.

With the indoor player, conservative treatment of hallux rigidus includes the use of a stable, stiff-soled shoe and orthotics with a firm first metatarsal support. On the beach, taping is the mainstay. Surgical treatment for hallux rigidus may be necessary if conservative measures fail.

Hyperflexion injuries to the toes are rare indoors. It is common to have the toes fold plantarly when landing following a jump on uneven terrain (sand). Initial treatment is PRICEMM. Appropriate taping to prevent hyperflexion is used to prevent reexacerbation (Fig. 20-5). Capsulitis and synovitis of the MTP joint may become chronic in addition to joint laxity. In chronic, symptomatic cases that do not respond

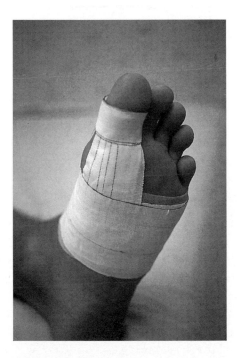

Fig. 20-4 *Turf Toe.* To limit extension of the great toe, the following steps may be followed:
1. Anchor the forefoot.
2. Anchor the great toe.
3. Place vertical strips on the plantar surface from the great toe to the forefoot.
4. Anchor the vertical strips.

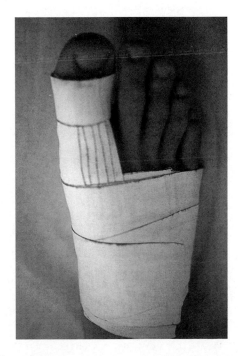

Fig. 20-5 *Turf Toe.* To limit flexion of the great toe, the following steps may be followed:
1. Anchor the forefoot.
2. Anchor the great toe.
3. Place vertical strips on the dorsal surface from the great toe to the forefoot.
4. Anchor the vertical strips.

to conservative treatment, surgery is recommended. A synovectomy or ligament or capsular repair may be indicated.[2]

Bibliography

1. Bonney G, McNab I: Hallux valgus and hallux rigidus: critical survey of operative results, *J Bone Joint Surg* 34B:366, 1952.
2. Coughlin MJ: Lesser toe deformities, *Orthopedics* 10:63, 1987.
3. DeLee JC, Evans R, Julian J: Stress fractures of the fifth metatarsal, *Am J Sports Med* 11:349, 1983.
4. Inglis AE et al: Ruptures of the tendo Achilles: an objective assessment of surgical and non-surgical treatment, *J Bone Joint Surg* 58A:990, 1976.
5. Jack EA: The etiology of hallux rigidus, *Br J Surg* 27:492, 1940.
6. Kavanaugh JH, Brown TD, Mann RV: The Jones fracture revisited, *J Bone Joint Surg* 60A:776, 1978.
7. Lambrinudi C: Metatarsus primus elevatus, *Proc R Soc Med* 31:1273, 1938.
8. McMurray TP: Treatment of hallux valgus and rigidus, *BMJ* 2:218, 1936.
9. Stewart IM: Jones fracture: fractures of the base of the fifth metatarsal, *Clin Orthop* 16:190, 1960.

Rehabilitation of the Athlete's Foot and Ankle

21

Assessment of the Dancer's Foot and Ankle for Rehabilitation

Marika Molnar

The uniqueness of dance as an art form needs to be considered in order to construct a meaningful rehabilitation program. Dancers are often compared to elite athletes because the physical requirements are similar. Indeed, the modalities required to rehabilitate the dancer are much the same as those required for other athletes. Additionally, therapy must also include perfecting dance technique as well as understanding the particular requirements of the type of dance performed. This chapter describes a total body approach to the assessment of the dancers foot and ankle with special insight into functional dance technique.

Dancers are a unique population of people to work with. They come in a variety of sizes, shapes, skills, and levels of achievement. They range in age from the prepubescent student to the mature teacher/choreographer, with the great majority of professional dancers in the 20 to 40 year age range.

Certain injuries afflict students of dance due to their growth and development, such as metatarsal stress fractures and Achilles tendonitis; the professional dancer is plagued by microtraumas due to repetitive motion or overuse injuries; the mature dancer has "wear-and-tear" types of injuries such as hallux rigidus or tarsometatarsal joint arthritis.

For a professional dancer, complete recovery from an injury to the foot and ankle means that they are able to return to full and active participation in class, rehearsals, and performance. A comprehensive rehabilitation program requires that the clinician have:

- An understanding of the physical demands of dance for full functional return
- Confident use of the dance vocabulary and awareness of the repertoire of movement
- Knowledge of extrinsic and intrinsic factors that affect healing time and the pathomechanics of injury
- A solid understanding of the biomechanical integration of the foot and ankle into the locomotor system and the consequences of abnormal movement
- The ability to teach dynamic alignment for re-education of dance skills as well as normal motor patterns
- Good clinical reasoning skills to determine ap-

propriate treatment based on history, observation, evaluation, and assessment
· A responsible and motivated patient

The rehabilitation program should therefore include a total body screen with components to address the above needs.

Screening the Dancer

It has been established that the physical demands of dance are equal to those of professional football,[12] yet the dancer cannot go on stage with protective taping and bracing to prevent injury. A dancer must have full confidence that the strength, flexibility, and stability required will be there so that the focus can be on the performance.

In the ankle, the anterior talofibular ligament is the most vulnerable to injury due to its line of pull and the stresses and strains placed on it during dancing of any style.[6] Flexor hallicus longus (FHL) tendonitis and posterior impingement syndromes affect ballet dancers more often because of their extreme plantarflexion/ hallux dorsiflexion range and the wearing of *pointe* shoes. Fractured or bruised sessamoids and anterior impingement syndromes are more commonly seen in the modern or Broadway dancer.

A total body screen, with an *emphasis* on the foot and ankle, is a good way to gather essential subjective and objective information. This is useful for prevention as well as for establishing specific guidelines to evaluate and treat dancers so that their special needs can be met.

The total body screen that we use is outlined in Box 21-1.

The *Dance/Performance History* is the first part of a total body screen. This is the clinician's introduction to the dancer and is a useful way to gather insight into the precipitating and predisposing factors that could have led to the present injury. *The History of Present and Past Injury* is covered next. Weakness and instability are often the result of past injuries that were not properly treated and therefore affect the dancer's present condition.

The *Posture Assessment* is a general overview of the organization of the neuromusculoskeletal system. Observing distal to proximal can give information about lower extremity relationships, muscle hypertonicity or hypotonicity, and spinal alignment. Areas that require more detailed examination can be noted.

The *Hip Range of Motion* and *Manual Muscle Testing*[8,10,11] screens are used specifically to get detailed information about muscle balance around the pelvis and lower extremity. Deficits in strength or flexibility may be picked up that can predispose the dancer to injury, or residual dysfunction from a past injury may be uncovered, which must be rectified.

The *Foot Evaluation*[2,13,14] is a specific biomechanical examination to determine the normal and abnormal motions and compensations of the foot and ankle. This is done in nonweight-bearing.

Observing the *Gait Patterns*[3] can reveal muscle weakness, leg length discrepancies, and abnormal compensations.

Proprioception[4] tests are used to evaluate how well the receptors in the peripheral joints are relaying and receiving the messages to and from the central nervous system.

Motion testing of the spine is used to determine abnormalities such as scoliosis, kyphosis, and flat areas as well as where the restrictions are coming from. Spinal rotation greater in kneeling than standing could implicate the tibiofibular joint and below as the cause of limitation in segmental motion.

Technique Assessment

Dancers execute thousands of pliés and relevés during the course of their day. If they are performing these basic steps with faulty alignment, they are susceptible to overuse injuries due to repetitive motion microtrauma. Keep in mind also that most preparations for turns and jumps, as well as all landings, pass through the plié position. A form such as that shown in Box 21-2 can be used to assess the dancer's performance of these basic steps.

Box 21-1   Total Body Screen

Dance/Performance History

Age began dancing and type of dance (ballet, jazz, modern, etc.)

Age began *pointe* work

Formal dance training (include school and number of years)

Present dance training and number of classes per week

Years of professional dancing

Name of company you are performing with now and style of dancing

Type of shoes worn and size (street and ballet)

Orthotics

Type of floor surface

Do you teach or choreograph and what amount?

Do you generally warm up before class? For how long? What do you do?

Special Questions for Women

Age of onset of menses

Regularity or absence

Any history of scoliosis or stress fractures?

From a biomechanical perspective, a plié can be considered closed kinetic chain pronation and a relevé is similar to closed kinetic chain supination. Both have an external rotation component superimposed when the dancer is turned out. The sagittal plane movements of plantarflexion and dorsiflexion are now transverse and frontal plane movements with an anteriorly directed force of gravity often complicating matters.

Box 21-1 Total Body Screen—cont'd

History of Present Injury

Diagnosis _____ M.D. _____ Date _____
Date of Birth _____ Height _____ Weight _____
Date of Injury _____
Describe injury and how it occurred (positions, symptoms, etc.) _____
_____
_____
_____

Place of occurrence _____
Precipitating factors (e.g., not warmed up, hard floor, cold studio) _____
_____
Prior treatment (M.D., chiropractors, physical therapy, massage, etc.) _____
_____
Assistive devices used _____
Medical tests performed (X-rays, magnetic resonance imaging, blood tests, urinalysis, etc.) _____

Major Injuries or Illnesses Throughout Dance Career

Date	Type of Injury	Whom Seen	Course of treatment	Recovery (includes setbacks)

Posture Assessment

Posterior View

Left   Right

Ear levels
Shoulder height
Inferior scapular angle
Waist creases
Iliac crests
Popliteal creases
Rearfoot varus/valgus
Muscle tone:
   Trapezius
   Paravertebrals
   Hamstrings
   Gastroc-soleus

Box 21-1   Total Body Screen—cont'd

Anterior View

Right   Left

Clavicle (angle)
Acromioclavicular joint
Iliac crest
Knees: genu valgum/varum
Q angle
Tibial torsion
Forefoot varus/valgus
Hallux valgus
Dorsal calluses
Muscle tone
    Pectorals
    Quads
    VMO
    Adductors
    Anterior calf
    Gastroc-soleus
Lateral View

Left   Right

Forward head (+/−, normal)
Cervical lordosis (+/−, normal)
Thoracic kyphosis (+/−,
    normal)
Lumbar lordosis (+/−, normal)
Genu recurvatum (Y/N)
Anterior leg-foot angle (+/−,
    normal)
Navicular height
Hip Range of Motion

Right   Left

Hip external rotation (supine)
Hip internal rotation (supine)
Hip external rotation (prone)
Hip internal rotation (prone)
Total rotation (passively turning
    out feet)
Hip flexion (supine)
Hamstring range of motion
Hip extension (prone)
Firing patterns: extensors, abduc-
    tors
Janda Screen:
    Psoas
    Rectus
    Adductors
    Tensor fascia lata
    Hip capsule

Continued.

Assessment of the Dancer's Foot and Ankle for Rehabilitation   Chapter 21

Box 21-1 Total Body Screen—cont'd

Manual Muscle Testing

Right   Left

Back extensors
Gluteus maximus
Abdominals
Hip abduction (parallel and
Hip adduction turned out)
Hip external rotation
Hip internal rotation
Quads
Hamstrings
Gastroc-soleus
Peroneals (all foot and ankle
    muscles tested at short, mid,
    and end range)
Posterior tibialis
Anterior tibialis
Intrinsics

Foot Evaluation

Right   Left

Malleolar position
Ankle plantarflexion
Ankle dorsiflexion (knee straight)
Ankle dorsiflexion (knee bent)
Subtalar neutral
Subtalar range of motion
    (inversion)
Subtalar range of motion
    (eversion)
Midtarsal motion: Tarsometatar-
    sal joint pronation
Midtarsal motion: Tarsometatar-
    sal joint supination
Forefoot relationship
First ray position
Plantar lesions
Toe positions
Arch height
Hallux dorsiflexion
Leg length (prone)
Leg length (supine)

Box 21-1   Total Body Screen—cont'd

Gait Patterns

_____

Proprioception

Modified Rhomberg test _____
BAPS _____

Motion Testing of Spine

Forward, sideward, and backward bending
  Standing _____
  Sitting _____
Standing, seated, and kneeling rotation
_____

Box 21-2   Technique Assessment

Posterior view, parallel stance facing barre

1. Parallel first position turned out

_____
_____
_____

2. Parallel demi-plié

_____
_____

3. Parallel relevé

_____
_____

4. First position demi-plié

_____
_____

5. First position relevé

_____
_____

6. Second position relevé

_____
_____

7. Second position grande plié

_____
_____
_____

Continued.

Box 21-2   Technique Assessment—cont'd

8. Tendu

   Front _____
   _____

   Side _____
   _____

   Back _____
   _____

9. First position coupé (single leg stance)
   _____
   _____
   _____

The passive range of motion at the foot and ankle in plantarflexion is measured at 50 degrees and in dorsiflexion at 20 degrees[2] (Fig. 21-1**A**). Most professional dancers can plantarflex to a position greater than 90 degrees but lose at least 10 degrees range in dorsiflexion.[7]

Parallel to first position turned out (Fig. 21-1**B**) evaluates the ability of the lumbar spine to remain neutral with a stable pelvis as the hip joints maximally externally rotate. This rotation continues distally to the feet.

The movement should be symmetrical, with abdominal stabilization and contraction of the deep external rotators and adductors rather than the gluteus maximus. The forefoot and hindfoot should be in line without excessive forefoot abduction or hallux valgus.

Parallel demi-plié and relevé (Fig. 21-2) is evaluated for correct alignment and range of mo0 tion at the talocrural joint. Height of the heel and position of the heel should be symmetrical.

Decreased range of motion in demi-plié can imply an anterior impingement or tight posterior soleus. Observe muscle bulk for symmetry; decreased calcaneal height in relevé can result from weakness of the triceps surae, chronic Achilles tendonitis, or posterior impingement.

Observe the eversion and inversion of the calcaneus from plié to relevé. Normally, 10 degrees of eversion and 20 degrees of inversion are available at the subtalar joint.[14] Often dancers have a deficit of eversion due to their overuse of plantarflexion, which causes more inversion of the calcaneus. The forefoot may abnormally compensate for lack of calcaneal eversion by "rolling in" or flattening the medial arch.

Often dancers will relevé too high and appear to "sickle in," placing excessive stress on the anterior talofibular ligament. Dancers may also shift their weight laterally if they have a hallux limitus or rigidus or weak peroneals.

First position demi-plié and relevé (Fig. 21-3) evaluates the integration of lumbar, pelvic, and lower extremity alignment. Depth of demi-plié and height of relevé should be even with the center of gravity directly in the midline.

Second position relevé (Fig. 21-4**A**) should demonstrate a straight line down the front of the leg to the toes without a change at the ankle.

Second position grande plié (Fig. 21-4**B**) checks for hip, knee, and ankle flexion with center of gravity in the midline. There should be no shifting of weight to either side.

The *tendu* (Fig. 21-5) is the first step that requires a transfer of weight from two feet to one

Text continued on p. 323.

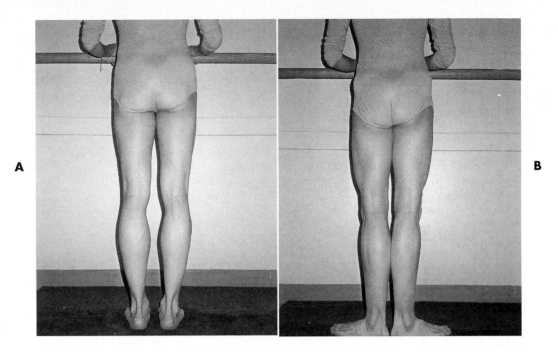

Fig. 21-1   A, Parallel starting position. B, Parallel to first position turned out.

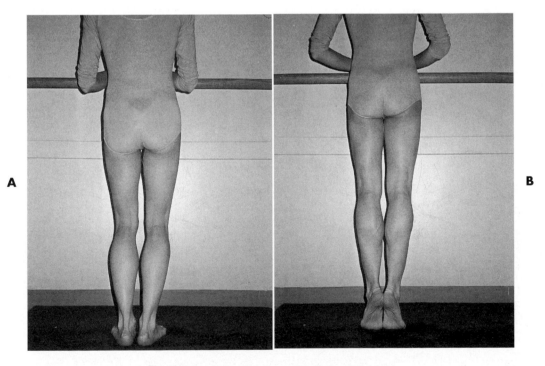

Fig. 21-2   A, Parallel demi-plié. B, Parallel relevé.

Assessment of the Dancer's Foot and Ankle for Rehabilitation   Chapter 21   319

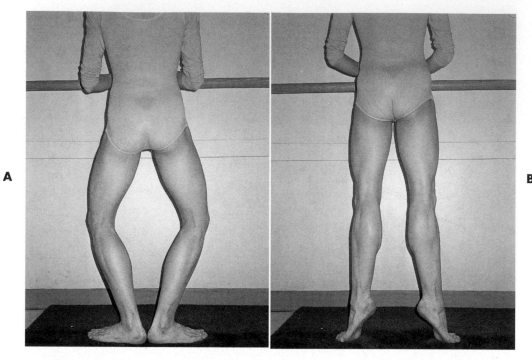

Fig. 21-3 **A,** First position demi-plié (turned out). **B,** First position relevé (turned out).

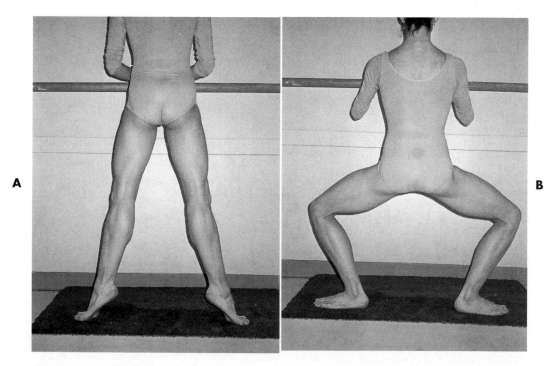

Fig. 21-4 **A,** Second position relevé. **B,** Second position grand plié.

Rehabilitation of the Athlete's Foot and Ankle

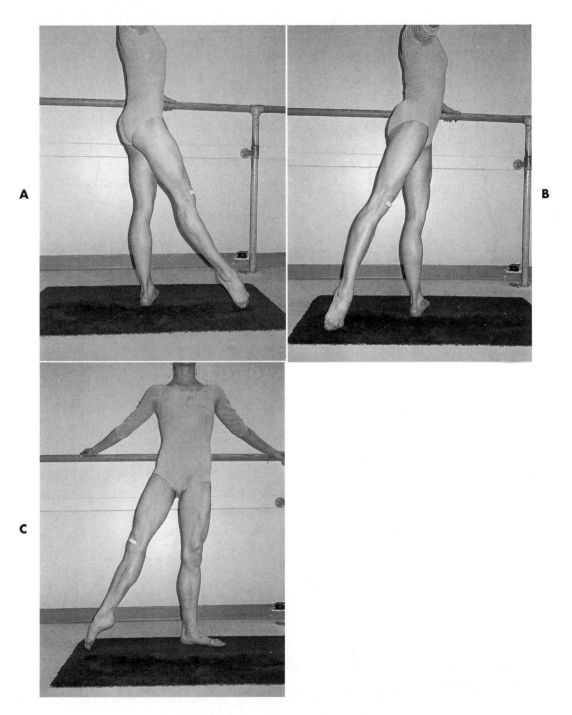

Fig. 21-5 Tendu. **A,** Front. **B,** Back. **C,** Side.

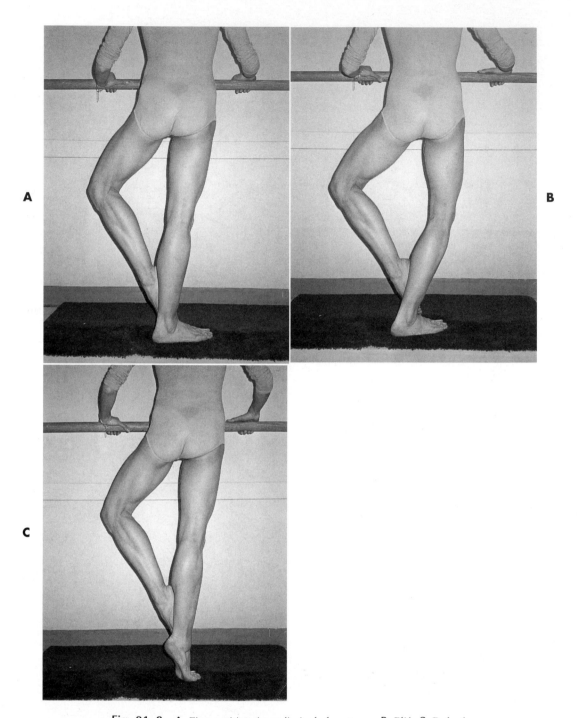

Fig. 21-6 **A,** First position (coupé) single leg stance. **B,** Plié. **C,** Relevé.

foot. The standing leg is the supporting leg and the other one is referred to as the "gesture" leg or working leg.

The shoulders and the pelvis should remain level and the face squarely to the front during the front and side tendu. In the back tendu, once the leg has taken up the full hip extension range of motion, the pelvis on that side will move slightly backward with it to maintain the turn-out of the leg.

Both the supporting and the working leg must maintain their turn-out position. There should be no weight borne on the toes of the gesture leg, and there should be no rolling in or out on the supporting foot.

First position (coupé) single leg stance (Fig. 21-6) evaluates the weight shifting in the trunk, pelvis, and lower extremity as well as the range of motion in dorsiflexion/plantarflexion as the dancer moves from demi-plié to relevé on one leg. Compare right and left sides for muscle usage, range of motion, alignment, and coordination.

Both legs should be *equally* turned out and maintained in that position. There are more compressive stresses on the joints as well as increased torque due to single leg stance that may predispose to injury if there are inherent weaknesses or instability.

Special Tests for Foot and Ankle

Nonweight-bearing

1. Examine *accessory movements*[1,5,9] of the foot and ankle joints:
   Superior and inferior tibiofibular
   Talocrural
   Subtalar
   Calcaneocuboid
   Talonavicular
   Intercuneiform
   Tarsometatarsal
   Intermetatarsal
   Metatarsophalangeal
2. *Palpate* the above joints and surrounding tissues while the foot points and flexes to determine tissue tensions, painful arcs, crepitus, and to differentiate tendons involved.

   Place the foot in a *fully plantarflexed position* and ask the dancer to flex and point the big toe. Palpate behind the medial malleolus and feel for thickening, crepitus, and pain response to your pressure. This differentiates flexor hallucis longus dysfunction from posterior tibial or Achilles involvement.

   Palpate behind the lateral malleolus and move the finger in deep to find the os trigonum while the foot is in relaxed plantarflexion. If palpable and painful, it could be a cause of dysfunction.

   Passively plantarflex the foot by aggressively moving the heel toward the tibia to test for posterior impingement; extreme pain is a positive response.

3. Place the patient prone and passively plantarflex all toes to slacken the plantar aspect of the foot. Palpate through soft tissues to feel for cuboid subluxation, which will be painful and have a boney feel. (This technique can be used to find other "dropped" bones as well.)

4. *Seated talar glide:* With the patient sitting at the edge of the table with knees straight, hold the feet and place your thumbs on the talus in between the tibia and fibula. Glide the talus posteriorly as you bend the knees and dorsiflex the ankles symmetrically. An uneven return to 90 degrees of knee flexion implies possible soleus tightness or anterior displacement of talus (inability to glide posteriorly) or dysfunction of the tibiofibular joint.

5. Talocrural stress tests: anterior drawer sign and talar tilt for lateral ligaments; dorsiflexion/abduction test for medial ligaments.

Weight-bearing

1. With the patient standing, palpate motion of the superior tibiofibular and inferior tibiofibular joints during parallel and turned out plié and relevé. There should be distinct cephalad and caudad movements.

2. With the patient standing, palpate the medial and lateral borders of the talus during plié and relevé. Place the subtalar joint into neutral position and maintain it while the dancer again performs a plié and relevé. Notice the effects proximally and distally when the subtalar joint is in neutral alignment as compared to the dancer's habitual pattern. This can be corrected by realignment and proprioceptive exercises.

The outcome of these tests often indicates the treatment choices. For example, if the soleus is tight, restricting talar posterior glide or maintaining inversion of the calcaneus, a soft tissue release approach to the soleus muscle and fascia should proceed joint mobilization and reeducation.

Summary

It is of paramount importance that the strength, flexibility, stability, and proprioception of the dancer's foot and ankle be fully rehabilitated. The treatment of dance injuries includes the use of manual therapy skills, therapeutic exercises, modalities, and alignment/technique reeducation. The aesthetic and athletic qualities of dance as well as the longevity of a dancer's career depend on the therapist's knowledge and skill.

From the results of the total body screen and technique assessment, the clinician will be able to determine the treatment philosophy. Short- and long-term goals will be based upon the dancer's needs as well as the physical evaluation. Correction of faulty foot and ankle biomechanics during basic dance steps is one way to reduce injuries due to repetitive microtrauma or poor movement patterns. It also enables dancers to take responsibility for their health and maintenance as they learn how the body can move more efficiently without trauma.

Bibliography

1. Corrigan B, Mailand CD: 1983. *Practical orthopaedic medicine: part I—peripheral joints,* London, 1983, Butterworth.
2. Donatelli R: *The biomechanics of the foot and ankle,* Philadelphia, 1990, FA Davis.
3. Donatelli R, Wikes JS: Lower kinetic chain and human gait, *J Back Musculoskeletal Rehab* 2:4, 1992.
4. Freeman MAR, Wyke BD: Articular reflexes at the ankle joint: an electromyographic study of the normal and abnormal influences of ankle joint mechanoreceptors upon reflex activity in the leg muscles, *Br J Surg* 64:990, 1967.
5. Greenman PE: Lower extremity technique. In *Principles of manual medicine,* Baltimore, 1989, Williams & Wilkins.
6. Hamilton WG: Foot and ankle injuries in dancers, *Clin Sports Med* 7:143, 1988.
7. Hamilton WG et al: A profile of the musculoskeletal characteristics of elite professional ballet dancers, *Am J Sports Med* 20:267, 1992.
8. Janda V: *Muscle function testing,* London, 1983, Butterworths.
9. Kaltenborn FM: Manual therapy for the extremity joints, ed 2, Oslo, 1976, Olaf Norlis Bokhandel.
10. Kendall FP, McCreary EK: *Muscle testing and function,* ed 3, Baltimore, 1983, Williams & Wilkins.
11. Kessler RM, Hertling D: *Management of common musculoskeletal disorders: physical therapy principles and methods,* Philadelphia, 1983, Harper & Row.
12. Nicholas JA: Risk factors in sports medicine and the orthopedic system: an overview, *J Sports Med Phys Fitness* 3:243, 1975.
13. Root ML: *Biomechanical examination of the foot,* vol I, Los Angeles, 1971, Clinical Biomechanics.
14. Root ML, Orien WP, Weed JN: *Clinical biomechanics,* vol II: *Normal and abnormal function of the foot,* Los Angeles, 1977, Clinical Biomechanics.

4

Taping, Shoe Modifications, Orthoses, Arthrodeses

22

Taping and Padding of the Foot and Ankle

Thomas J. Herrmann

Rehabilitation

When discussing the rehabilitation of the foot and ankle it makes sense to approach them as one since it is unlikely that an injury to one will not affect the other. Most rehabilitation and sports medicine practitioners use a phased approach[1] when constructing any rehabilitation program, and the approach to the foot and ankle is no different. The protocol that follows is broken down into five phases.

Phase I: Maximum Protection/Control of Acute Responses

Goals

Protection and anatomic reduction

Pain control

Swelling control

Minimize neuromotor loss

Maintain general conditioning

Components

Removable splint or other orthosis

Limited weight-bearing

Antiinflammatory medications if warranted

Ice, compression, elevation

Electrical stimulation around injury for pain control

Muscle stimulation along muscles that control the joint

Isometric muscle strengthening in neutral position in concert with the stimulation

Active range of motion in safe plane and range

Stationary cycling as tolerated

Weight training as tolerated

Application

In the orthosis at all times except during therapy

Non or partial weight-bearing per pain

Nonsteroidal antiinflammatory drugs (NS-AIDs) if warranted

Cold whirlpool or immersion baths (10 to 15 minutes)

Active motion in cold water

Immediate elevation out of cold with active motion per limits for 5 minutes in compression wrap

Use of cold or compression device with elevation (e.g., Cryotemp by Jobst or Cryo-cuff[R] by Aircast) (20 to 30 minutes)

Interferential or high-voltage stimulation at joint for pain control[7]

VMS or Russian stimulation on gastrocnemius, anterior tibialis, peroneals, and posterior tibialis for neuromotor response[9] (all

327

stimulation can be done inside cold or compression device)

Stationary cycle and weight training of upper and lower body as tolerated

Frequency

Minimum 3 times a week (weekend warrior in clinical setting)

Maximum 3 times a day (high-caliber athlete in training room setting)

Phase II: Moderate Protection and Basic Function

Goals

Maintain protection of injury

Increase weight-bearing as tolerated in orthosis

Early strengthening

Early proprioception

Eliminate swelling

Maintain fitness

Components

Continue orthosis

Continue modality applications as in Phase I

Rhythmic isometrics in neutral position

Short-arc manual resistance exercises in plantarflexion and dorsiflexion and proprioceptive neuromuscular facilitation (PNF) patterns

Passive stretching to pain (plus a little) in plantarflexion and dorsiflexion

Cardiovascular and weight training as tolerated

Application

In orthosis at all times except during therapy

Modalities as in Phase I

Stretch gastrocsoleus complex and plantar fascia passively and nonweight-bearing

Randomly and rhythmically applied force to foot by therapist/trainer while foot is held in neutral position by athlete

Manual resistance exercises in the pain-free arcs of plantarflexion and dorsiflexion and D1/D2 PNF patterns[11]

Biomechanical Ankle Platform System (BAPS) board activities at level 1 and 2, no weight and nonweight-bearing

Seated lower extremity closed kinetic chain activities (e.g., Kinetron, leg press)

Stationary cycling and weight training

Frequency

Minimum 3 times a week

Maximum 2 times a day

Phase III: Minimum Protection/Normal Function

Goals

Wean to full weight-bearing

Wean from orthosis

Restore strength

Proprioception training

Introduction to functional activities of sport

Maintain general fitness

Components

Pain as guide to discontinuation of orthosis

Replace orthosis with a functional brace

Pain as guide to progression to full weight-bearing

BAPS and Kinesthetic Awareness Trainer (KAT) board activities

Static balancing activities

Push to full range of motion plantarflexion and dorsiflexion (still limit inversion to pain)

Straight-ahead functional activity in brace/tape

Application

Orthosis off for activities of daily living (ADL), on for high-risk terrain or surfaces

Lace-up brace or pneumatic stirrup for ADL

Wean from crutches P.A.G (Pain As Guide).

Aggressive stretching of gastroc-soleus complex

Aggressive stretching into dorsiflexion

Modalities continue as in Phase I and II

Joint mobilizations to reduce capsular tightness

Cross-friction massage at joint lines

Ultrasound therapy, pulsed 10% or 20% along joint lines to promote capsular flexibility[9]

Walking/jogging/running program in tape/brace straight ahead; acceleration/deceleration activities in tape/brace straight ahead

Balancing activities with eyes closed

BAPS board and KAT board activities full weight-bearing at moderate levels in tape/brace

Manual resistance exercises full active range of motion in plantarflexion and dorsiflexion and PNF patterns D1/D2

Progressive resistance exercises (e.g., toe raises)

Continue general fitness training

Frequency

Minimum 3 times a week

Maximum 2 times a day

Phase IV: Return to Activity

Goals

Full strength

Full range of motion

Full neuromotor control

Return to play

Components

Progressive resistance exercises

Manual resistance exercises

Running to full speed, including directional changes

Hopping, jumping activities including directional changes (plyometric activities)

Backward running

BAPS and KAT board activities, full weight-bearing

Challenged balance activities

Controlled return to sport activities

Tape/functional brace

Continue modalities as necessary

Continue general fitness training

Application

Aggressive manual resistance exercises in straight and PNF patterns, full range of motion

Aggressive progressive resistance exercises (e.g., three-position toe and heel raises, leg press)

Balancing on affected foot while tossing foam ball or while therapist/trainer gently pushes on shoulders (eyes open or closed)

BAPS and KAT board activities, full weight-bearing with eyes closed

Progressive running activities in tape/brace: straight forward and backward to full speed, Ss, figure eights, Zs to full speed (large to small based on gait and pain)

Jumping/hopping on grid, clockwise, counterclockwise, zig-zag in tape/brace

Sport-specific drills in tape/brace with trainer/therapist

Controlled return to sport activity in tape/brace, begin at 50% of practice activity, increase as tolerated

Cold whirlpool or cold soaks, ultrasound, soft tissue mobilization as indicated

General conditioning with team

Frequency

Minimum 3 times a week

Maximum daily

Phase V: Full Return/Maintenance Program

Goals

Unrestricted return to activity

Maintain strength and function

Components

Gradual return to full activity

Continue strength and functional training

Modalities as indicated

Tape/brace

Application

Return to activity in tape/brace, increased pain as guide

Continue strengthening, especially BAPS and KAT board activities

Continue modalities as indicated

Frequency

Minimum 3 times a week

Maximum daily

There are a few comments that are worth making regarding the rehabilitation of the foot and ankle. The first is that, unlike most other joints susceptible to injury in sport, the ankle/foot complex seems to respond favorably to being "overtreated." That is, the ankle/foot seems to respond quickly when treatment/rehabilitation bouts are pushed to 2 or 3 times a day. The second is that cryokinetics can have a dramatic effect on the initial swelling and the elimination of inappropriate scar formation.[1,6] Combining cold and motion activates the vascular/lymphatic pump to move the swelling and helps minimize the formation of scar tissue that is not along the functional axis of the healing tissue. This helps ensure a comfortable and functional range of motion. The third is that the ankle can be well protected as the athlete is returned to activity, which is of tremendous assistance when pushing for an early return.

The demands of the sport have considerable effect on the success of an early return to sport after injury. Athletes whose sport contains a significant vertical component, such as basketball and volleyball, seem to have less success in early return attempts. The proprioceptive challenge and the impact/deceleration problem of landing from repeated jumps is a confounding factor. From the trainer's perspective, it is usually easier to control the torsional forces of more horizontal sports such as football and soccer.

To risk proposing a time line for return to activity requires determining a starting point in the rehabilitation/treatment protocol. Generally, Grade I injuries fall into Phase III in the protocol and can be fully returned to activity in 5 days to 2 weeks depending on the demands of the sport and the response of the athlete to pain. Grade II injuries usually start in Phase I but don't spend a great deal of time there before moving

on, with the usual return to activity in 1 to 3 weeks, again depending on the demands of the sport and the athlete's response. Grade III injuries begin in Phase I and can spend as long as 3 or 4 weeks in Phases I and II. It is overly optimistic to expect an athlete to return to full activity in fewer than 4 weeks after a Grade III ankle injury. A successful return in about 6 weeks is more typical, but the athlete should be braced for the fact that the ankle may still be sore for months (see box).

In my experience, the quickest athlete to rehabilitate and return to sport from a Grade III ankle sprain did so in 5 weeks from the date of injury. Suprisingly, this athlete was a male intercollegiate volleyball player. The slowest was 10 weeks, after a Grade III inversion injury with a syndesmosis injury and a medial capsular impingement (for practical purposes, the athlete subluxed his talus). Again suprisingly, this athlete was an intercollegiate pole vaulter, and the injury was to his drive foot during his pole plant. Persistent pain along the anterior/medial joint

---

Graded Injuries and Phased Rehabilitation

Grade III—Complete tissue disruption
    Severe swelling
    Near complete loss of function
    (70- 100%)
    Severely limited ROM
    Marked decrease in stability

Long–Term Rehab Program →

Grade II—Partial tissue disruption
    Moderate/severe swelling
    Moderate loss of function (30-70%)
    Moderate/severe loss of ROM
    Moderate decrease in stability

Moderate–Term Rehab Program →

Grade I—No real tissue disruption
    Mild/moderate swelling
    Mild loss of function (0-30%)
    Mild loss of ROM
    No decrease in stability

Short –Term Rehab Program →

Phase I—Rest/immobilization, PWB to NWB, ICE, pain control, ROM in safe planes, isometrics, rest of body conditioning, modalities as indicated.

Phase II—Continue Phase I PRE's in safe planes, AROM in all planes with pain as guide, increase weight-bearing, modalities.

Phase III—Continue Phase II, AROM in plantar and dorsiflexion to full, isotonic exercises to FROM, full weight-bearing, neuromotor training, proprioception, modalities.

Phase IV—Continue Phase III, isokinetic training, skill training, flexibility training, high-speed training, high-resistance training, limited practice.

Phase V—Continue Phase IV as maintenance, gradual return to full activity.

ROM = range of motion, PWB = partial weight-bearing, NWB = nonweight-bearing, ICE = ice, compression, elevation, PRE = progressive resistance exercises, AROM = active ROM, FROM = full ROM.

line restricted his ability to fully dorsiflex and drive off his foot. In general, athletes who are able to return quickly are those that can perform in a semirigid orthosis that offers considerable support and range of motion restrictions[2,5] (e.g., offensive linemen in football).

Finally, it is important to recognize that pain and swelling equal disability. The inhibitory effects of pain and swelling on the proprioceptive mechanism and muscular recruitment and strength are real and can be deleterious to the athlete's return.[3,11] Pain is also a major distraction and can be a behavioral preoccupation for an athlete. There is nothing wrong with allowing an athlete to admit that the injury "hurts too much to play."

Taping and Padding

The value of taping and padding the foot and ankle lies in the ability of the athletic trainer to customize a support system for each athlete.

Taping

While many studies suggest that the effects of tape are temporary and that the support offered quickly diminishes,[2,10] taping remains a mainstay for many athletes. The proprioceptive enhancement derived from the tactile stimulation of the tape and the relative comfort when compared to a brace provide the athlete with a sense of security and control.[1]

The standard ankle tape has undergone many variations and improvements over the years, but the "basketweave" developed by Gibney still represents the fundamental approach to ankle taping.[1] In essence, the ankle is surrounded by a series of interlocking strips known as *stirrups and horseshoes,* applied alternately to form a basketweave pattern from inferior and posterior to superior and anterior of the joint (Fig. 22-1). This weave is followed by a figure eight and heel locks, or an interrupted figure eight with a heel lock interposed, in order to approximate with tape the capsular and extracapsular ligament pattern around the joint (Figs. 22-2, 22-3, 22-4). Once closed with circular and semicircular strips,

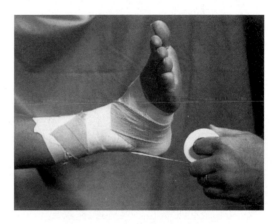

Fig. 22-2   Initiating the figure eight with heel locks.

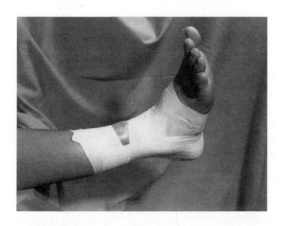

Fig. 22-1   The basic basketweave pattern.

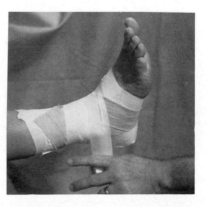

Fig. 22-3   Continuing the figure eight with heel locks.

this forms a customized ankle orthosis, which limits the extremes of motion in most planes while still permitting a functional range of motion (Fig. 22-5).

Variations on ankle taping include the addition of buttressing strips to add support along specific movement patterns or adding checkreigns in order to more severely limit a specific motion. The use of elastic tape is helpful when working to limit inversion while not severely restricting plantarflexion. By using 2-inch elastic tape, the trainer can create a high-tension restraint to inversion along the path of the anterior talofibular ligament while permitting some retained flexibility in the system (Fig. 22-6).

Using 2- or 3-inch elastic tape to create a "spartan" strip allows the trainer to add compression at the joint lines (Fig. 22-7) or at the distal tibiofibular joint (Fig. 22-8) in order to control torsional forces at the ankle mortise. These strips are helpful with syndesmosis injuries, tibiofibular ligament sprains, and in general with any ankle sprain that an athlete is pushing to an early return. Spartan strips seem especially helpful with

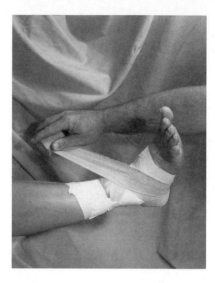

Fig. 22-6   A high-tension, dynamic inversion/plantarflexion restraint using elastic tape: apply before figure eight/heel locks, beginning on the medial side at the proximal anchor strips.

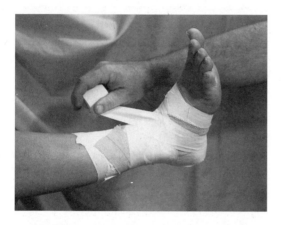

Fig. 22-4   Finishing the figure eight with heel locks.

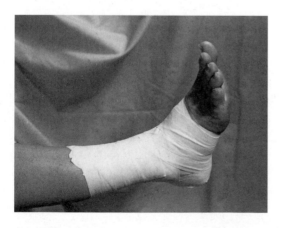

Fig. 22-5   The completed ankle tape.

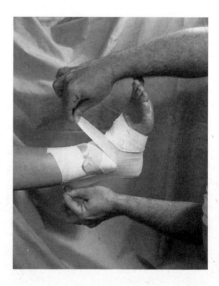

Fig. 22-7   A low spartan strip for joint line compression.

Taping, Shoe Modifications, Orthoses, Arthrodeses

jumping athletes, adding to their comfort and confidence.

Adding a dorsal checkrein to the ankle tape will act to limit plantarflexion (Fig. 22-9). While it may rob the athlete of some power, it adds considerable stability to the support system by not allowing the talus to rotate too far out of its tightly mortised neutral position. With Grade II or greater ankle injuries, this addition is very helpful. Combined with the spartan strips, many athletes participate with considerable security when their plantarflexion is aggressively limited.

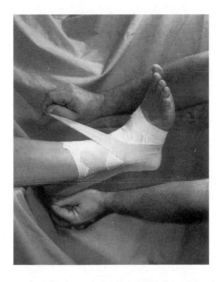

Fig. 22-8 A high spartan strip for tibiofibular compression.

The "sideline tape job," which often gets mentioned by the media during the course of a contest, where an athlete limps off the field or the court only to return to the contest a few minutes later with a "good tape job," is generally a combination of all of the above-mentioned variations. After assessment of the injury and determination of its severity, many athletes with mild injuries want to attempt a return to play. Shoring up the ankle for all potential stresses by creating a system with more-or-less omnidirectional support and significant range of motion limitations provides the athlete with the best chance. With a Grade I injury, it is likely that the athlete can finish the contest, though jumping athletes seem to have less success playing on a mildly sprained ankle than do athletes in primarily horizontal sports.

Taping the foot presents challenges for the athletic trainer, though there are a few standard approaches that are always a good place to begin. The standard X-pattern longitudinal arch tape is a good support system for many foot and leg complaints (Fig. 22-10). At its simplest, it is an external system designed to shore up the plantar ligaments and the plantar fascia, adding an extra string to the bow, if you will. For many injuries to the midfoot, this is the system of choice since the amount of tension can be customized and there is no pad to push up against the tender foot. In order to effectively control the ten-

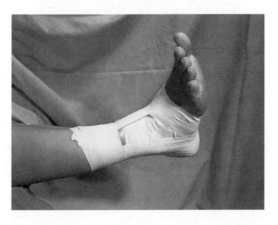

Fig. 22-9 A dorsal checkrein to limit plantarflexion: apply before figure eight/heel locks.

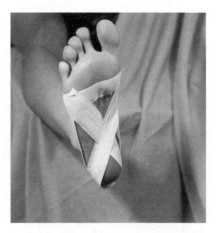

Fig. 22-10 The X-style longitudinal arch tape: apply each side of the X separately to control tension.

sion of the tape, however, it is helpful to apply each half of the X separately, with one piece going from the head of the first metatarsal and returning to the first metatarsal and the crossing piece going from the head of the fifth metatarsal and returning to the fifth metatarsal. By using this technique, the arch is supported but not cinched. Finishing with semicircular strips transversely helps support the transverse arch and midfoot (Fig. 22-11).

It is important to note that in most cases the arch should be taped with the ankle and foot in neutral. To tape the arch with the ankle plantarflexed and the foot relaxed allows the trainer to generate a great deal of leverage with the tape but generally causes the athlete considerable discomfort when weight-bearing by restricting normal foot movements. If a tremendous amount of control is the desired effect, then having the athlete slightly plantarflex and relax the foot produces the desired position.

One instance where a tremendous amount of leverage is required is when applying the low-dye tape. This tape job is intended to limit the amount of pronation during the stance phase of gait and to maintain a more rigid foot. It is especially helpful with athletes who have a pronated foot or valgus heel. It is also helpful when working with athletes who suffer from midfoot injuries (e.g., a Lisfranc sprain or a navicular stress fracture).

Unlike other arch taping, the low-dye tape is applied with the ankle and foot relaxed, which basically allows some plantarflexion and slight inversion. Strips of tape are then applied from the lateral side of the head of the fifth metatarsal, parallel to the bottom of the foot, around the heel to the medial side of the head of the first metatarsal. Before fixing the tape to the first metatarsal, the trainer must depress the head of the first metatarsal and elevate the head of the fourth metatarsal (Fig. 22-12). The tape must then be pulled tight, then placed on the first metatarsal. It usually necessary to do this three or four times, retracing the same path, depending on the size of the athlete and the amount of correction desired. The tape is then anchored in the same manner as the longitudinal arch tape, with semicircular strips applied transversely.

If this is done properly, when the athlete pulls the foot to neutral the first metatarsal should move medially and inferiorly, causing the big toe to move away from the second toe and toward the floor (Fig. 22-13). An aggressive move of the first metatarsal will allow the trainer to put one finger between the first and second toes. What is accomplished is the creation of a stiffer foot, where the midfoot is held in some supination, the first ray of the foot posts on the ground sooner, and the posterior tibialis receives a mechanical assist in elevating the midfoot during propulsion. At first many athletes will tell the

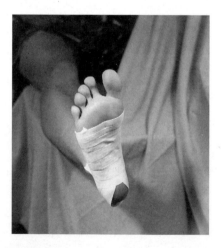

Fig. 22-11 The completed X-style longitudinal arch tape with transverse anchor strips applied.

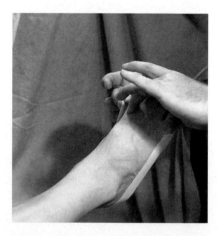

Fig. 22-12 Initiating the low-dye tape: depress the head of the first metatarsal; elevate the head of the fourth metatarsal; avoid pronating the entire foot.

trainer that they feel pigeon-toed or that they are falling to the outside of their feet. This sensation diminishes some as the tape loosens and is less noticeable when they put on their shoes.

Among its many applications, such as diverting force from the midfoot, diverting force from the posterior tibialis and medial tibia, or diverting force from the first metatarsophalangeal (MTP) joint in cases of turf toe, the low-dye tape is an excellent trial of function for orthotics. In many cases, if the athlete's complaints are relieved by the low-dye, then a soft, or semisoft orthotic system will work.

Padding

Padding of the foot generally falls into one of two categories, pads for pressure relief and pads for mechanical support. Occasionally a padding system may fall into both categories. In these circumstances, a mechanical problem causes abnormal pressures, presenting a double-edged sword.

Donut pads for focal pressure relief are helpful when dealing with blisters, painful calluses, or painful bony prominences (e.g., metatarsal heads, bunions). Very simply, the hole in the pad must be just slightly larger than the tender area. The width of the body of the pad is variable, but in general the larger the surface area over which

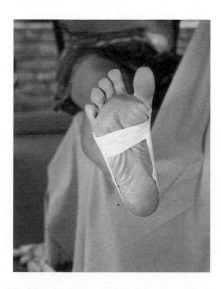

Fig. 22-13 Completed low-dye tape: note the medial and plantar deflection of the first metatarsal when the foot is pulled into neutral.

force is distributed, the better the relief. In the case of relieving pressure under an individual metatarsal head, the body of the pad should cover the entire forefoot. The edges of the pad must be beveled at about 45 degrees so that the force of the pad gradually diminishes rather than abruptly ends. A sharp drop-off at the edge of a pad can cause pressure and pain, adding to rather than diminishing the athlete's complaints.[1]

One of the most common and useful pads is the teardrop-shaped metatarsal pad (Fig. 22-14). Used to post the middle metatarsals, the larger end of the pad should be placed just behind the metatarsal heads with the narrow end of the pad trailing back into the distal end of the longitudinal arch. This pad is best used when the desire is to relieve pressure at the second, third, and fourth metatarsal heads, to restore the metatarsal arch, or to divert pressure from a middle metatarsal stress fracture. In effect, the pad requires that the pressures be distributed in the desired three-point weight-bearing pattern, those points being the calcaneous, the first metatarsal, and the fifth metatarsal.[4]

A soft longitudinal arch pad is often helpful when addressing problems related to pronation, overpronation, the plantar fascia, or the medial tibial structures (Fig. 22-15). It should be noted, however, that, when placing the pad, the athlete should feel the majority of the pressure from the support below the navicular. The navicular is the anatomic apex of the medial longitudinal arch and should be the point where the medial longitudinal arch pad produces its maximum support. The pad should be beveled steeply to the posterior so as not to elevate the medial side

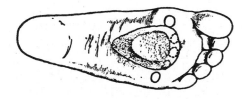

Fig. 22-14 The teardrop-shaped felt metatarsal pad: note that the bulk of the pad is just proximal to the heads of the metatarsals and that the edge is beveled. (From Cramer Corp. Athletic training in the seventies. Cramer Corp., Gardner KS, 1971.)

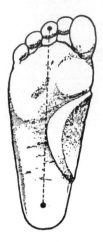

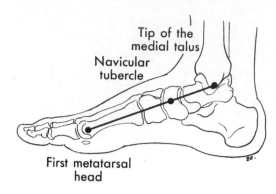

Fig. 22-16 The normal Feiss line.[3]

Fig. 22-15 The felt longitudinal arch pad. (From Cramer Corp. Athletic training in the seventies. Cramer Corp., Gardner KS, 1971.)

of the calcaneous (unless a medial heel post is going to be incorporated into the system) and gradually to the anterior so that it ends just posterior to the head of the first metatarsal head.

To assess the height of the arch support, the trainer can draw a line from the inferior tip of the medial malleolus to the medial aspect of the head of the first metatarsal while the athlete is weight-bearing. The posterior tibial tubercle of the navicular should fall on this line (Fig. 22-16). In a pronated or flat foot, the tubercle is below the line and the arch should be elevated or supported in some manner. In a cavus or high-arched foot, the tubercle is above the line, creating a rigid midfoot and an entirely different set of problems for the athlete.

Padding the cavus foot generally focuses on energy attenuation. The impact forces in a cavus foot are abnormally high due to the rigidity of the foot.[8] Forefoot pain, metatarsalgia, medial leg pain, shin splints, and heel pain are common in athletes with cavus feet. Many of these complaints can be addressed with commercial shoe inserts that are designed to attenuate force.[7] These inserts can be made from different materials, including Plastozote, high-density foams, and viscoelastic materials. Many can also be padded and posted, as has been discussed, in order to divert and relieve focal points of pressure and pain. The very nature of a rigid foot, however, makes changing its mechanical properties difficult.

A taping/padding system that addresses pain or dysfunction at or around the first MTP joint has to perform two basic functions. The first is to preserve good joint alignment so that the athlete can transfer force efficiently through the joint. The second is to relieve pressure and pain so that the athlete is not required to change weight-bearing patterns to avoid the joint.

The problems created by "turf toe" and its sequellae are sometimes best addressed by taping the toe in slight extension, 10 to 15 degrees, then holding it there using long strips of tape extending from the bottom of the toe well back into the foot and securing them with semicircular anchor strips (Fig. 22-17). If bunionlike problems accompany the turf toe, which is a common complaint, then some long strips along the medial aspect of the toe and back into the foot that pull the toe into slight varus may also be helpful in aligning the proximal phalanx with the long axis of the first metatarsal (Fig. 22-18). If bony spurring or hypertrophic bone formation has occurred, this is not always possible and may actually cause impingement and more discomfort.

In advanced cases, creating a felt rocker pad that ends just posterior to the MTP joint may allow the athlete to transfer weight across the joint without actually going through the joint. The rocker pad elevates the forefoot just posterior to the MTP joint, causing the athlete to fall across the joint and land on the toe. If this pad is used in conjunction with a taping system that holds the toe in slight extension, the athlete can transfer weight to the big toe without the benefit of a great deal of extension at the MTP joint.

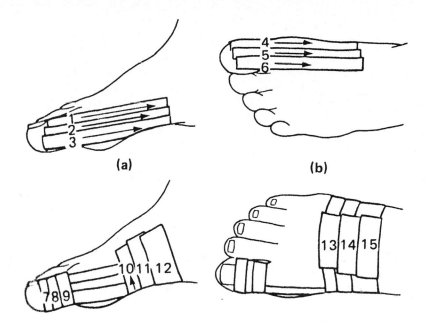

Fig. 22-17   Turf toe taping: apply with the toe in neutral or in slight extension and varus.[1]

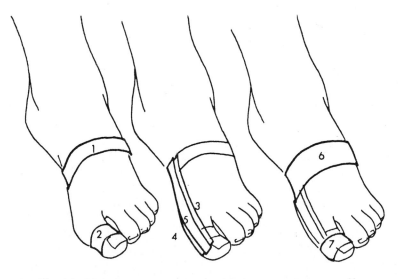

Fig. 22-18   Bunion taping: apply with the toe in slight varus.[11]

(This type of system is also helpful with athletes suffering from a painful or fractured sesmoid.)

In general, taping and or padding the foot/ankle complex provides the athlete with a customized support system that can be adapted to them and their needs. In contrast, a commercial or over-the-counter support system requires that the athlete conform to it to some extent. While the commercial systems work well and their efficacy is well documented and defended,[2,5,10] my experience is that the high-performance athlete seems to prefer the "feel" of being taped. While much of this preference may be purely psychological, one must never downplay the importance of "feeling right" during athletic performance. Many athletes link their trip to the training room to get taped with their mental preparation for the activity to follow. Getting taped is a very personal event for the athlete and for many marks the beginning of getting ready to play.

Bibliography

1. Arnheim D: *Modern principles of athletic training,* ed 7, St Louis, 1989, Mosby.
2. Gross MT et al: Comparison of support provided by ankle taping and semirigid orthosis, *J Orthop Sports Phys Ther* 9:33, 1987.
3. Hartley A: *Practical joint assessment,* St. Louis, 1990, Mosby.
4. Hicks JH: The three weightbearing mechanisms of the foot. In Evans FG, editor: *Biomechanical studies of the musculoskeletal system,* Springfield, Ill, 1972, Charles C Thomas.
5. Kimura IF et al: Effects of the airstirrup in controlling ankle inversion stress, *J Orthop Sports Phys Ther* 9:190, 1987.
6. Konradsen L, Holmer P, Sondergaard L: Early mobilizing treatment for grade III ankle ligament injuries, *Foot Ankle* 12:69, 1991.
7. Milgrom C, Finestone A, Shlamkovitch N: Prevention of overuse injuries of the foot by improved shoe shock attenuation, a randomized prospective study, *Clin Orthop* Aug (281):189, 1992.
8. Nachbauer W, Nigg BM: Effects of arch height of the foot on ground reaction forces in running, *Med Sci Sports Exerc* 24:1264, 1992.
9. Nelson RM, Currier DP: *Clinical electrotherapy,* East Norwalk, Conn, 1987, Appleton-Century-Crofts.
10. Rovere G et al: Retrospective comparison of taping and ankle stabilizers in preventing ankle injuries, *Am J Sports Med* 16:228, 1988.
11. Roy S, Irvin R: *Sports medicine: prevention, evaluation, management and rehabilitation,* Englewood Cliffs, NJ, 1983, Prentice-Hall.

23

The Shoe in Rehabilitation of the Foot and Ankle

Dennis J. Janisse

Special care must be taken when providing footwear in the rehabilitation of the foot and ankle. The foot that has recently undergone surgery or trauma may have changed significantly in size and shape. It may be prone to edema or have areas of delicate skin due to skin grafts or scar tissue. It may have lost flexibility or become hypermobile as a result of lost motor function. It may require the use of an ankle-foot orthosis (AFO) or prosthesis. All of these factors must be considered when providing footwear for the rehabilitation process. The use of an appropriate, properly fitted shoe can be a key component in speeding rehabilitation; the wrong shoe could slow the process or even cause additional complications. A Board Certified Pedorthist (C.Ped.) or experienced shoe fitter should be included in the team of health care professionals involved in rehabilitation of the foot and ankle.

In this chapter, the role of the shoe in the rehabilitation of the foot and ankle is considered, with respect first to shoe construction and second to shoe fitting. Finally, the particular types of shoes used in rehabilitation are discussed. (For a detailed explanation of shoe modifications and specific applications, see Chapter 24.)

Shoe Construction

To choose footwear appropriate for rehabilitation, it is first necessary to have a basic understanding of shoe construction. This section begins with a description of the parts of the shoe in order to develop a terminology for future discussion. The three primary aspects of shoe construction are then covered: (1) shoe shape, which is determined by the last, or mold over which the shoe is constructed; (2) sole attachment, which can be done in a variety of ways, depending on the type and purpose of the shoe; and (3) shoe materials, including those used in construction of both the shoe upper and the sole.

Parts of the Shoe

The important parts of a shoe are illustrated in Fig. 23-1. Terms useful in describing the

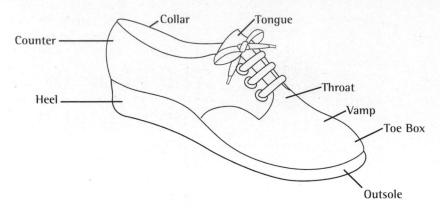

Fig. 23-1 Parts of a shoe. (From Janisse DJ: Pedorthic care of the diabetic foot. In Levin ME, O'Neal LW, Bowker JH, editors: *The diabetic foot,* ed 5, St Louis, 1993, Mosby–Year Book, p 551; with permission.)

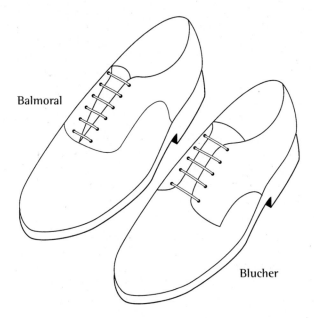

Fig. 23-2 Two types of throat openings: *left,* balmoral; *right,* blucher. (Redrawn from Rossi WA, Tennant R: *Professional shoe fitting,* New York, 1984, National Shoe Retailers Association; with permission.)

shoe upper include (1) *toe box,* the part of the shoe that covers the toe area; (2) *vamp,* the part that covers the instep; (3) *counter,* the part behind the heel; and (4) *throat,* the place where the vamp meets the tongue. There are two basic types of throat openings: the blucher and the balmoral (Fig. 23-2).

Figure 23-3A is a cross-sectional view of the shoe, showing the parts of the sole. The *insole* is the uppermost layer of the sole, upon which the foot directly rests. In terms of shoe construction, the insole is perhaps the most vital part of the shoe because virtually every other part of the shoe is attached to it.[6] The *outsole* is the bottom layer of the sole, that part which comes in contact with the ground. A shoe may also be made with a *midsole,* a layer of material between the insole and outsole. A midsole can provide extra support and comfort, help retain the shape and stability of the sole, and is often used to give the shoe a more rugged look. Figure 23-3B illustrates the *shank,* or bridge between the heel and

    Taping, Shoe Modifications, Orthoses, Arthrodeses

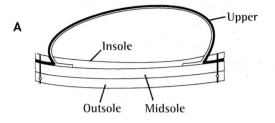

A

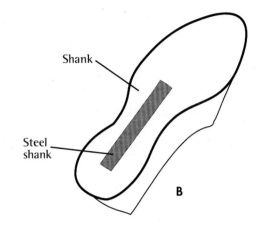

Upper

Insole

Outsole   Midsole

Shank

Steel
shank

B

Fig. 23-3   **A,** Cross-section of a shoe, illustrating the parts of the sole. **B,** Plantar view of the sole, with reinforced shank. (Redrawn from Rossi WA, Tennant R: *Professional shoe fitting,* New York, 1984, National Shoe Retailers Association; with permission.)

ball area of the shoe. The shank may be reinforced with a thin strip of spring steel added between the outsole and insole, often referred to as a steel shank.

Shoe Shape

The first aspect of shoe construction is determination of the overall shape of the shoe, including both the sole and the upper.[3] The shape of a shoe is dependent primarily upon the *last,* or the mold over which the shoe is made. Lasts are made in an unlimited variety of shapes and sizes; however, most popularly priced, mass-produced shoes are made from a single, basic last shape called the *standard last.* It comes in limited sizes and often only in a single "medium" width.

On the other hand, lasts used in the manufacture of prescription footwear, and increasingly in athletic footwear, are made not only in a wide

range of sizes and widths but in many shapes. A commonly used orthopedic last is the *combination last,* which has a heel that is narrower than the forefoot, providing room for the metatarsals and toes while maintaining a good heel fit. For example, a typical B width shoe made on a combination last might have a triple A heel. Additional orthopedic last shapes include the inflare, outflare, straight, short-toed, and long-toed.

It is important to remember that the last determines not only the shape of the sole but the shape of the upper as well. Most prescription and athletic footwear is now made from an *in-depth last,* which results in a shoe whose upper is shaped to allow extra volume for the foot inside the shoe and provides enough room for a generic insole or a custom insert. (Use of in-depth shoes is discussed in further detail below.)

Types of Sole Attachments

The second primary component of shoe construction is the manner in which the sole is attached to the upper.[6] The type of sole attachment used for a given shoe determines its functional character, appearance, performance, and the fit and feel of the shoe on the foot. In this section, six major types of sole attachments are considered (Fig. 23-4).

Goodyear Welt

This type of sole attachment takes its name from the Goodyear sole-stitching machine invented about a century ago. The distinguishing factor of this construction is the use of a *welt,* a flat, narrow strip of leather or other material chainstitched to the insole and upper (Fig. 23-4**A**). The outsole is then lockstitched to the welt, forming a very strong, sturdy shoe. The space between the outsole and insole is layered with a filler material (ground cork or other material) for a flat tread surface. Goodyear welt shoes tend to be heavier, less flexible, and more expensive than the other types. In addition, they are the easiest type of shoe to use in attaching an AFO. (AFO attachment is described below.)

Stitchdown

In the stitchdown type of construction, the edge of the upper is flanged outward and stitched

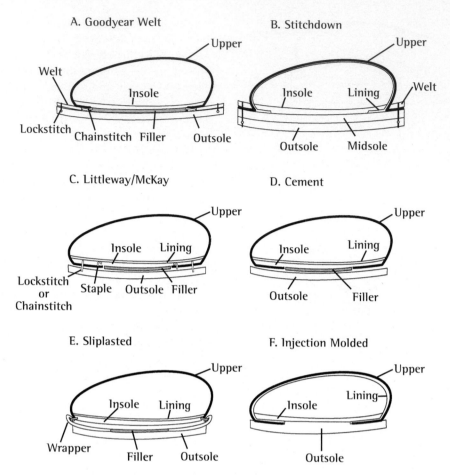

Fig. 23-4 Types of sole attachments. **A,** Goodyear welt. **B,** Stitchdown. **C,** Littleway/McKay. **D,** Cement. **E,** Sliplasted. **F,** Injection molded. (Redrawn from Rossi WA, Tennant R: *Professional shoe fitting,* New York, 1984, National Shoe Retailers Association; with permission.)

to the outsole (Fig. 23-4**B**). This simple, relatively inexpensive type of construction may also make use of a welt and a midsole.[1]

Littleway/McKay

In each of these types, the upper is fastened to the insole with staples; the outsole is then attached with either lockstitches (Littleway) or chainstitches (McKay).[5] This type of construction is typically found in moccasins or deck shoes and results in a very flexible shoe (Fig. 23-4**C**).

Cement

In the cement process the outsole is attached to the insole and upper using a firm-bonding glue or cement (Fig. 23-4**D**). As in the Good-

year welt, a thin layer of filler material is included between the outsole and insole. Shoes made in this way are lightweight and flexible; most athletic shoes currently use the cement type of sole attachment.

Sliplasted

In a sliplasted shoe (Fig. 23-4**E**), the upper is sewn to an insole that is made of a similar material. The outsole is then attached with the cement process. A wrapper made of rubber or other similar material may be added to improve the appearance of the shoe. Sliplasting is used in many athletic shoes and results in a shoe that is flexible and can provide maximum shock absorption.

Injection Molded

Injection molded shoes are constructed with a heat-sealing process; no stitching is used (Fig. 23-4**F**). The outsole is made of a thermoplastic material, which liquefies when heated. Using a special molding machine, it is then heat-sealed to the upper. It quickly hardens to become the shoe bottom. Injection molded shoes are less expensive than the other types but come in a smaller range of sizes and widths and are generally more difficult to modify.

Materials

The third primary aspect of shoe construction is the choice of materials.[1,6] Given the variety of materials available, it would be impossible to cover all of those currently used in shoe construction. In this section, discussion will therefore be limited to those upper and sole materials most commonly found in shoes suitable for rehabilitation.

Upper

The material used in the shoe upper affects the fit, comfort, and performance of the shoe. Cowhide is probably the most durable of the commonly used upper materials, and it can be stretched and/or molded but with some difficulty. Deerskin, on the other hand, is a softer, more accommodative upper material but is less durable and scuffs easily. Some shoe uppers are made with a heat-moldable lining material, which allows the upper to be molded to the individual foot, especially useful for severe deformities or unusual foot shapes. Shoe uppers can also be made from fabric; for example, many athletic shoes are currently made from a combination of leather and fabric, typically nylon or canvas.

Sole

Materials used in the sole vary widely in terms of weight, shock absorption, durability, and flexibility. Following are the most commonly used sole materials.

Leather

Once the most common sole material, leather is now used primarily in high-quality men's dress shoes made with the Goodyear welt construction. Leather soles are long wearing and moderately flexible but tend to be heavy, offer little shock absorption, and can be very slippery when wet. Although AFOs can now be used with a variety of shoes, leather soles allow AFO attachment with minimal shoe modifications.

Hard Rubber

A good alternative to leather, especially for use with an AFO, is hard rubber. It is generally longer wearing than leather and does not become slippery and when used on a welt shoe still allows for easy AFO attachment.

Crepe

A rubber compound containing additives that give it a cellular structure, crepe (also called microcellular rubber) offers excellent shock absorption and traction. Shoes with crepe soles are lightweight and lend themselves well to external shoe modifications such as flares. (See Chapter 24, Pedorthics in the Rehabilitation of the Foot and Ankle, for a complete description of shoe modifications.) An AFO may be added to a crepe-soled shoe, but more extensive modifications will be necessary than with a leather or hard rubber sole.

Vibram[R]

A denser microcellular rubber sold under the brand name Vibram has all of the good qualities of crepe but is more durable and shock absorbent and even lighter in weight. It is found in hiking boots, walking shoes, and in the newer "comfort" dress shoes.

Ethyl Vinyl Acetate (EVA)

A chemical blend of ethylene and vinyl acetate, EVA is probably the most popular sole material used in good quality running shoes. It is lightweight, flexible, and highly shock absorbent.

Shoe Fitting

Providing a shoe that is well constructed and made from appropriate materials is important in the rehabilitation of the foot and ankle. It is even more important that the shoe fit properly; in fact, properly fitting footwear is considered the most important factor in good foot health.[4] This section covers the two basic components of shoe fit, namely, shoe shape and shoe size, and ends with a set of guidelines for achieving proper shoe fit.

Shoe Shape

Proper shoe fit is attained when shoe shape is matched to foot shape.[2,3,6] As rehabilitation progresses, the shape of the foot may change; subsequent adjustments must then be made in shoe fit. These could be accomplished with the use of a shoe that has built-in adjustability or with shoe modifications or may require the use of different shoes during the various stages of rehabilitation.

Both the shape of the sole and the shape of the upper must be considered. The patient undergoing rehabilitation may require a shoe made from a combination last in order to provide adequate metatarsal and toe room yet maintain a good heel fit. If any shoe inserts are needed, then an in-depth shoe will most likely be required.

The specific parts of the shoe upper—in particular, the counter, toe box, vamp, and throat—are key factors in shoe fit.[3] The counter controls the heel and is important to heel fit. Many in-depth shoes have extended medial counters to help support the medial arch. A shoe that has a high toe box and a rounded, or oblique, toe provides the best fit by allowing the toes to fit comfortably inside the shoe. A shoe with a tapered toe box and a pointed toe applies pressure to the toes and forces them into an unnatural shape, causing calluses and discomfort and eventually leading to deformity. This could be disastrous for the foot undergoing rehabilitation.

As with the toe box, the vamp should be high enough to prevent pressure on the instep. In addition, a shoe with laces generally provides the best fit because (1) the laces allow adjustability and (2) the shoe can be fit properly without any danger of its slipping off. Pumps and slip-ons often have virtually no vamp so that they must be

fitted too snugly or they will fall off. Of the two types of throat openings, the blucher is generally preferred over the balmoral, especially in rehabilitation, since the blucher allows for greater adjustability and easier entry.

Shoe Size

Once the properly shaped shoe has been found, the next step in fitting shoes is to determine the proper size. There are three essential measurements in determining shoe size: (1) overall foot length (heel to toe), (2) arch length (heel to arch, or first metatarsal), and (3) width. The proper shoe size is the one that accommodates the first metatarsophalangeal joint (i.e., the widest part of the foot) in the widest part of the shoe.[3] It is for this reason that shoes must be fit by arch length rather than by overall foot length. The feet in Fig. 23-5 have the same overall foot length but require different size shoes because of the difference in arch length.

The Brannock measuring device is commonly used to determine foot size. The measurements obtained offer a good starting point to use when fitting shoes. It is very important to realize, however, that shoe sizes (e.g., 6A, 10D) are not absolute measurements. The actual size of a 6A, for

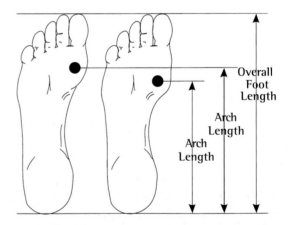

Fig. 23-5 Overall foot length vs. arch length. These feet have the same overall foot length, but the foot on the left requires a larger size shoe because it has a longer arch length. (Redrawn from Rossi WA, Tennant R: *Professional shoe fitting*, New York, 1984, National Shoe Retailers Association; with permission.)

example, varies from one shoe manufacturer to another and may even vary within the same manufacturer for different shoe styles. The meaning of "6A" can only be considered in relative terms. For one specific style made by one specific manufacturer, a 6A will always be longer in arch length than a 5A and shorter than a 7A; similarly, it will be wider than a 6AA and narrower than a 6B. Shoe fitting should never be done on the basis of numbers. It should be done by a competent professional, such as a certified pedorthist, who can evaluate the fit of the shoe on the foot.

Achieving Proper Fit

Determining the correct shoe shape and the right size are the primary components in achieving proper shoe fit. In addition, a properly fitting shoe should have ⅜ to ½ inch of toe room between the end of the shoe and the longest toe, and may allow some movement of the heel in the counter since the foot will stretch during gait. Following is a set of guidelines that can be used to achieve proper shoe fit.[3]

Guidelines for Attaining Proper Shoe Fit

1. Measure both feet with an appropriate measuring device; the Brannock measuring device is recommended.
2. Fit shoes on *both* feet while weight-bearing.
3. Check for the proper position of the first metatarsophalangeal joint. It should be in the widest part of the shoe.
4. Check for the correct toe length. Allow ⅜ to ½ inch between the end of the shoe and the longest toe.
5. Check for the proper width, allowing adequate room across the ball of the foot.
6. Look for a snug fit around the heel.
7. Determine that proper fit over the instep has been achieved by an appropriately high vamp, preferably with laces to allow adjustability.

Shoe fit should be monitored throughout the rehabilitation process. Proper shoe fit is crucial during rehabilitation and can be a key factor in maintaining good foot health and preventing future injury.

Shoes Used in Rehabilitation

Many types of shoes are used in the rehabilitation of the foot and ankle, since the patient's footwear requirements vary as rehabilitation progresses. Immediately following surgery or other trauma, the patient may require some type of postoperative or healing shoe or a postoperative appliance such as a night splint. Later on, there may be a need for a shoe to which an AFO can be attached or for a moldable or even custom-made shoe to accommodate a severe deformity associated with a fracture, skin graft, or muscle flap. Eventually, the patient may require some type of in-depth shoe, possibly an athletic shoe, to be used in conjunction with a special insole or other shoe insert. This section covers the four major types of shoes used in rehabilitation: in-depth, custom-made, AFO shoes, and postoperative or healing shoes. Other postoperative appliances, such as night splints and controlled ankle motion walkers, are also briefly discussed.

In-Depth Shoes

The basic shoe used in rehabilitation is the in-depth shoe. It is designed with an additional ¼ to ⅜-inch depth throughout the shoe, allowing extra volume for the foot inside the shoe and providing enough room for a generic insole or a custom insert.[4] In-depth shoes usually come in a basic oxford style, are available for men and women in a wide range of shapes and sizes, and are currently made by several shoe manufacturers. They are made with a variety of upper materials, including cowhide and deerskin, are generally lightweight, and have shock-absorbing soles and strong counters. An in-depth shoe, with any necessary modifications, is usually sufficient for most patients undergoing rehabilitation.

Three types of specialized in-depth shoes are particularly appropriate for use in rehabilitation: athletic, moldable, and lace-to-toe shoes.

Athletic Shoes

Many athletic shoes are now being made with removable insoles and therefore have enough added volume inside the shoe to be used as an in-depth shoe. Athletic shoes also tend to be lightweight, with shock-absorbing soles and strong counters, and are cosmetically appealing to many patients. In addition, most running and walking shoes are made with a rocker sole, which helps to rock the foot from heel to toe, assisting in gait. (See Chapter 24 for a more complete description of rocker soles.)

Moldable Shoes

Some in-depth shoes have uppers that can be molded to the individual foot shape. The upper is made of an outer layer of thin, soft deerskin laminated to a lining made of heat-moldable polyethylene foam. The upper can be heated and stretched and will then hold this shape, accommodating severe deformities. The softness of the deerskin upper is particularly useful for patients with a high potential for skin breakdown, as in skin grafts or muscle flaps. Moldable shoes can be easily modified, and the heat of the foot in the shoe allows the shoe to continue to conform to the shape of the foot.[4]

Lace-to-Toe Shoes

As its name indicates, the lace-to-toe shoe has lace stays that extend all the way to the toe. It has a blucher type of throat opening and is available as either a shoe or boot. Lace-to-toe shoes are made from a variety of lasts to accommodate many foot shapes and have uppers made of cowhide or deerskin. The lace-to-toe shoe is particularly useful for patients who have difficulty getting the foot into a shoe, either because of a lack of flexibility or a loss of motor control. The extra long lacing area also allows for greater adjustability throughout the rehabilitation process. Many regular in-depth shoes can be modified to become lace-to-toe.

Custom-made Shoes

A custom-made shoe is constructed from a cast or model of the patient's foot and is needed only in rare cases when extremely severe deformities prohibit the use of an in-depth shoe, even with extensive modifications. For instance, a muscle flap may be too bulky to be properly accommodated in an in-depth shoe. Custom-made shoes

are also sometimes used to incorporate an extreme modification that would otherwise be cosmetically unappealing. In the case of a leg length discrepancy, for example, a large shoe extension can be built into a custom-made shoe and be much less noticeable than if it were simply added onto the bottom of an in-depth shoe.

AFO Shoes
Metal AFOs

Until recently it was generally thought that a metal AFO could only be attached to a Goodyear welt shoe with a leather or hard rubber sole and a separate heel. Although this is still the easiest shoe for AFO attachment, a metal AFO can be attached to virtually any shoe that has a steel shank or to which a steel shank has been added, when properly modified by a certified pedorthist. Athletic shoes of all kinds, deerskin in-depth shoes, and even crepe-soled casual shoes can all be made strong enough to handle a metal AFO with the addition of a steel shank.

The procedure for modifying a nontraditional shoe is fairly simple. The pedorthist first cuts off all but $\frac{1}{16}$ to $\frac{1}{8}$ inch of the existing outsole. After consulting with the orthotist to determine the type of AFO to be attached, the proper steel shank is added—generally a regular shank is used with a free ankle motion AFO and an extended shank with a fixed ankle AFO (see Chapter 24). Next, a thin midsole ($\frac{1}{8}$ to $\frac{3}{16}$ inch) is cemented over the entire bottom of the shoe. Care must be taken to maintain the shape of the shoe so that the original outsole can be reattached after the AFO has been added; some sanding may be necessary to maintain proper alignment.

Gaining patient acceptance of a metal AFO is often difficult. It can be made easier, however, if the AFO is attached to a more cosmetically appealing shoe. This modification procedure increases the likelihood of patient acceptance since it can be performed on such a wide variety of shoes.

Plastic AFOs

Most plastic (in-shoe) AFOs can be accommodated simply by using an in-depth shoe (with no insole). The patient should not use a larger sized shoe, since the AFO requires extra *depth,* not extra length. Good fit is especially important with an AFO; an oversized shoe will have neither the proper arch length nor a good heel fit.

Healing Shoes

Immediately following surgery or other trauma, the presence of swelling, edema, or bulky dressings may necessitate the use of some type of healing shoe before a regular in-depth or custom-made shoe can be worn.[4] Healing shoes are made in a variety of styles by several manufacturers but fall into the following two basic categories.

Heat-moldable Healing Shoe

Made from a nylon-covered moldable polyethylene foam (Plastazote), this closed-toe, soft, extra-wide healing shoe can be molded directly to the patient's foot (Fig. 23-6**A**). It also has a removable Plastazote insole, a Velcro strap closure, and a crepe sole. It is most commonly used following amputation or skin grafting but can be used whenever a soft, flexible, accommodative healing shoe is needed.

Postoperative Shoe

This shoe is generally open-toed, with uppers made of canvas or nylon mesh; the upper may be padded for additional comfort (Fig. 23-6**B**). It has a wide forefoot opening with either Velcro straps or lace closures and can accommodate extreme swelling and the bulkiest dressings. The postoperative shoe can be made with a flexible crepe sole but is most often found with a more rigid sole made of firm crepe or lightweight wood. This is particularly helpful for allowing ambulation while limiting motion and is used following pin insertion, fusion, or other similar procedures.

Postoperative Appliances

Following surgery, some patients may require a type of postoperative appliance designed to limit ankle motion. Following are two such appliances.

Night Splint

Designed primarily to prevent contractures in patients confined to bed rest, a night splint consists of a rigid polyethylene outer shell with a soft, cushioning foam inner liner (Fig. 23-7**A**).

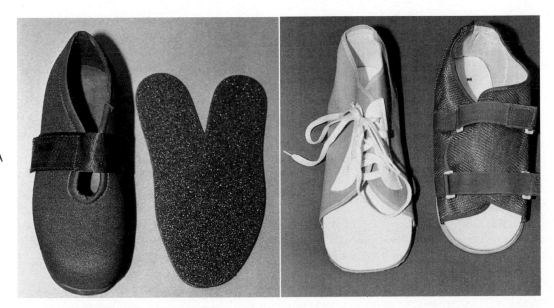

A   B

Fig. 23-6 Healing shoes. **A,** Heat-moldable healing shoe, with removable Plastazote insoles. **B,** Postoperative shoes: *left,* canvas upper with lace closure; *right,* nylon mesh upper with Velcro closure.

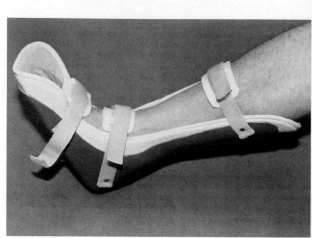 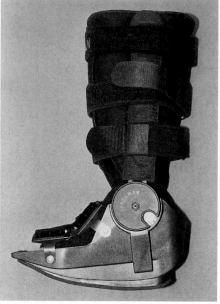

Fig. 23-7 Postoperative appliances. **A,** Night splint. **B,** Controlled ankle motion walker.

The foot and leg are held in place with Velcro straps, and the cushioned liner is designed to prevent heel ulceration with either a heel cut-out or an air pocket between the liner and outer shell in the heel area. Night splints are especially helpful for patients with spinal cord injury or stroke but can also be used to maintain ankle position following a variety of surgical procedures.

Controlled Ankle Motion Walker

For the patient who can be mobile but must maintain a fixed ankle position or limited ankle motion, the controlled ankle motion walker can provide the necessary stability and support while allowing a comfortable, natural gait pattern. This appliance is essentially a postoperative shoe to which medial-lateral uprights and a posterior Achilles plate have been added (Fig. 23-7**B**). The foot and ankle are held in place with wide Velcro straps, and the ankle joint may be held in a fixed position or allowed to move within a limited (up to 45 degrees) range of motion. A cushioned liner provides pressure relief, and a rocker sole allows a natural walking gait. The controlled ankle motion walker is

useful following such procedures as ligament and tendon repair, osteotomy, pinning procedures, stress fractures, and hallux valgus surgery.

Summary

The use of appropriate, properly fitting footwear is an essential component in rehabilitation of the foot and ankle. Factors to be considered in choosing an appropriate shoe are the type of sole attachment, materials used in the shoe upper and sole, shoe shape and size, and the desired purpose of the rehabilitative footwear. Shoes available for rehabilitation include indepth, custom-made, AFO footwear, healing shoes, and other postoperative appliances. A certified pedorthist can provide valuable assistance in selecting appropriate footwear for rehabilitation of the foot and ankle.

Bibliography

1. Cheskin MP, Sherkin KJ, Bates BT: *The complete handbook of athletic footwear,* New York, 1987, Fairchild Publications.

2. Gould N: Shoes and shoe modification. In Jahss MH, editor: *Disorders of the foot and ankle,* vol 3, Philadelphia, 1991, WB Saunders.
3. Janisse DJ: The art and science of fitting shoes, *Foot Ankle* 13:257, 1992.
4. Johnson JE: Prescription footwear. In Sammarco GJ, editor: *Foot and ankle manual,* Philadelphia, 1991, Lea & Febiger.
5. Prescription Footwear Association: *Directory of pedorthics,* Columbia, Md, 1992, Prescription Footwear Association/Board for Certification in Pedorthics.
6. Rossi WA, Tennant R: *Professional shoe fitting,* New York, 1984, National Shoe Retailers Association.

24

Pedorthics in the Rehabilitation of the Foot and Ankle

Dennis J. Janisse

Role of the Board Certified Pedorthist

The Board Certified Pedorthist (C.Ped.) is an important member of the team of health care professionals involved in the rehabilitation of the foot and ankle. Before discussing the specific role of the C.Ped., a brief description of pedorthics and the C.Ped.'s specialized training is in order.

A pedorthist is a health professional who provides prescription footwear, including shoes, shoe modifications, and orthoses, to patients referred by the medical profession.[11] In order to achieve the status C.Ped., a candidate must complete the certification process established by the Board for Certification in Pedorthics (BCP). The C.Ped. designation is intended to provide the prescribing physician with the assurance of competence in dispensing prescription footwear. The BCP works in cooperation with the Pedorthic Footwear Association (PFA) to establish standards and provide educational opportunities for individuals involved in the practice of pedorthics.[11]

To become certified, candidates must pass a comprehensive written examination covering the relevant medical aspects of patient evaluation, footwear and foot orthoses, and certain business considerations. They must have references attesting to their ability to fill footwear prescriptions. To maintain certification, a C.Ped. must participate in continuing education programs.[11]

The C.Ped. plays an important role in the rehabilitation of the foot and ankle.[3,4] First, he or she can provide the necessary footwear, including shoes, modifications, and orthoses. The C.Ped. maintains or can order an extensive shoe inventory to ensure that the patient receives the specific footwear prescribed. The C.Ped. has been trained in all aspects of shoe fitting and can therefore see that shoes fit properly, a critical factor in achieving good foot health.[6] He or she can also take foot impressions and provide any needed external shoe modifications, total contact inserts (TCIs), or other orthoses. If necessary, the C.Ped. can also construct custom-made shoes.

The second part of the C.Ped.'s role is in the area of patient education. The C.Ped. is a valuable resource for instructing patients in all aspects of footwear: shoe selection, criteria for proper fit, purpose of modifications and orthoses, and the role of footwear in rehabilitation. In addition, the C.Ped. can reinforce the information presented by other team members, emphasizing the team approach to treatment and helping the patient to realize that footwear is only one part of the overall rehabilitation program.

Finally, the C.Ped. is able to assist in follow-up care. In most cases, patients come to the C.Ped. with a written prescription from their physician; this initial prescription will often require routine adjustments and eventual modification as rehabilitation progresses. The C.Ped. therefore serves as a valuable link in communication between the physician, patient, and other team members. In return visits to the C.Ped., the patient can report success or problems experienced with the prescription footwear. The C.Ped. should inspect both the footwear and the patient's feet, looking for problems or signs of trouble. The overall effectiveness of the prescription footwear should then be noted and reported to the prescribing physician, with recommendations for additional modifications or adjustments. The C.Ped. sees patients several times, until certain that the prescription is filled correctly and functioning properly.

In monitoring patient progress, the C.Ped. is able to accommodate changes in the foot and ankle as rehabilitation continues. Immediately following surgery or trauma, the purpose of the prescription footwear is to promote healing; later, any necessary long-term modifications can be determined. In the case of a chronic illness such as rheumatoid arthritis or diabetes, the C.Ped. can provide prescription footwear that responds to the changing needs of the patient. In addition, C.Peds. maintain detailed footwear records for all patients, facilitating effective follow-up and long-term management of foot and ankle problems.

Shoes used in rehabilitation of the foot and ankle are covered in detail in Chapter 23. In this chapter, the focus is on prescription footwear. Both external shoe modifications and TCIs are described; the rest of the chapter is devoted to specific applications, including surgery, trauma, and chronic disorders.

Shoe Modifications

External Shoe Modifications

The outside of the shoe can be modified in a variety of ways. The following external shoe modifications are covered in this section: rocker soles, stabilization, extended steel shank, cushion heel, and extensions.

Rocker Soles

The rocker sole is one of the most commonly prescribed shoe modifications. As its name suggests, the basic function of a rocker sole is literally to rock the foot from heel-strike to toe-off without bending the shoe. However, the actual shape of the rocker sole varies according to (1) the patient's specific foot problems and (2) the desired effect of the rocker sole. In general, the biomechanical effects of a rocker sole are (1) to restore lost motion in the foot and/or ankle related to pain, deformity, or stiffness, resulting in an overall improvement in gait, and (2) to relieve pressure on some area of the plantar surface.[3]

There are two terms relevant to a discussion of rocker soles. These are (1) the *midstance,* or the portion of the rocker sole that is in contact with the floor when in a standing position, and (2) the *apex,* or high point, of the rocker sole, located at the distal end of the midstance. These points are illustrated in Fig. 24-1**A**. It is important to note that the apex must be placed *behind* any area for which pressure relief is desired.

In general, rocker soles are custom made for each patient; however, the following basic types of rocker soles can be identified.[3]

Mild Rocker Sole

The most widely used and most basic of the rocker soles has a mild rocker angle at both the heel and the toe (see Fig. 24-1**A**). This type of rocker sole can relieve metatarsal pressure and may assist gait by increasing propulsion and reducing the amount of energy expended in the

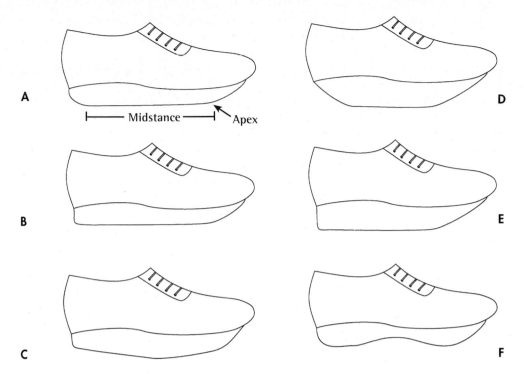

Fig. 24-1 Rocker soles. **A,** Mild rocker sole, with midstance and apex indicated. **B,** Heel-to-toe rocker sole. **C,** Toe-only rocker sole. **D,** Severe angle rocker sole. **E,** Negative heel rocker sole. **F,** Double rocker sole.

effort of walking. It is appropriate for the foot that is not at risk and is typically found on athletic walking shoes. The other types of rocker soles are essentially variations of this basic, mild rocker sole.

Heel-to-Toe Rocker Sole

This type of rocker sole is shaped with a more severe angle at both the heel and the toe (Fig. 24-1**B**). It is intended to aid propulsion at toe-off, decrease heel-strike forces on the calcaneus, and decrease the need for ankle motion. The heel-to-toe rocker sole would be appropriate for the patient who has undergone a triple arthrodesis.

Toe-Only Rocker Sole

As the name suggests, the toe-only rocker sole has a rocker angle only at the toe, with the midstance extending to the back end of the sole (Fig. 24-1**C**). The purpose of this type of rocker sole is to increase weight-bearing proximal to the metatarsal heads, to provide a stable midstance,

and to reduce the need for toe dorsiflexion on toe-off. Indications for the toe-only rocker sole include hallux rigidus and metatarsal ulcers associated with diabetes.

Severe Angle Rocker Sole

This type of rocker sole also has a rocker angle only at the toe, but it is a much more severe angle than that found on the toe-only rocker sole (Fig. 24-1**D**). The purpose of the severe rocker angle at the toe is to eliminate the weight-bearing forces anterior to the metatarsal heads.

Negative Heel Rocker Sole

Shaped with a rocker angle at the toe and a negative heel, this type of rocker sole results in the patient's heel being at the same height or lower than the ball of the foot when in a standing position (Fig. 24-1**E**). The purpose of the negative heel rocker sole is to accommodate a foot that is fixed in dorsiflexion or to relieve forefoot pressure by shifting it to the hindfoot and midfoot (e.g., following surgery for Morton's neuroma). Also, because forefoot pressure relief is accomplished through the use of a negative heel, the depth or height of the sole itself can be minimized, thereby increasing overall stability of the shoe. It is therefore indicated for patients who feel unstable with the normal height of a rocker sole. The negative heel rocker sole is to be used with caution, however, since inability to attain the necessary ankle dorsiflexion will cause discomfort and may increase pressure on the problem area.

Double Rocker Sole

This type of rocker sole is a mild rocker sole with a section of the sole removed in the midfoot area, thereby giving the appearance of two rocker soles—one at the hindfoot and one at the forefoot—and two areas of midstance (Fig. 24-1**F**). Since the thinnest area of the double rocker sole is at the midfoot, it is used to relieve a specific midfoot problem area, such as the Charcot foot deformity associated with diabetes.

Clearly, there are many types of rocker soles, and each must be individualized for a given patient's foot condition and the desired effect. A poorly or improperly designed rocker sole can actually worsen the problem it was supposed to

help correct.[3] When prescribing a rocker sole, it is essential that the physician clearly specify the desired effect or purpose of the rocker sole. A C.Ped. is trained to know which type of rocker sole will best achieve that purpose. The C.Ped. can also provide follow-up care to make sure that the rocker sole is performing properly for the individual patient.

Stabilization

A second type of external shoe modification involves the addition of material to the medial or lateral portion of the shoe in order to stabilize some part of the foot (Fig. 24-2).

Flare

A flare is an extension to the heel and/or sole of the shoe. Flares can be medial or lateral, and their purpose is to stabilize a hindfoot, midfoot, or forefoot instability. For example, a medial heel flare might be used to support a foot with a valgus heel deformity.

Stabilizer

A stabilizer is an extension added to the side of the shoe, including both the sole and upper. Made from rigid foam or crepe, a stabilizer pro-

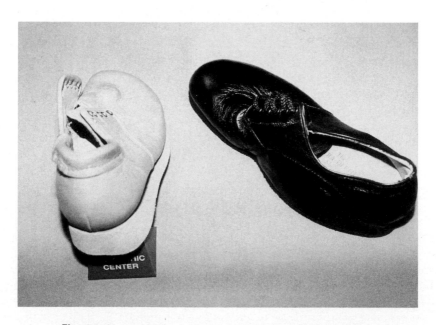

Fig. 24-2 Stabilization: *left,* lateral flare; *right,* medial stabilizer.

vides more extensive stabilization than a flare and is used for more severe medial or lateral instability of the hindfoot or midfoot. Before a stabilizer is added, the patient must wear the shoe for a few weeks until it is "broken in" (i.e., has taken on the shape of the deformed foot). Adding a stabilizer to a new shoe can lead to excessive pressure build-up, blistering, or serious skin breakdown.

Fiberglass Counters

A third type of stabilization is the addition of fiberglass to reinforce the counter of the shoe (i.e., the part of the shoe that is behind the heel). (See Chapter 23 for a complete description of the parts of a shoe.) The inside of the counter is lined with fiberglass and covered with moleskin. This type of stabilization is essentially invisible and is therefore more cosmetically acceptable for many patients. As with the stabilizer, the shoe should be worn before fiberglass counters are added.

Extended Steel Shank

An extended steel shank is a strip of spring steel that is inserted between the layers of the sole, extending from the heel to the toe of the shoe (see Chapter 23). It is most commonly used in combination with a rocker sole and in fact will often make the rocker sole more effective. An extended steel shank can also prevent the shoe from bending, limit toe and/or midfoot motion, aid propulsion on toe-off, and strengthen the entire shoe and sole. It is indicated for hallux limitus or rigidus or when ankle motion is limited.

Cushion Heel

A cushion heel is a wedge of shock-absorbing material that is added between the heel and sole of the shoe (Fig. 24-3). Its purpose is to provide a maximum amount of shock absorption at heel strike (in addition to that provided by a TCI) while maintaining a stable stance (e.g., following a calcaneal fracture).

Extensions

An extension is material added to the sole of a shoe to increase the height or thickness of the sole (Fig. 24-4). Extensions may be added to the heel area only or to the entire sole and heel.[7]

Heel-Only Extension

When an extension is added only to the heel area of the sole, its purpose is to accommodate a fixed deformity or to relieve hindfoot pressure.

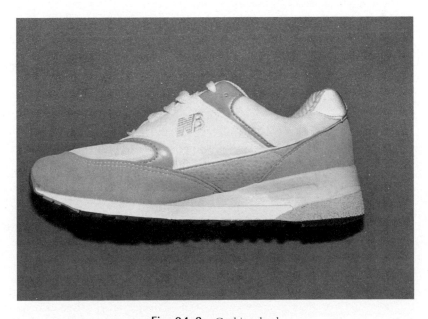

Fig. 24-3 Cushion heel.

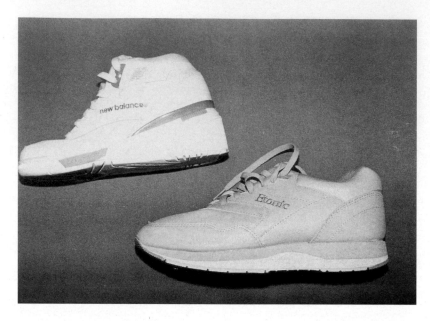

Fig. 24-4   Extensions: *left,* high-top shoe with heel-only extension; *right,* heel and sole extension. Note that extensions are added between midsole and outsole, resulting in a more cosmetically appealing shoe.

A heel-only extension is useful in accommodating a foot that is fixed in a plantarflexed position and for Achilles tendinitis.

Heel and Sole Extension

A complete heel and sole extension is used to eliminate a leg-length discrepancy. Depending on its height, the extension is generally made of crepe, leather, or Bock foam and should be used in conjunction with a rocker sole to compensate for the loss of flexibility in the sole when the extension is added. Extensions can be used with a wide variety of shoes, including athletic footwear and dress shoes, and can be covered with matching upper material to achieve cosmetically pleasing results.

Total Contact Inserts

A total contact insert (TCI) is a custom-made shoe insert that is made from a model of the patient's foot, thereby achieving total contact with the plantar surface of the foot (Fig. 24-5).[3,4,5,12] The TCI is composed of a shell, the layer of material next to the foot and in total contact with the foot, and the posting, the material that fills in the space between the shell and

the shoe. The TCI can be further customized by adding small amounts of additional materials to specific areas, such as a sponge rubber metatarsal pad or viscoelastic polymer under the heel.

Objectives

Achieving total contact with the proper choice of materials means that the TCI can achieve the following objectives[3,5]:

1. Relieve areas of excessive plantar pressure by evenly distributing pressure over the entire plantar surface
2. Reduce shock through the use of shock-absorbing materials in the TCI
3. Reduce shear since total contact minimizes horizontal foot movement
4. Stabilize and support the joints of the foot with the use of more rigid, supportive materials in the TCI posting
5. Limit the motion of joints, also through the use of supportive materials.

Foot Impression Techniques

As noted above, the TCI is made from a model of the patient's foot. Three principal techniques are used to take a foot impression, the choice of

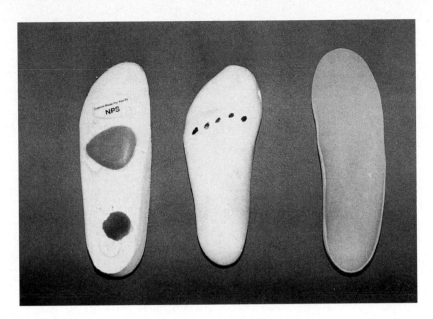

Fig. 24-5 Total contact insert (TCI) and plaster model of foot: *left,* plantar view of TCI—note addition of a metatarsal pad and viscoelastic polymer at the heel; *center,* plantar view of plaster model, with position of metatarsal heads indicated; *right,* top view of TCI.

technique determined by the desired function of the TCI. In terms of function, there are two basic types: (1) *accommodative,* whose primary function is to accommodate a rigid foot or one that is particularly at risk, and (2) *functional,* which is designed to control a more flexible foot by providing support and/or stability. Following are the three basic foot impression techniques.[3,5]

1. *Plaster cast.* A traditional plaster cast is applied to the foot, and a model is then made from that cast. This technique, when maintaining the foot in a neutral position, is most useful when the purpose of the TCI is primarily functional.

2. *Wax.* A thin sheet of wax is heated in warm water and then molded to the foot. This procedure gives a good clean impression and is a general purpose technique that can be used for both functional and accommodative TCIs.

3. *Foam box.* The patient's foot is pushed into a box of crushable rigid foam, while maintaining the foot in as neutral a position as possible. This technique is best used with a more rigid foot and results in a TCI with passive

support and localized accommodation. It is also a more convenient, portable, and less time-consuming technique.

Materials

As with impression techniques, the selection of materials for the TCI is determined by the desired function. TCI materials can be described in terms of their function and can be divided into three types[3,5,12]:

1. *Soft.* Cross-linked polyethylene foams (e.g., Plastazote) are the most common soft materials currently in use. They are made by a large number of manufacturers and are rapidly being developed and improved. They are generally moldable with the application of heat (250 to 300°F) and come in a variety of densities. Their function is accommodative, and they are generally used in the TCI shell. Studies show, however, that they decrease in thickness rather quickly, a phenomenon referred to as "bottoming out."[2]

2. *Semiflexible.* Leather and cork fall into this category. Many of the cork materials are now being combined with plastic compounds to

make them moldable when heated. Semi-flexible materials are somewhat accommodative but provide more functional support than the soft type and do not bottom out as quickly.

3. *Rigid.* Acrylic plastics and thermoplastic polymers are considered rigid materials. They are moldable at very high temperatures and are primarily functional in nature. They are the most durable and most supportive of the three types.

A study of five commonly used insole materials by Brodsky et al[2] confirmed the characteristic properties described above. The study found that while the soft polyethylene foams had better pressure distribution characteristics when new, repeated exposure to the types of pressures TCIs must withstand resulted in more rapid bottoming out than the more durable polymers. Other studies give similar results and show additionally that loss of thickness of the moldable polyethylene foam is inversely related to its density.[9,10]

These studies would seem to suggest that in order to provide maximum moldability (essential for total contact) along with the necessary shock absorption and control, a TCI should be made from a combination of materials. Most TCIs have a soft, moldable shell and a more rigid, nonmoldable posting; they may also have additional layers. The specific design and materials vary according to the needs of the individual patient.

Writing Footwear Prescriptions

A complete written prescription from the physician is necessary to ensure that the C.Ped. will be able to achieve the desired treatment results.[6] Unfortunately, it is often the only communication between the physician and the pedorthist. Even if a patient's footwear needs have been ideally determined in consultation with the physician in a clinic setting, a written prescription becomes a permanent part of the C.Ped.'s patient records, serving as a valuable resource for providing follow-up care, monitoring patient progress, and obtaining insurance reimbursement.

The written footwear prescription should include the following[3,4]:

1. *Complete diagnosis.* It is important to provide the patient's complete diagnosis; the physician should never rely on the patient to communicate diagnoses to the C.Ped. It is also important that the diagnosis be as specific as possible; for example, a diagnosis of "heel pain" might more appropriately read "calcaneal stress fracture."

2. *Desired effect.* The prescription should include a precise description of the desired effect or function of the footwear. For the above diagnosis, this might be "to relieve excessive pressure on calcaneus."

3. *Specific footwear required to produce the desired effect.* The physician should give the C.Ped. some direction on how to accomplish the desired effect, such as type of shoes, external shoe modifications, and inserts. Because the physician may not be familiar with the specific shoes, modifications, or inserts available, he or she may find it desirable to give the C.Ped. some latitude in this area.

Applications

In this section, pedorthic solutions for specific rehabilitative situations involving the forefoot, mid/hindfoot, and ankle are covered, including surgery, trauma, and chronic or long-term disorders. Following the format for footwear prescriptions described above, each application is presented as follows: (1) diagnosis, (2) desired effect or objectives, and (3) specific footwear required. The focus is on external shoe modifications and TCIs; however, it is important to remember that every footwear prescription must begin with a properly fitting, appropriately chosen shoe (see Chapter 23). Recommendations for external shoe modifications and TCIs are exhaustive. Most patients will not require all of the modalities described; depending on the individual foot, any or all of the recommendations may be used.

Surgery

Prescription footwear following surgery in the forefoot, mid/hindfoot, and ankle is discussed in this section.

Forefoot
Bunions

Initially, the objective following bunion surgery is to maintain toe position. A variety of appliances are available for this purpose (Fig. 24-6). The hallux valgus night splint, made from rigid plastic, is designed to be used immediately following surgery. A more flexible version is the hallux valgus day splint, which still maintains toe position but can be worn inside a shoe. A less bulky alternative is the toe spacer, which can be used later in the rehabilitation process, possibly even over the long term. In addition, a TCI may be used to decrease any pronation, thereby relieving pressure in the first metatarsophalangeal (MTP) joint. An important factor in long-term success of any bunion surgery is a properly fitted shoe with adequate toe room.

First MTP Fusion

The chief objectives following a first MTP fusion are to relieve pressure on the affected joint and to compensate for the lost motion. These objectives can be achieved through the use of a TCI designed to decrease any pronation and therefore relieve pressure on the first MTP joint; the addition of an extended steel shank and rocker sole can provide additional support to the joint and assist in gait. For women who want to continue to wear a dress shoe with a heel, a rocker sole can be added to the forefoot portion of a dress shoe, creating a platform effect and decreasing the effective heel height.

Hammertoes

Immediately following hammertoe surgery, the primary objective is to maintain the position of the affected toe(s) while healing. This can be achieved with the use of a hammertoe shield, which consists of a foam pad that rests under the metatarsal heads and a strap that holds the toe(s) down (Fig. 24-7). A less bulky alternative, which may be worn inside a shoe, is the toe crest, consisting of a smaller strap and a narrow pad that fits under the sulcus area (see Fig. 24-7). Also important, especially in the long-term rehabilitation of hammertoes, is a shoe that has adequate toe room to allow extension of the toes.

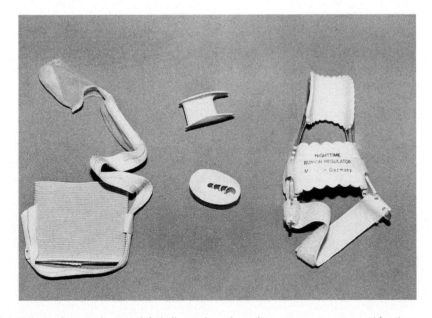

Fig. 24-6 Hallux valgus appliances: *left,* hallux valgus day splint; *center,* toe spacers, side view and top view; *right,* hallux valgus night splint.

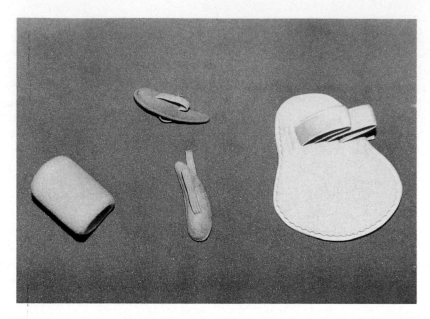

Fig. 24-7 Toe appliances: *left,* toe cap; *center,* toe crests; *right,* hammertoe shield.

Toe Nails

Following toe nail surgery, such as toe nail removal or ingrown toe nail surgery, protection of the affected toe(s) is of primary importance. Immediately following surgery, the toe can be protected with the use of a foam toe cap (see Fig. 24-7); these are available premade or can be fashioned from a piece of tube foam. To ensure continued comfort for the affected toe(s) over the long term, a shoe that has adequate height in the toe area is essential.

Morton's Neuroma

The primary objective following surgery for Morton's neuroma is to relieve any pressure at the surgery site. A TCI with a metatarsal pad carefully placed just proximal to the two involved metatarsal heads can result in the spreading apart of the webspace upon weight-bearing and achieve the needed pressure relief. A rocker sole and extended steel shank can also be helpful. The pain caused by the entrapped and damaged nerve in patients with Morton's neuroma is aggravated when the toes are pinched together— for example, by wearing shoes with inadequate toe room.[1] A shoe with adequate forefoot and toe space is therefore essential.

Mid/Hindfoot

Posterior Tibial Tendon Reconstruction

Following posterior tibial tendon reconstruction, it is necessary to provide adequate medial arch support while protecting the sensitive surgery site. A supportive TCI with cork posting and viscoelastic polymer added at the surgery site may be used. A shoe with a long medial counter, possibly reinforced with fiberglass, can also be helpful.

Kidner Procedure

Objectives following a Kidner procedure are similar to those for posterior tibial tendon reconstruction: support in the medial area and protection of the surgery site. A TCI with viscoelastic polymer added at the surgery site and a shoe with a long medial counter are recommended.

Tarsal Tunnel

Medial arch support and protection of the tender surgery site are important following the nerve release surgical procedure for tarsal tunnel. A TCI with support in the medial arch and viscoelastic polymer at the surgery site can be helpful. Additional medial support can be provided with fiberglass reinforcement of the medial counter.

Taping, Shoe Modifications, Orthoses, Arthrodeses

Triple Arthrodesis

Providing balance and stability as well as compensating for the loss of motion (i.e., inversion/eversion) are the objectives following a triple arthrodesis. A shoe with an extended steel shank and rocker sole can assist in gait and provide some added stability; flares can also help with stability and improve the patient's ability to walk on uneven ground. In addition, a supportive TCI can help balance the foot.

Plantar Fascia

Following surgery to release the plantar fascia, the primary objective is to relieve any tenderness at the surgery site and along the medial plantar surface. It is also important to reduce any excessive pressure in that area and reduce any tendency toward pronation. A shoe with a long medial counter and good arch support is helpful. A TCI may also be used, with viscoelastic polymer placed at the tender area or with a well or depression made on the top of the TCI. The addition of a cushion heel can also relieve shock on heel strike.

Retrocalcaneal Bursitis

Following surgery to remove the prominence or "pump bump" associated with retrocalcaneal bursitis, the primary objective is to relieve any pressure on that area. This is particularly important because it is at the site of the Achilles tendon. It may be necessary to stretch the counter of the patient's shoe and possibly to remove any reinforcement from the counter. A TCI with a high heel cup may also be helpful. Pressure relief can be achieved by adding viscoelastic polymer to the tender area or by building a well into the TCI at the site of the prominence.

Ankle
Fusion

Following ankle fusion, the objectives are to help replace the lost motion (i.e., dorsiflexion or plantarflexion) and to provide any needed stability since the foot may end up slightly inverted or everted after surgery. A heel-to-toe rocker sole with an extended steel shank is recommended, and a flare may be added for additional stabilization. It is also important, when adding the rocker sole, to be sure that the shoe's heel height matches the fused ankle position.

Fracture

The primary objective following surgery for an ankle fracture is to provide support and stability. A high-top shoe and a supportive TCI can be helpful. The addition of a rocker sole and extended steel shank can assist in gait and provide additional support.

Trauma

Prescription footwear for fractures and soft tissue trauma are covered in this section. It should be noted that, in general, TCIs for fractures are more functional in nature in order to provide the stability and control that are needed to promote healing.

Fractures
Sesamoid Fracture

The primary objective following a sesamoid fracture is to relieve pressure on the sesamoid and the area under the first MTP joint. This can be accomplished with the use of a TCI in which a well has been created under the first MTP joint, effectively transferring pressure to the second through fifth metatarsal heads. Additional pressure relief of the sesamoid can be achieved with the addition of a soft viscoelastic polymer under the first metatarsal head or by adding a small pad to the TCI just behind the first MTP joint.

Metatarsal Stress Fracture

Following a metatarsal stress fracture, it is essential to provide support and to immobilize the affected area so that healing can occur. The total contact made possible with a TCI can be an effective way to minimize motion; the TCI can also provide support. An extended steel shank in conjunction with a rocker sole can also assist in providing support and decreasing motion. Another option is to use a TCI with a built-in plate made of a lightweight graphite material, which when added to a TCI can take the place of an extended steel shank. The use of this special TCI in a walking shoe that comes with a mild rocker sole is a less expensive alternative when a custom rocker sole is not necessary.

Calcaneal Fracture

The objective following a calcaneal fracture is to protect the heel area by relieving any excessive pressure. A rocker sole with a more severe angle on the heel will help to decrease shock on heel strike; a cushion heel can provide additional pressure relief. A TCI to help contain the heel, made with a high heel cup and a soft viscoelastic polymer added to the heel area, can also be helpful.

Soft Tissue Trauma
Posterior Tibial Tendinitis

The pedorthic solution for posterior tibial tendinitis is essentially the same as for posterior tibial tendon reconstruction. A medial flare or stabilizer may also be used if the condition is particularly severe or the tendon has ruptured.

Plantar Fasciitis

Prescription footwear for plantar fasciitis is the same as that for plantar fascia surgery except that it may be desirable to drill or cut a hole in the insole of the shoe, in addition to that on the TCI, and fill it with viscoelastic polymer for additional cushioning. A TCI that provides medial arch support is still recommended, and it should have a high heel cup to contain any fatty tissue.

Achilles Tendinitis

Objectives for Achilles tendinitis include providing support, decreasing pronation, and minimizing any tension on the Achilles tendon during the rehabilitation process. A supportive TCI with strong medial support is recommended. Tension on the Achilles tendon can be relieved by elevating the heel. A small amount of elevation can be added to the TCI; however, it may also be necessary to add a heel-only extension to the shoe. The size of this extension may be gradually decreased as rehabilitation progresses. Two cautions are in order regarding the extension. First, it is important that the extension not have a posterior flare, because this will cause premature heel strike and aggravate the problem area. Second, the counter of the shoe must not

strike the Achilles tendon; protection of the tendon is crucial.

Free Tissue Transfer

When providing prescription footwear for free tissue transfer, also referred to as free flaps, the following objectives must be met[7]: (1) stabilize and protect free tissue transfer by reducing shock and shear; (2) protect the insensitive area on the plantar aspect of the foot; and (3) contain the transferred tissue.

An in-depth shoe can provide the necessary room for a multiple layer TCI. A specialized type of TCI, the hindfoot containment orthosis (HCO),[8] with the following layers is recommended (Fig. 24-8): (1) a soft material such as Plastazote next to the skin; (2) a soft-density viscoelastic polymer under the heel for maximum shock absorption and to replace a soft tissue or bony deficit; (3) fiberglass surrounding the heel to contain the transferred tissue; and (4) a rigid material, such as cork, used for posting. Because of the bulk of the HCO, especially in the early stages of rehabilitation, it may be necessary to use mismated shoes (i.e., a larger size shoe on the affected foot). This will change as rehabilitation progresses, as swelling decreases and eventual atrophy occurs. It may also be necessary to reconstruct the HCO one or more times during rehabilitation as these changes in the foot occur.

External shoe modifications for free flaps include a rocker sole designed to decrease shock on heel strike and a cushion heel for extra shock absorption at the heel (since many free flaps are on the heel).

Chronic or Long-Term Disorders

Providing pedorthic care for chronic disorders is very different from the short-term rehabilitation involved in the applications discussed above. While these patients may occasionally undergo surgery or trauma, long-term management of the disease process is the primary concern. The C.Ped.'s ability to monitor patients over time and keep careful records can be very helpful, not only in providing footwear that adapts to the changing foot but in helping to prevent injury or deformity through appropriate footwear, careful foot examination, and continuing patient

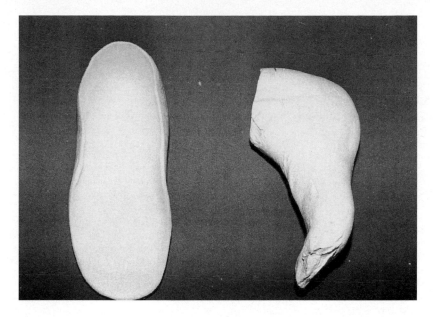

Fig. 24-8 *Left,* top view of hindfoot containment orthosis; *right,* plaster model of foot.

education. In this section, the following chronic/long-term disorders are covered: rheumatoid arthritis (RA), diabetes, and cerebrovascular accident (CVA).

Rheumatoid Arthritis

Prescription footwear for the patient with RA has both accommodative and functional aspects. It is accommodative in that it must be designed for an often painful, even hypersensitive, foot. However, it must also be functional in order to support unstable, painful joints and replace painful motion.

TCIs for RA patients generally have a shell that is made from a soft, moldable material to accommodate a loss of fatty tissue as well as any plantar prominences, including dropped metatarsal heads, nodules, or other bony prominences. It may be necessary to use a more rigid material in the TCI shell to provide any needed stability or support. Flares or stabilizers may also be helpful, and rocker soles are often used to replace painful motion and assist in gait. Shoes for the RA patient must provide adequate room for hammertoes, dorsal nodules, or hallux valgus. Involvement in the knees, hips, or even the hands can also affect footwear design. For example, pa-

tients may have difficulty reaching their feet because of hip involvement or may not be able to tie their shoes because of painful joints in the hand, and therefore require shoes with Velcro closures.

Diabetes

Prescription footwear for the patient with diabetes must also be both accommodative and functional to some degree; however, unlike the very painful, hypersensitive RA foot, the diabetic foot may be insensate. Serious foot problems may occur very quickly without the patient being aware of them because of the lack of sensation. Foot inspection, patient education, and careful follow-up are crucial in order to prevent serious complications in the diabetic foot. Applications for prescription footwear in the diabetic patient include accommodating deformities, maintaining healed ulcers and preventing their recurrence, and providing custom footwear following amputation.

Cerebral Vascular Accident

The primary objective of prescription footwear for patients following a CVA is to provide control and stability. Many patients require an ankle foot orthosis (AFO); a rocker sole is usually necessary with a fixed ankle AFO. (AFO attachment to shoes is covered in Chapter 23.) Medial and/or lateral flares can help provide additional stability. A shoe with adequate depth to accommodate resulting hammertoes may be necessary, and a Velcro closure can help if only one hand is useful.

Summary

Prescription footwear is an essential component in the rehabilitation of the foot and ankle. The C.Ped. can provide the needed shoes, external shoe modifications, total contact inserts, and other foot appliances. The C.Ped. can also be important in providing patient education and follow-up care. The C.Ped. is a valuable member of the treatment team involved in the rehabilitation process.

Bibliography

1. Alexander IJ: *The foot: examination and diagnosis,* New York, 1990, Churchill Livingstone.
2. Brodsky JW et al: Objective evaluation of insert material for diabetic and athletic footwear, *Foot Ankle* 9:111, 1988.
3. Janisse DJ: Pedorthic care of the diabetic foot. In Levin ME, O'Neal LW, Bowker JH, editors: *The diabetic foot,* ed 5, St Louis, 1993, Mosby–Year Book.
4. Janisse DJ: Indications and prescriptions for orthotics in sports, *Orthop Clin North Am* 25:95, 1994.
5. Janisse DJ: A scientific approach to insole design for the diabetic foot, *Foot* 3:105, 1993.
6. Johnson JE: Prescription footwear. In Sammarco GJ, editor: *Foot and ankle manual,* Philadelphia, 1991, Lea & Febiger.
7. Johnson JE, Janisse DJ, Kaczmarowski J: Modern pedorthic and orthotic management of complications in the foot and ankle. In Johnson JE, Brennan MJ, Gould JS, editors: *Complications of foot and ankle surgery,* Baltimore, Williams & Wilkins (in press).
8. Johnson JE et al: Pedorthic management of bone and soft tissue defects of the heel. Paper presented at American Orthopaedic Foot and Ankle Society Summer Meeting, Napa Valley, Calif, July, 15-19 1992.
9. Kuncir EJ, Wirta RW, Golbranson FL: Load-bearing characteristics of polyethylene foam: an examination of structural and compression properties, *J Rehabil Res Dev* 27:229, 1990.
10. Leber C, Evanski PM: A comparison of shoe insole materials in plantar pressure relief, *Prosthet Orthot Int* 10:135, 1986.
11. Prescription Footwear Association: *Directory of pedorthics,* Columbia, Md, 1992, Prescription Footwear Association/Board for Certification in Pedorthics.
12. Riegler HF: Orthotic devices for the foot, *Orthop Rev* 16:293, 1987.

25

Orthoses for Impaired Foot and Ankle Function

John H. Bowker

Orthoses* (braces) have been used to support weakened limbs over many centuries in many cultures. European master bracemakers brought the field to a high state of development in the nineteenth and early twentieth centuries as a result of repeated epidemics of poliomyelitis. With the virtual disappearance of new poliomyelitis cases in the developed world, most major lower limb orthoses are used currently in cases of hemiplegia due to cerebrovascular accident or traumatic brain injury, posttraumatic arthritis, and paraplegia secondary to spinal cord injury or myelomeningocele. In addition, with growing interest in disorders of the foot, a variety of specific foot orthoses have been developed in recent years.

Orthoses may be described according to their physical and functional attributes. They are primarily named for the segments they encompass, such as an ankle-foot orthosis (AFO) or foot orthosis (FO). Secondary description includes the degree of motion permitted by the device. Examples are an AFO with a 90-degree posterior stop to prevent foot drop, a 90-degree

anterior stop to prevent excessive foot dorsiflexion in the case of a paralyzed triceps surae, or a fixed orthosis that allows no ankle motion.[2]

There are two major reasons for the orthopedic foot and ankle surgeon to be knowledgeable regarding orthotic indications and prescription. One is the wide applicability of orthoses both as definitive treatment and as adjuncts to surgery. The second is the indifferent result of orthotic prescription that often results from lack of physician communication with the specialist making the orthosis regarding the specific indications and special requirements of the individual patient.

As stated in the title, the devices to be discussed here are limited to various forms of AFO that affect the ankle and subtalar joints, and foot orthoses that are designed to variably control the hindfoot, midfoot, or forefoot.

The Roles of Orthoses

Before proceeding further, it is useful to review briefly what an orthosis can be reasonably

*Orthosis = singular noun, orthoses = plural noun, orthotic = adjective, orthotics = the discipline.

expected to accomplish in the foot–ankle region and what it cannot do. The most common need for an orthosis is to support a weakened limb by controlling abnormal motion. A flaccid drop foot paralysis exemplifies a common condition of this type that can be effectively controlled by an AFO, preferably a lightweight custom-molded plastic one. Another example is hypermobility of the subtalar joint, manifested as flexible pes planus, which if uncontrolled will often lead to shortening of the triceps surae with the heel in valgus. This may also contribute to eventual attrition of the posterior tibial tendon leading to a severe fixed valgus deformity. Mildly lax subtalar joints can be controlled with a submalleolar foot orthosis (UCBL type), but more severe cases may require proximal extension to the supramalleolar level or even a mid- to full-length AFO with anterior trim lines if the patient's superincumbent weight is a major factor (Fig. 25-1).

An orthosis can also be used to control pain effectively in the ankle or foot. Effective prescription depends on an understanding of the two major factors in pain production in weight-bearing joints damaged by disease or trauma that may be amenable to orthotic relief. One is joint motion, and the other is weight-bearing itself. They may also coexist in varying proportions, making it sometimes difficult to determine which factor is predominant from the history and physical examination alone. In doubtful cases, a well-fitted weight-bearing short leg cast should be applied as a trial. If pain is relieved, an orthosis that restricts joint motion is in order. If pain continues in the face of rigid immobilization, however, an orthosis that transfers weight to the upper calf and patellar tendon can be prescribed. This design is a derivation of the patellar-tendon bearing (PTB) prosthesis for transtibial amputees. The proximal molded plastic PTB portion is attached to the shoe with double steel uprights, which fork at the ankle level to securely attach to a sole plate incorporated in the shoe. With the necessary limitation of ankle and foot motion in these designs, provision must be made for normal forward progression in gait by modifying the shoe with a cushion heel and rocker sole (see Chapter 24).

What an Orthosis Cannot Accomplish

Having reviewed some conditions for which an orthosis can be helpful, it is equally important to recognize situations for which an orthosis is inappropriate. It is often assumed, for example, that an orthosis can control an increasing deformity or correct a fixed deformity. While the device may have a role in preventing further deformity in very early cases, it should not be expected to control forces of the magnitude of body weight in the face of major limb segment malalignment. Severe valgus following posterior tibial tendon rupture or Charcot neuroarthropathy, for example, cannot be safely controlled or reduced by an AFO. Attempts to brace with three-point force systems virtually always result in ulceration over the medial foot and ankle, a condition especially dangerous in insensate limbs (Fig. 25-2). It follows that if a deformity is fully reducible, a properly designed orthosis has a much better chance of controlling the problem.

The Orthosis as a Complement to Surgery

On occasion, an orthosis is prescribed to enhance or protect a surgical procedure. For example, in the treatment of severe spastic equinovarus deformity following brain injury, a split anterior tibial transfer (SPLATT), frequently combined with a percutaneous fractional Achilles tendon lengthening, will restore balanced dorsiflexion to the foot.[3] The procedure, however, will require temporary or permanent protection by an AFO to prevent recurrent deformity. In other words, the surgery has made the foot braceable, while the orthosis complements the surgery, helping to assure a permanent good result.

A second example is severe flexible pes planus with occult shortening of the triceps surae secondary to years of walking with the heel in pronation. The contracture is noted when an attempt is made to dorsiflex the foot while the sub-

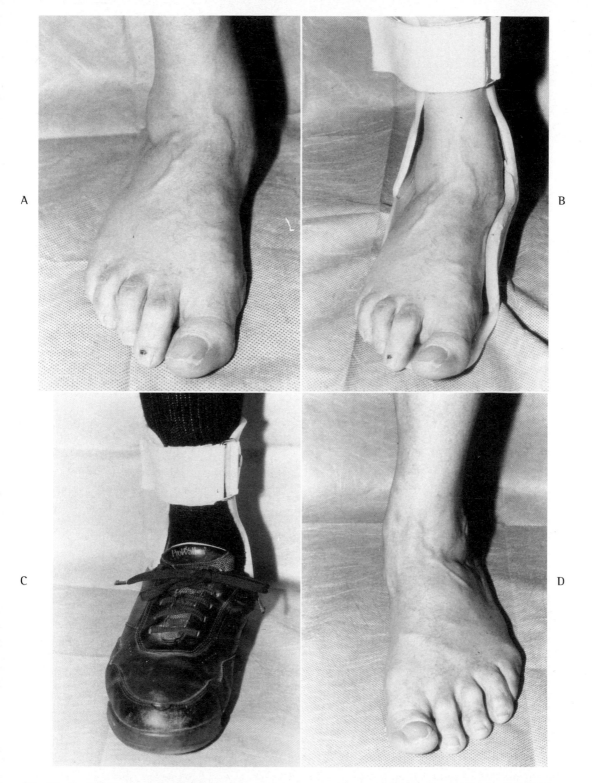

Fig. 25-1 **A,** Unsupported right foot of man with symptomatic hypermobile flat foot with severe discomfort along course of posterior tibial tendon. **B,** Midlength ankle-foot orthosis (AFO) relieved symptoms by controlling motion. **C,** Orthotic system completed by use of lace shoe. **D,** Unsupported left foot of same person with similar but milder symptoms. **E,** Supramalleolar orthosis relieved the complaints for this active man. **F,** Orthotic system completed by lace shoe. Cosmesis is enhanced by trousers and/or use of additional stocking to cover orthosis. *Continued.*

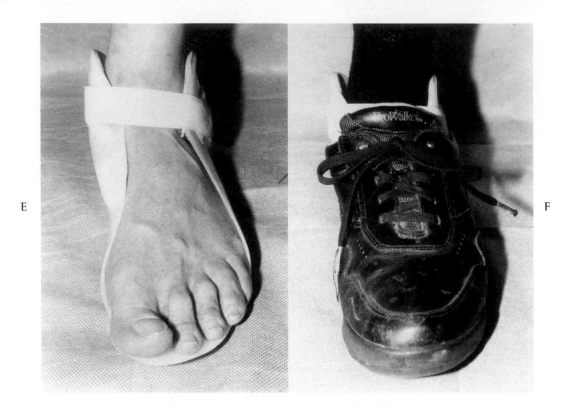

E   F

Fig. 25-1 cont'd. For legend, see p. 367.

talar joint is passively held in a neutral position. Following a fractional percutaneous heel cord lengthening, the unstable hind foot can be held plantigrade in a neutral valgus/varus position by a supramalleolar orthosis, which fits nicely in a standard shoe and is easily disguised by an extra stocking.

The Orthosis as an Alternative to Surgery

When a patient is opposed to surgical intervention, is severely debilitated or malnourished, or the affected limb is dysvascular, an orthosis can serve as a reasonable permanent alternative to surgery. For example, a patient with a fracture of the talar neck resulting in nonunion or avascular necrosis of the talar body may be placed in a PTB orthosis to reduce painful distal weight-bearing. A patient with Charcot neuroarthropa-

thy who presents subacutely many weeks to months after a midfoot fracture may be a poor candidate for surgery due to disintegration of the bony structure associated with a marked inflammatory response. Nonetheless, stable bony healing will usually be attained with prolonged casting followed by a clam-shell orthosis with an integral walking sole (Fig. 25-3). The orthosis may be replaced with a custom-molded shoe following bony consolidation of the fractured areas.

Prescription

Rote prescription by disease category is to be avoided; for example, prescribing a postpolio, spina bifida, stroke, or cerebral palsy orthosis is meaningless. In addition, although the etiologies of drop foot may include trauma to lumbosacral roots or peripheral nerves, diabetic neuropathy, or anterior horn cell disease such as poliomyeli-

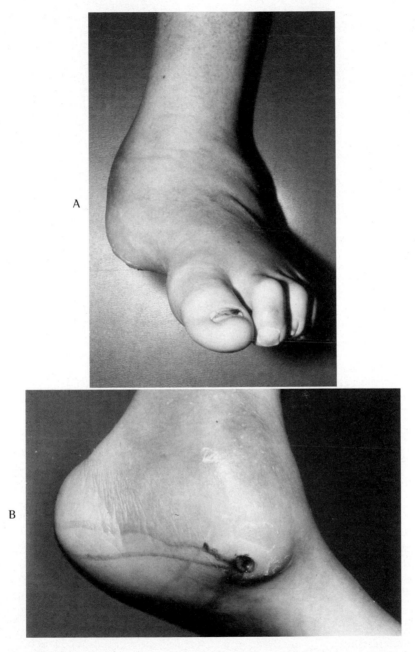

Fig. 25-2 **A,** Anterior view, left foot, of diabetic man with severe midtarsal Charcot neuroarthropathy. Note large medial prominence of talar head. **B,** Attempt to control this severe deformity with an AFO resulted in a large ulcer and abscess over the talar head area. Successful salvage required a Syme ankle disarticulation.

Orthoses for Impaired Foot and Ankle Function   Chapter 25   369

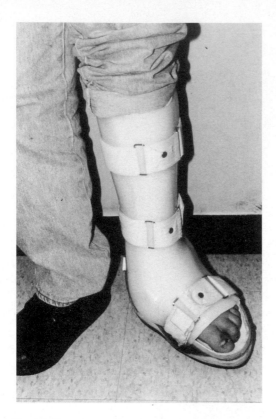

Fig. 25-3 Clam-shell orthosis consisting of anterior and posterior halves with an integral walking sole used in case of Charcot neuroarthropathy following initial bony consolidation in serial casts.

tis or Guillain-Barré syndrome, the orthotic prescription is relatively generic.

Prescription should begin with a careful history and a complete evaluation of joint stability, range of motion, relative muscle strength, and sensory function.[1] This is followed by a detailed visual gait analysis from which the observer will form a biomechanical synthesis of the segments to be braced. By performing this detailed evaluation and biomechanical synthesis prior to the design and fitting of an orthosis, costly and potentially harmful errors in design and application can be averted. The device prescribed should be designed to provide the desired effect while limiting normal function as little as possible.

Because the majority of patients requiring an orthosis have an underlying neurologic disorder, it is extremely important to determine if the body segments encompassed have at least "protective" sensation. This is defined as the ability to sense excessive pressure that will lead to eventual skin ulceration. If the history and initial examination suggest that sensation may be impaired, confirmation is easily obtained by use of the simplified three-filament Semmes-Weinstein filament set. In this concise test, the filaments identifying normal, protective, and absent sensation are applied to the skin in turn. Each filament tip is pressed on the skin with the least force required to bend it, while the patient tries to sense each one with eyes closed.

In designing an orthosis for a paralyzed limb, it is also important to note if the paralysis is flaccid or spastic. Flaccid limbs, in the absence of contractures, are easily supported by an orthosis in a weight-bearing posture. Severely spastic limbs, in contrast, may be difficult or impossible to brace until the spasticity is controlled. This can frequently be accomplished with antispastic drugs, such as baclofen. The degree of residual spasticity will then determine the orthotic approach. In hemiplegic gait, for example, if the foot is held in equinovarus during swing phase and then becomes plantigrade at midstance, the spasticity is considered mild and an AFO with midline trim lines will hold the foot plantigrade throughout gait. In contrast, if the foot remains in equinovarus throughout the gait cycle, it is unlikely that the heel will remain seated in an orthosis, leading to unsteady, unsafe ambulation. In this case, a percutaneous fractional lengthening of the Achilles tendon, coupled with a SPLATT procedure, will make effective orthotic fitting possible.[3]

Perhaps the most difficult foot to safely brace is the insensate foot with Charcot neuroarthropathy. If bracing is attempted when the foot or ankle is rigidly deformed, skin ulceration is to be expected. If treated early by prolonged casting, deformity can often be limited. As explained above, this is followed by long-term circumferential bracing for up to a year, followed by fitting with a custom-made shoe with a custom-molded foot orthosis.

An AFO is best fabricated, fitted, and serviced by a Certified Orthotist (C.O.), while foot orthoses are provided by either the orthotist or a

Certified Pedorthist (C.Ped.). Either professional is well qualified to provide shoe modifications or custom shoewear. The best results can be expected if the orthotist and/or pedorthist are part of the treatment team with the patient and surgeon, actively participating in the design of the device.

Bibliography

1. Bowker JH: Neurologic aspects of prosthetic/orthotic practice, *J Prosthet Orthot,* 5:52, 1993.

2. McCollough NC III: Biomechanical analysis systems for orthotic prescription. In *Atlas of orthotics: biomechanical principles and application,* ed 2, St Louis, 1985, The CV Mosby Co.

3. Waters RL, Perry J, Garland D: Surgical correction of gait abnormalities following stroke, *Clin Orthop* 131:54, 1978.

Suggested Reading

Hoppenfeld S: *Orthopaedic neurology: a diagnostic guide to neurologic levels,* Philadelphia, 1977, JB Lippincott.

26

Rehabilitation Following Arthrodesis in the Foot and Ankle

Thomas C. Skalley

Lew C. Schon

Arthrodesis is a commonly performed procedure in the treatment of foot and ankle disorders. The primary goals of arthrodesis include enhanced stability, elimination of painful motion, and restoration or maintenance of normal biomechanical alignment.[40]

The foot and ankle lend themselves well to arthrodesis, as a system of multiple linked joints with some overlap in function. The mobility lost following an arthrodesis is partially compensated for by adjacent joints.[9,40] Stress transfers occur within the foot and also proximally to the knee and hip.[24]

Solid bony union at the arthrodesis site requires rigid immobilization while the bones heal, which may take a long period of time. To achieve functional success, preservation of motion in the surrounding joints and strength in the musculotendinous structures is critical. The goal of rehabilitation following arthrodesis about the foot and ankle is to achieve a stable, painless weight-bearing platform with functional mobility in nonfused joints and a near normal gait pattern without compromise of strength.

In general, arthrodesis in the foot and ankle joints is accomplished surgically by removal of articular surfaces down to well-vascularized bone.[17] The surfaces should be flush to permit maximum contact area and stability. Bone graft obtained from the iliac crest, tibia, fibula, or bones in the foot may be used to augment the fusion. Compression and stability are obtained through internal or external fixation devices.

Postoperatively, the foot and ankle are immobilized in a bulky compression dressing and a plaster splint. In midfoot, hindfoot, and ankle arthrodesis, a short leg cast or "off-the-shelf" walker brace (ankle foot orthosis) (Fig. 26-1) is applied once the postoperative edema has decreased. The patient is kept partial or nonweight-bearing for a period of time depending on the site of arthrodesis and the technique used. During this time, the patient will require ambulation training with crutches, a walker, or a wheelchair as necessary. A foot pump may be

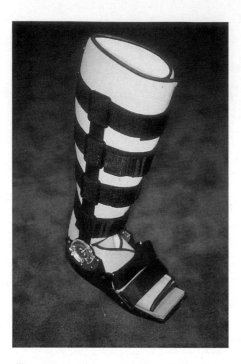

Fig. 26-1 "Off-the-shelf" walker brace.

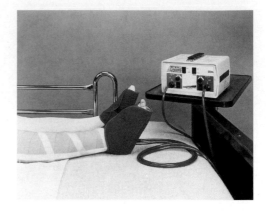

Fig. 26-2 Foot pump.

useful in select cases to decrease swelling (Fig. 26-2). During recovery, it is imperative to maintain overall body strength and range of motion in the nonimmobilized joints of the involved extremity.

Once adequate healing and stability of the arthrodesis is certain, at 6 weeks in routine cases, weight-bearing is commenced in the short leg cast or walker brace if internal fixation was used. Initially, we recommend 20 pounds of weight-bearing on the involved extremity (the patient can determine the amount of weight by placing the foot on a scale). An additional 20 to 30 pounds of weight per week can be added as tolerated up to full weight-bearing. The patient can then be weaned out of the walker brace or the short leg cast removed by 12 weeks postoperatively.

In cases where external fixation is used, weight-bearing may or may not be commenced prior to removal of the external fixation device (Fig. 26-3). Factors such as supplemental internal fixation, the design of the external fixation system, and the degree of stability noted intraoperatively all must be considered.

In arthrodesis of the forefoot, which is discussed in more detail later in the chapter, either a cast or a hard sole postoperative shoe (Fig. 26-4) may be used postoperatively. Weight-bearing on the heel and uninvolved side of the foot is allowed, often from the onset. Crutches, a cane, a walker, or a wheelchair may occasionally be required.

When rigid fixation has been achieved surgically, gentle active and passive range of motion exercises in the surrounding joints can be instituted early in the postoperative period if no cast is used. In cases in which cast immobilization is used, range of motion is obviously postponed until the cast is removed.

When bone graft is used, additional consideration must be given to the donor site in designing a postoperative rehabilitation program. Bone graft taken from the calcaneus or tibia may occasionally delay unprotected full weight-bearing until the donor site is fully healed to prevent fractures through these areas. Bone graft from the iliac crest is often quite painful postoperatively, but weight-bearing can be commenced as soon as the pain begins to subside.

Hallux Interphalangeal Joint Arthrodesis

Arthrodesis of the hallux interphalangeal (IP) joint involves fusion of the proximal and distal

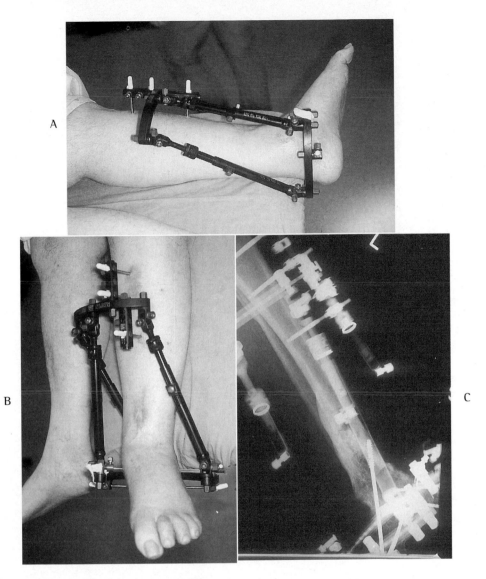

Fig. 26-3 External fixator(s).

phalanx. Indications include painful degenerative joint disease, inflammatory arthritis, and severe deformity involving the IP joint.[13] Arthrodesis has also been reported in conjunction with an extensor hallucis longus tendon transfer for the treatment of hallux varus[17,18] and for a claw hallux deformity (Jones procedure).[13]

Surgical correction entails removal of the remaining joint surfaces until well-vascularized cancellous bone is obtained. The hallux is brought into the corrected position and secured with Kirschner wires (K-wires) or a screw. The recommended position of IP arthrodesis is 15 to 20 degrees of dorsiflexion to allow smooth roll-off during gait and 5 to 10 degrees of valgus to conform to normal shoe curvature.[13]

Postoperatively, weight-bearing as tolerated is permitted in a postoperative shoe with weight allowed only on the heel and lateral border of the foot. When the Jones procedure is performed, a short leg cast may be used. Full weight-bearing may be commenced at approximately 6 weeks if the arthrodesis site is healing well.

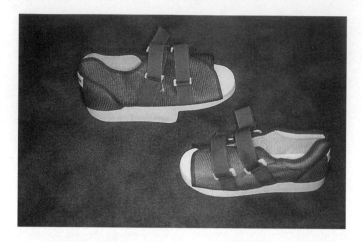

Fig. 26-4 Postoperative shoe with and without wedge.

First Metatarsophalangeal Joint Arthrodesis

Arthrodesis of the first metatarsophalangeal (MTP) joint involves fusion of the first metatarsal to the proximal phalanx (Fig. 26-5). Indications for arthrodesis of the first MTP joint include posttraumatic degenerative joint disease, advanced hallux rigidus, osteoarthritis, gouty arthritis, rheumatoid arthritis, severe hallux valgus, severe hallux varus, avascular necrosis of the first metatarsal head, severe instability, and as a salvage for failed surgery (i.e., infection, silicone synovitis from an implant, or unsuccessful resection arthropathy).[13,17,47]

Many different techniques have been described. Most commonly the surgery involves removal of the remaining articular cartilage with remodeling of the bony surfaces and internal fixation using screws, staples, plates and screws, K-wires, or Steinmann pins (Fig. 26-6). Occasionally, bone graft is used, especially in the case of a significantly shortened hallux that requires interposition corticocancellous iliac crest bone graft to restore length.[17] The recommended position of the arthrodesis ranges from 15 to 30 degrees of dorsiflexion and 10 to 25 degrees of hallux valgus.[2,13,17,28] Women who routinely wear heels higher than ½ inch may be fused in slightly more dorsiflexion.[28]

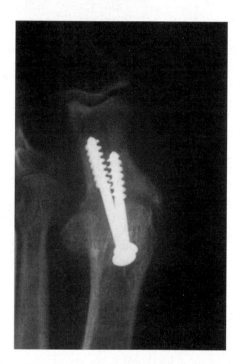

Fig. 26-5 X-ray of first metatarsophalangeal fusion.

Following first MTP arthrodesis, no motion is present at the first MTP joint. Gait is usually fairly normal.[24] Patients may tend to roll off the lateral side of their forefoot, especially if the hallux is not adequately dorsiflexed. A return to nearly all activities and most sports with few limitations can generally be expected following

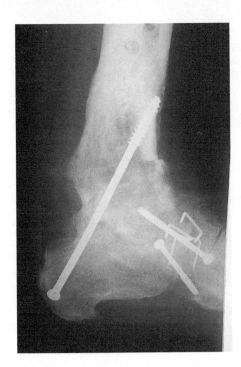

Fig. 26-6 Screws, Kirschner wires, staple and Steinmann pins are used for internal fixation.

successful arthrodesis and rehabilitation.[13] Squatting activities will be altered. Some forms of dance and sprinting will be restricted.

Postoperative rehabilitation includes weight-bearing as tolerated on the heel and lateral border of the foot in a hard-soled postoperative shoe. Crutches, a cane, a walker, or a wheelchair may be used as necessary. Excessive ambulation should be avoided to decrease edema and secondary musculoskeletal injuries due to altered gait mechanics. Gentle passive range of motion of the hallux IP joint can be instituted fairly early after surgery. Full weight-bearing is commenced once the patient is pain free and good radiographic evidence of healing is present, usually at 6 to 16 weeks. Alternatively, a short leg walking cast or walker brace may be used postoperatively. If percutaneous pins are used, full weight-bearing is usually not instituted until the pins are removed. In cases of interpositional bone graft arthrodesis, poor bone quality, or less than optimal stability obtained intraoperatively, nonweight-bearing is usually maintained for 4 to 8 weeks.

Although normal shoes may be worn after healing, some patients may require a metatarsal bar to improve the roll-off of the forefoot during ambulation. Other patients may benefit from an extra-depth wide-toe-box shoe to accommodate the dorsiflexed hallux and limit rubbing against the shoe at the dorsal IP joint. An accommodative orthotic device may be useful to decrease symptomatic lateral stress transfer.

Tarsometatarsal Joint Arthrodesis

Indications for arthrodesis of the tarsometatarsal (TMT) joints (Lisfranc's joint) is done for local posttraumatic degenerative joint disease and instability, osteoarthritis, neuropathic fracture dislocation (Charcot neuroarthropathy), pes cavus with forefoot equinus, and severe metatarsus adductus* (Fig. 26-7). The first TMT joint[34,36] or first TMT and second metatarsal[19-21] may be fused as part of a bunionectomy (Lapidus procedure).

Most commonly, surgery consists of removal of the joint surfaces, contouring of the bone to achieve proper position, and internal fixation with screws or K-wires. Bone graft is often utilized. Occasionally, an Achilles tendon lengthening is performed when correcting a rocker bottom deformity with an equinus contracture of the hindfoot.[32]

The functional impairment following first, second, and third TMT joint arthrodesis is slight due to the small amount of motion normally found in these joints (3.5, 0.6, and 1.6 degrees of sagittal plane motion, respectively, from in vitro studies[41]). If the arthrodesis includes the more mobile fourth and fifth TMT joints (9.6 and 10.2 degrees of sagittal plane motion, respectively, from in vitro studies[41]), functional loss is increased significantly.

Postoperatively, a compressive dressing and splint are used initially and changed to a short leg cast once postoperative edema has decreased. Nonweight-bearing or 20 pounds of partial

*References 5-17,26,33,35,40,49,53.

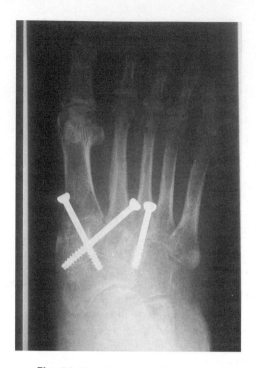

Fig. 26-7 X-ray of midfoot fusion.

weight-bearing with crutches, a walker, or a wheelchair is maintained for approximately 6 weeks. Progressive partial weight-bearing in a cast or brace is then started and increased by 20 to 30 pounds per week until full weight-bearing is achieved by 12 weeks. The cast or brace is discontinued if clinical and radiographic healing is progressing well. In some cases a postoperative shoe may be used immediately following surgery, circumventing a cast or brace. Range of motion exercises in the surrounding joints are instituted as soon as possible following removal of external immobilization devices. Isometric strengthening exercises are recommended to maintain strength in the affected lower extremity.[33] and extra-depth shoes with a rigid and rocker bottom sole may be required.

TMT arthrodesis for a neuropathic fracture dislocation (Charcot neuroarthropathy) requires nonweight-bearing in a short leg cast for 8 weeks followed by a short leg walking cast or an ankle foot orthosis for an additional 6 to 12 months (Fig. 26-8).[48] An extra-depth shoe with a rigid sole, rocker bottom, and accommodative or-

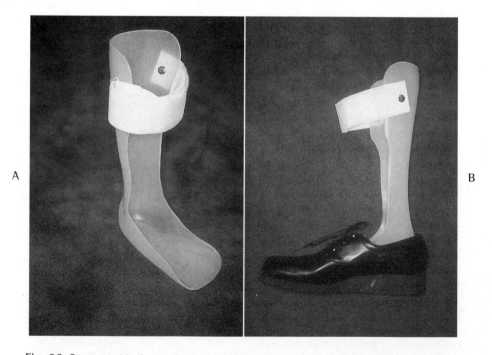

Fig. 26-8 **A,** Ankle foot orthosis (AFO). **B,** AFO with extra depth high toe box shoe.

Taping, Shoe Modifications, Orthoses, Arthrodeses

thotic is then recommended. Continued observation for skin breakdown or activation of a neuropathic fracture elsewhere in the foot is necessary.

Isolated Talonavicular or Calcaneocuboid Arthrodesis

An isolated talonavicular (TN) or calcaneocuboid (CC) arthrodesis is performed infrequently for posttraumatic degenerative disease, rheumatoid arthritis, or osteoarthritis involving only the TN or CC joints.[40] Occasionally, TN arthrodesis is used in conjunction with a flexor digitorum longus tendon transfer for posterior tibial tendon reconstruction following planovalgus collapse at the TN joint.[35] Because of the complex interactions of hindfoot and midfoot articulations,[27] arthrodesis of one joint limits motion in adjacent joints.[40] Additionally, most disease processes in the hindfoot and midfoot involve more than one joint.[10] As a result, a double—TN and CC—or triple—TN, CC, and talocalcaneal (subtalar)—arthrodesis is more commonly indicated than an isolated arthrodesis at the TN or CC joint (Fig. 26-9).

Arthrodesis at the TN or CC joint involves removal of the remaining articular surface down to well-vascularized cancellous bone and internal fixation with screws, K-wires, or staples. Proper alignment must be achieved for clinical success. Bone graft may be used to counteract unbalanced shortening of the foot.

Range of motion lost as a result of CC or TN arthrodesis includes a reduction in subtalar motion,[14] forefoot abduction/adduction, and pronation/supination of the foot.

As a result of this limited supination and pronation, patients may have difficulty walking on uneven terrain. Walking on rocky ground or slanted and banked surfaces may lead to instability and may increase the tendency to fall. Some sports will not be manageable, especially those that involve cutting and rapid running.

Postoperatively, a compressive dressing and splint are applied initially and then changed to a short leg nonweight-bearing cast or walker brace for 6 weeks. Partial weight-bearing is then begun in a short leg walking cast or ankle foot orthosis and advanced by 20 to 30 pounds of weight per week as tolerated. The cast or brace may be discontinued once bony union is complete, usually approximately 12 weeks after surgery. As described for TMT arthrodesis, range of motion exercises in the surrounding joints can be commenced following discontinuation of external immobilization devices. Isometric strengthening of the involved extremity should be maintained postoperatively.

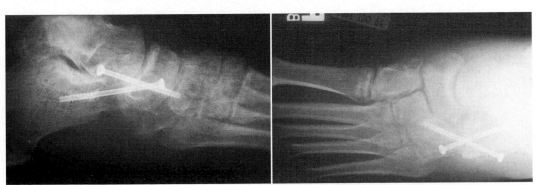

B

Fig. 26-9 Calcaneocuboid orthoses was performed for a patient with a severe painful pes planovalgus following chronic posterior tibialis tendon rupture. **A**, Lateral. **B**, X-ray of foot.

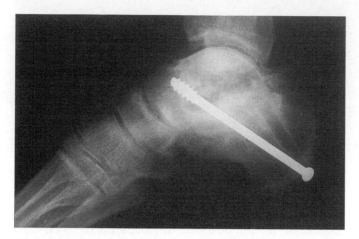

Fig. 26-10   X-ray of isolated subtalar fusion.

Double (Talonavicular and Calcaneocuboid) Arthrodesis

Arthrodesis of the transverse tarsal joints (Chopart's joint) includes the TN and CC joints. Indications include local posttraumatic degenerative joint disease,[40] osteoarthritis, symptomatic flexible pes planovalgus deformity unresponsive to conservative treatment,[26] and posterior tibial tendon dysfunction in the presence of a pain-free, mobile subtalar joint.[29]

The surgical procedure and postoperative rehabilitation program are similar to that described previously for isolated TN or CC joint arthrodesis.

Limitations following double arthrodesis include a reduction of subtalar, abduction/adduction, and pronation/supination motion.

Isolated Subtalar Arthrodesis

Subtalar, or talocalcaneal, joint arthrodesis is the most common isolated fusion performed in the hindfoot[40] (Fig. 26-10). Indications include posttraumatic degenerative joint disease as often seen following calcaneal fractures,[8,37] localized osteoarthritis and rheumatoid arthritis,[40] planovalgus deformity from posterior tibial tendon dysfunction,[17] and severe valgus hindfoot deformities in children as seen in cerebral palsy and paralytic conditions such as poliomyelitis.[4,10,11]

Surgical fusion of the subtalar joint can involve intraarticular, extraarticular, or bone block interposition techniques. Internal fixation is used, employing compression screws, staples, or K-wires, following removal of the articular surfaces in intraarticular arthrodesis. Extraarticular arthrodesis (i.e., Grice procedure),[10,11] performed more often in children, fuses the talus to the calcaneus at a site adjacent to, but not part of, the joint. Interposition bone graft with corticocancellous bone graft from the iliac crest is used when restoration of hindfoot height is required.[8,37] This is often seen following displaced and depressed intraarticular calcaneus fractures (Fig. 26-11). The recommended position of the arthrodesis is 3 to 5 degrees of valgus.[46]

Inversion and eversion of the hindfoot are lost following subtalar arthrodesis, which can cause some problems for the patient on uneven ground,[46] such as walking transversely on hills. Some pronation and supination remain at Chopart's joint,[45] enabling minimal compensation on uneven ground. As previously discussed, there is a close interrelationship between Chopart's joint and the subtalar joint,[27] resulting in some loss of motion at the TN and CC joints after subtalar arthrodesis.[40,45]

Taping, Shoe Modifications, Orthoses, Arthrodeses

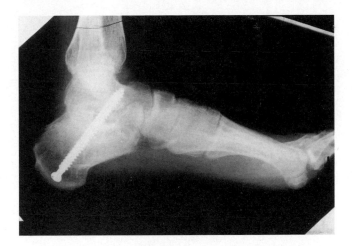

Fig. 26-11 X-ray of interposition bone block subtalar fusion, following calcaneal fracture malunion.

Following initial immobilization in a compressive dressing and splint, a nonweight-bearing cast or walker brace is worn for 6 weeks. Partial weight-bearing is then instituted at 20 pounds and increased by 20 to 30 pounds per week over the next 6 weeks, at which time the cast or brace can be discontinued if the arthrodesis is healing well. Once the arthrodesis is solid, range of motion exercises may be instituted for ankle and midfoot joints, but exercises such as the BAPS (Biomechanical Ankle Platform System, CAMP, Jackson, Mich) board should be avoided since the hindfoot is unable to invert and evert. Isometric strengthening should be maintained in the involved extremity during the postoperative period.

Triple (Talonavicular, Calcaneocuboid, and Subtalar) Arthrodesis

Triple arthrodesis involves surgical fusion of the subtalar, TN, and CC joints. Indications include posttraumatic degenerative joint disease,[9,24,40] rheumatoid arthritis,[1,9] tarsal coalition,[3] severe cavovarus deformity,[25,51,52] severe planovalgus deformity,[9,35,40] fixed equinovarus deformity,[3,23,40] and paralytic instability.[9,40]

Surgery incorporates the various techniques previously described for isolated arthrodesis of the TN, CC, and subtalar joints (Fig. 26-12). Bone graft may be used.

Functional changes following triple arthrodesis include loss of hindfoot inversion/eversion and a significant decrease in forefoot pronation/supination and abduction/adduction. Loss of dorsiflexion/plantarflexion at Chopart's joint is usually fairly well compensated for by the ankle and midfoot joints.[9] Jahss,[14] however, reported a 10-degree decrease in ankle motion following triple arthrodesis. Gait is fairly normal following triple arthrodesis,[23] although walking on uneven ground is difficult.[55] Difficulty with shoes, especially high heels, has been reported following this procedure.[9]

Postoperatively, the foot and ankle are immobilized in a compression dressing and splint, which is then changed to a short leg cast or walker brace. Nonweight-bearing is maintained for 6 weeks. Partial weight-bearing is then commenced at 20 pounds of weight and increased by 20 to 30 pounds per week. At 12 weeks postoperatively, full weight-bearing without the cast or brace may be instituted if the fusion is healing well.

Ankle and TMT joint range of motion exercises may be started once healing is progressing well. The BAPS board should be avoided following triple arthrodesis since no hindfoot inversion or eversion is present and pronation and su-

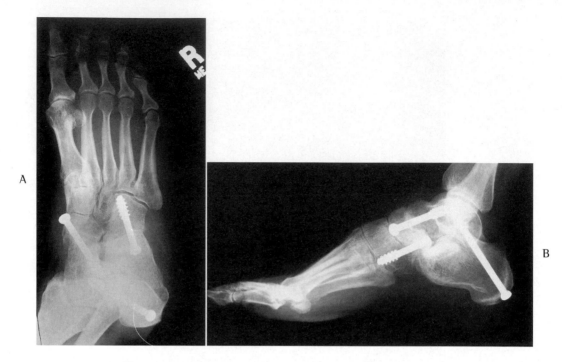

Fig. 26-12 Triple arthrodesis. **A**, Oblique view, **B**, lateral view.

pination are severely limited. Isometric strengthening exercises in the involved extremity should be maintained during the postoperative period.

Ankle Arthrodesis

Ankle arthrodesis involves surgical fusion of the tibiotalar joint. Indications include localized osteoarthritis, posttraumatic degenerative joint disease, rheumatoid arthritis, avascular necrosis of the talus, salvage of failed total ankle arthroplasty, severe fixed equinus deformity, severe crural varus or valgus deformities, and salvage following infection.[7,40,50] Ankle arthrodesis has also been reported for neuropathic fracture dislocation (Charcot neuroarthropathy) of the ankle.[44]

Surgical techniques include intra- or extraarticular fusion, open or arthroscopic techniques, and internal or external fixation.[7,40] Intraarticular fusion requires removal of the remaining articular cartilage from the ankle joint, while ex-

traarticular fusion utilizes bone graft between the tibia and talus adjacent to, but not involving, the joint itself. At times the two are used in combination.[7,40] In cases of minimal or no deformity, arthroscopic removal of articular cartilage can be performed followed by internal fixation.[38] In the presence of significant deformity, open procedures are required.[38] Internal fixation devices utilized include screws, K-wires, and plates and screws[40] (Fig. 26-13). External fixation may be used in certain situations such as infection,[40] malposition,[7] and neuropathic fracture dislocation associated with an open wound (Fig. 26-14).[44] The optimal position for ankle arthrodesis is neutral dorsiflexion, 5 to 10 degrees of external rotation, and 0 to 5 degrees of valgus.[7,40] Tibiotalar motion is lost following ankle arthrodesis, but clinically, 25% to 30% of tibiopedal motion remains.[12,31] Relative to the tibia, the foot can be plantarflexed to 20 degrees below neutral and dorsiflexed to neutral as a result of sagittal plane motion at Chopart's and Lisfranc's joints.[40] On visual gait analysis, gait appears normal in two thirds of patients following ankle fu-

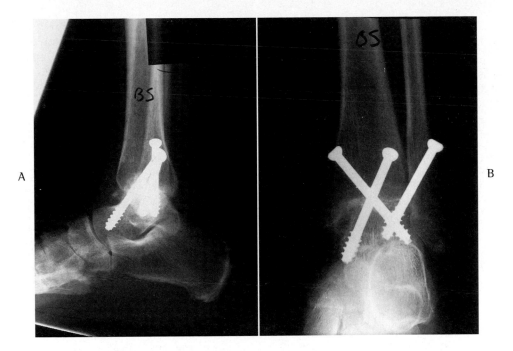

Fig. 26-13 Ankle fusion with three screws. **A**, lateral view. **B**, AP view.

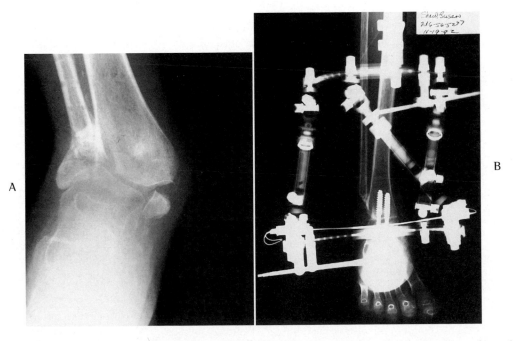

Fig. 26-14 X-ray of ankle fusion with internal and external fixation for a neuropathic nonunion of an ankle fracture. **A**, Preoperative, and **B**, postoperative x-ray of ankle.

sion.[40] Because of a shortened stride length, walking speed is decreased.[30] Limb shortening of 1 to 1.5 cm may be seen following intraarticular arthrodesis.[40] Calf atrophy and limitations in subtalar range of motion have been reported following ankle arthrodesis.[22,30]

Postoperatively, a compression dressing and splint are used followed by a short leg cast or walker brace. The patient is kept nonweight-bearing on crutches, a walker, or a wheelchair for 6 weeks.[39] Partial weight-bearing is then instituted at 20 pounds initially, followed by an increase of 20 to 30 pounds per week until full weight-bearing. At 12 weeks, the short leg walking cast or brace can be discontinued.[39]

If an external fixation device is utilized, nonweight-bearing is maintained for approximately 6 to 8 weeks. The external fixation device may be removed in some cases at this time, and a short leg walking cast or brace is applied for partial weight-bearing with advancement to full weight-bearing as previously described. The cast or brace can then be discontinued after 12 weeks if healing is progressing well. In some cases where there is a high risk of nonunion, the external fixation is left on until healing occurs. Weight-bearing can be initiated while the frame is left on.

In the case of neuropathic fracture dislocation treated with an ankle arthrodesis, nonweight-bearing is maintained for approximately 8 weeks, followed by protected weight-bearing in a cast or ankle foot orthosis for 6 months to a year.[54]

Once the ankle fusion is healing well, range of motion exercises for the subtalar joint as well as for Chopart's and Lisfranc's joints may be instituted. Most patients tolerate normal shoes,[39] but shoes with a rocker bottom sole and a cushioned heel may be prescribed to help accommodate the fused ankle.[5]

Tibiotalocalcaneal Arthrodesis

Tibiotalocalcaneal arthrodesis involves fusion of the tibiotalar (ankle) and talocalcaneal (subtalar) joints. Indications include posttraumatic degenerative joint disease,[43] rheumatoid arthritis

involving both the ankle and subtalar joints following poliomyelitis paralysis,[40] salvage after infection,[40] salvage after partial or total talectomy,[6] neuropathic fracture dislocation,[32,44] and avascular necrosis of the talus.[17]

The surgical technique involves a combination of that already described for isolated subtalar and ankle joint arthrodesis (Fig. 26-15). In cases such as severe neuropathic fracture dislocation of the talus, talectomy is sometime performed with arthrodesis of the tibia to the calcaneus.[44]

Following tibiotalocalcaneal fusion, no motion will be present in the ankle or subtalar joints, resulting in decreased tibiopedal motion and absent hindfoot inversion/eversion. As described earlier, some sagittal plane motion will be present due to motion at Chopart's and Lisfranc's joints.

Following surgery, a compression dressing and splint are used, followed by a short leg cast or walker brace. Nonweight-bearing with crutches, a walker, or a wheelchair is maintained for 6 weeks,[42,43] at which time partial weight-bearing is begun starting at 20 pounds and increasing by 20 to 30 pounds per week until full weight-bearing. The cast or brace can be discontinued after 12 weeks if good bony healing is present. Arthrodesis for neuropathic conditions is managed similarly to that described for neuropathic ankle arthrodesis. A cushioned heel shoe with a rocker bottom is usually necessary.[42,43] Leg length inequality following this surgery is treated with a shoe lift that keeps the affected extremity 0.5 cm shorter than the contralateral side.[42,43]

The BAPS board should not be used, since there is no longer any hindfoot inversion or eversion. Isometric strengthening of the involved lower extremity can be maintained postoperatively, as previously described for other arthrodeses.

Pantalar Arthrodesis

Pantalar arthrodesis includes fusion of the ankle, subtalar, TN, and CC joints. Indications include posttraumatic degenerative joint disease, rheumatoid arthritis involving the entire hind-

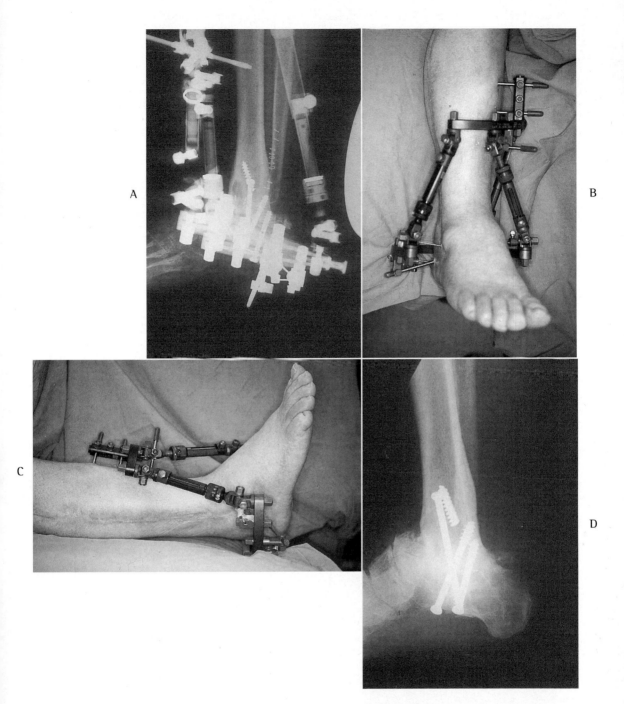

Fig. 26-15 Tibiocalcaneal fusion performed for avascular necrosis of the talus following open fracture dislocation. The patient had failed two previous attempts at fusion. **A**, Lateral x-ray during first 3 months. **B** and **C**, Leg with hybrid fixation. **D**, Lateral x-ray at 3½ months demonstrating solid fusion.

foot and ankle,[40] flail foot with paralysis,[40] neuropathic fracture dislocation,[44] and salvage following widespread infection involving the ankle and hindfoot.

The surgical technique combines that already described for ankle arthrodesis and triple arthrodesis (Fig. 26-16).

The functional motion loss following pantalar fusion is significant. Sagittal plane motion for tibiopedal motion occurs primarily at the TMT joint. No hindfoot inversion/eversion and virtually no forefoot pronation/supination remain, making uneven surfaces difficult to negotiate.

Postoperatively, the foot and ankle are immobilized in a compression dressing and splint, followed by a cast or brace. Nonweight-bearing is maintained with crutches, a walker, or a wheelchair for 6 weeks, at which time partial weight-bearing is begun starting at 20 pounds and increasing by 20 to 30 pounds per week until full weight-bearing. The cast or brace can be discontinued at 12 weeks if healing is progressing well.

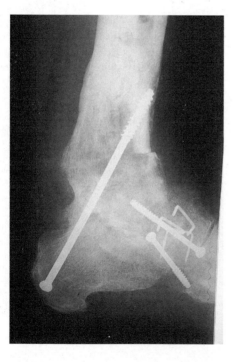

Fig. 26-16 Pantalar fusion with distal tibial osteotomy for severe varus malunion of the tibia and hindfoot.

Neuropathic conditions are managed postoperatively in a manner similar to that described for ankle arthrodesis in neuropathic conditions. A cushion-heeled shoe with a rocker bottom is nearly always required in the ambulatory patient following pantalar arthrodesis.

The BAPS board should be avoided due to the lack of hindfoot and Chopart's joint motion. Isometric strengthening can be instituted throughout the postoperative period in the involved extremity.

Bibliography

1. Adam W, Ranawat C: Arthrodesis of the hindfoot in rheumatoid arthritis, *Orthop Clin North Am* 7:827, 1976.
2. Alexander IJ: Arthrodeses of the metatarsophalangeal and interphalangeal joints of the hallux. In Myerson M, editor: *Current therapy in foot and ankle surgery,* St Louis, 1993, Mosby–Year Book.
3. Angus PD, Cowell HR: Triple arthrodesis, a critical long term review, *J Bone Joint Surg* 68B:260, 1986.
4. Baker LD, Hill LM: Foot alignment in the cerebral palsy patient, *J Bone Joint Surg* 46A:1, 1964.
5. Baker PL: SACH heel improves results of ankle fusion, *J Bone Joint Surg* 52A:1485, 1970.
6. Canale ST, Kelly FB: Fractures of the neck of the talus: long term evaluation of seventy one cases, *J Bone Joint Surg* 60A:143, 1978.
7. Carnesale PG: Arthrodesis of ankle, knee, and hip. In: Crenshaw AH, editor: *Campbell's operative orthopaedics,* ed 8, vol 1, St Louis, 1992, Mosby–Year Book.
8. Carr JB, Hansen ST, Benirschke SK: Subtalar distraction bone block fusion for late complications of os calcis fractures, *Foot Ankle* 9:81, 1988.
9. Graves SC, Mann RA, Graves KO: Triple arthrodesis in older adults, *J Bone Joint Surg* 75A:355, 1993.
10. Grice DS: Further experience with extra-articular arthrodesis of the subtalar joint, *J Bone Joint Surg* 37A:246, 1955.
11. Grice DS: An extra-articular arthrodesis for correction of paralytic flat feet in children, *J Bone Joint Surg* 34A:927, 1952.
12. Jackson A, Glasgow M: Tarsal hypermobility after ankle fusion—fact or fiction? *J Bone Joint Surg* 61B:470, 1979.
13. Jahss MH: Disorders of the hallux and first ray. In Jahss MH, editor: *Disorders of the foot and ankle,* ed 2, vol 1, Philadelphia, 1991, WB Saunders.
14. Jahss MH: The subtalar complex. In Jahss MH, editor: *Disorders of the foot and ankle,* ed 2, vol 2, Philadelphia, 1991, WB Saunders.
15. Jahss MH: Tarsometatarsal trucated-wedge arthrodesis for pes cavus and equinovarus deformity of the forepart of the foot, *J Bone Joint Surg* 62A:713, 1980.
16. Johnson JE, Johnson KA: Dowel arthrodesis for degenerative arthritis of the tartarsal metatarsal (Lis Franc) joints, *Foot Ankle* 6:243, 1986.

17. Johnson KA: Arthrodesis of the foot and ankle. In Johnson KA, editor: *Surgery of the foot and ankle,* New York, 1989, Raven Press.

18. Johnson KA, Spiegl PV: Extensor hallucis longus transfer for hallux varus deformity, *J Bone Joint Surg* 66A:681, 1984.

19. Lapidus PW: The author's bunion operation from 1931 to 1959, *Clin Orthop* 16:119, 1960.

20. Lapidus PW: A quarter of a century of experience with the operative correction of the metatarsus varus primus in hallux valgus, *Bull Hosp J Dis* 17:404, 1956.

21. Lapidus PW: Operative correction of metatarsus primus varus in hallux valgus, *Surg Gynecol Obstet* 58:183, 1934.

22. Lynch AF, Bourne RB, Rorabeck CH: The long term results of ankle arthrodesis, *J Bone Joint Surg* 70B:113, 1988.

23. McCauley JC: Triple arthrodesis for congenital talipes equinovarus deformities, *Clin Orthop* 34:25, 1964.

24. Mann RA: Biomechanics of the foot and ankle. In Mann RA, editor: *Surgery of the foot,* ed 5, St Louis, 1986, The CV Mosby Co.

25. Mann RA: Major surgical procedures for disorders of the ankle, tarsus, and midtarsus. In Mann RA, editor: *Surgery of the foot,* ed 5, St Louis, 1986, The CV Mosby Co.

26. Mann RA: Miscellaneous afflictions of the foot. In Mann RA, editor: *Surgery of the foot,* ed 5, St Louis, 1986, The CV Mosby Co.

27. Mann RA: Surgical implications of biomechanics of the foot and ankle, *Clin Orthop* 146:111, 1980.

28. Mann RA, Coughlin MJ: Hallux valgus and complications of hallux valgus. In Mann RA, editor: *Surgery of the foot,* ed 5, St Louis, 1986, The CV Mosby Co.

29. Mann RA, Miller R: Double arthrodesis in the adult. Paper presented at the American Orthopaedic Foot and Ankle Society 23rd annual meeting, San Francisco, Calif, Feb 21, 1993.

30. Mazur JM, Schwartz E, Simon SR: Ankle arthrodesis: long term follow-up with gait analysis, *J Bone Joint Surg* 61A:964, 1979.

31. Morgan CD et al: Long-term results of tibiotalar arthrodesis, *J Bone Joint Surg* 67A:546, 1985.

32. Myerson M: Arthrodesis for diabetic neuroarthropathy. In Myerson M, editor: *Current therapy in foot and ankle surgery,* St Louis, 1993, Mosby–Year Book.

33. Myerson M: Tarsometatarsal arthrodesis. In Myerson M, editor: *Current therapy in foot and ankle surgery,* St Louis, 1993, Mosby–Year Book.

34. Myerson MS: Metatarsocuneiform arthrodesis for treatment of hallux valgus and metatarsus primus varus, *Orthopedics* 13:1025, 1990.

35. Myerson MS: Acquired flatfoot in the adult, *Adv Orthop Surg* 22:155, 1989.

36. Myerson MS, Allon S, McGarvey W: Metatarsocuneiform arthrodesis for management of hallux valgus in metatarsus primus varus, *Foot Ankle* 13:107, 1992.

37. Myerson MS, Quill GE: Late complications of fractures of the calcaneus, *J Bone Joint Surg* 75A:331, 1993.

38. Myerson MS, Quill G: Ankle arthrodesis: a comparison of an arthroscopic and an open method of treatment, *Clin Orthop* 268:84, 1991.

39. Ouzounian TJ: Ankle arthrodesis. In Myerson M, editor: *Current therapy in foot and ankle surgery,* St Louis, 1993, Mosby–Year Book.

40. Ouzounian TJ, Kleiger B: Arthrodesis in the foot and ankle. In Jahss MH, editor: *Disorders of the foot and ankle,* ed 2, vol 3, Philadelphia, 1991, WB Saunders.

41. Ouzounian TJ, Shereff MJ: In vitro determination of midfoot motion, *Foot Ankle* 10:140, 1989.

42. Papa JA: Extended arthrodesis of the ankle and hindfoot for post-traumatic arthrosis. In Myerson M, editor: *Current therapy in foot and ankle surgery,* St Louis, 1993, Mosby–Year Book.

43. Papa JA, Myerson MS: Pantalar and tibiotalocalcaneal arthrodesis for post-traumatic osteoarthrosis of the ankle and hindfoot, *J Bone Joint Surg* 74A:1042, 1992.

44. Papa J, Myerson M, Girard P: Salvage of intractable diabetic neuroarthropathy of the foot and ankle with arthrodesis, *J Bone Joint Surg,* 75A:1056, 1993.

45. Prakash K et al: Ankle and foot biomechanics after subtalar fusion. Paper presented at the American Orthopaedic Foot and Ankle Society 23rd annual meeting, San Francisco, Calif, Feb 21, 1993.

46. Quill GE: Subtalar arthrodesis. In Myerson M, editor: *Current therapy in foot and ankle surgery,* St Louis, 1993, Mosby–Year Book.

47. Richardson EG: Disorders of the hallux. In Crenshaw AH, editor: *Campbell's operative orthopaedics,* ed 8, vol 4, St Louis, 1992, Mosby–Year Book.

48. Sammarco GJ: Neuropathic arthropathy. In Sammarco GJ, editor: *The foot in diabetes,* Philadelphia, 1991, Lea & Febiger.

49. Sangeorzan BJ, Veith RG, Hansen ST: Salvage of Lisfranc's tarsometatarsal joint by arthrodesis, *Foot Ankle* 10:193, 1990.

50. Schon LC, Ouzounian TJ: Adult ankle disorders. In Jahss MH, editor: Disorders of the foot and ankle, ed 2, vol 2, Philadelphia, 1991, WB Saunders.

51. Siffert RS, Forster RI, Nachamier B: "Beak" triple arthrodesis for correction of severe cavus deformity, *Clin Orthop* 45:101, 1966.

52. Siffert RS, Torto UD: "Beak" triple arthrodesis for severe cavus deformity, *Clin Orthop* 181:64, 1983.

53. Stephens R: Dorsal wedge operation for metatarsus equinus, *J Bone Joint Surg* 5:485, 1923.

54. Ullman B: In Sammarco GJ, editor: *The foot in diabetes,* Philadelphia, 1991, Lea & Febiger.

55. Williams PF, Menelaus MB: Triple arthrodesis by inlay grafting—a method suitable for the undeformed or valgus foot, *J Bone Joint Surg* 59B:333, 1977.

Index

Free tissue transfer, prescription
    footwear for, 362
Friction
    of activity surface, foot-ankle
        complex function and, 42
    in lateral movement, 49
Friction massage, 121
Functional examination. *See* Exami-
    nation, functional
Fungal infections, of toenails, 161

G

Gait
    assessment, in injury prevention
        evaluation, 203
    control theory, 222
    cycle, 229-230
        stance phase, 229
        swing phase, 229
    examination, 58
    normal, anterior compartment
        muscles in, 78-79
    patterns
        of idiopathic toe-walkers, 182
        injury risk and, 252-253
    running, 130
    steppage, 79
Gastrocnemius muscle, 13, 31, 80
Gastroc-soleus complex retraining,
    for basketball injuries, 273
Gate theory of pain, heat and, 217
Gate theory of pain modulation, 117
Glucose, requirements in diabetes
    mellitus, 164
Golf, foot and ankle function in,
    53-55
Golf shoes, 238
Golgi tendon apparatus, 96, 97
Goniometer, 62
Goniometry, 97
Goodyear welt sole attachment, 341,
    342
Great toe, hyperextension. *See* Turf
    toe
Greater saphenous vein, 22
Ground reaction forces (GRFs), 77,
    80
    in aerobic dancing, 52
    court shoe design and, 234
    in golf swing, 53
    at heel strike while walking, 230
    in landing from jump, 39-40
    in lateral movements, 38
    in running, 35-36, 37
    with structural abnormality, 245-
        246
Gymnasts, injury prevention, 203

H

Hallux interphalangeal joint, arthro-
    desis, 374-375
Hallux rigidus, 70, 287-288

Hallux synovitis
    from baseball, 287-288
    diagnosis, 287
    prevention, 288
    treatment, 287-288
Hallux valgus
    articular changes in, 94
    bunions and, 248
    etiology
        ligaments and, 92-94
        muscles and, 92-94
        metatarsophalangeal joint and,
            93-94
    orthosis
        fabrication technique, 197
        indications for use, 196
        outcome, 197
        rationale, 196
    postoperative footwear for, 359
Hammer toe
    etiology, 93
    postoperative footwear for, 359,
        360
Hamstring, tightness, examination,
    71
Hard rubber soles, 343
Head injury, reflex sympathetic dys-
    trophy and, 149
Healing shoes, for rehabilitation,
    347
Heat therapy
    alternating with cold therapy, 216
    blood flow and, 112, 113
    contraindications, 217
    deep, 218
    hot packs, 217-218
    indications, 112, 216, 217
    phonophoresis, 221
    shortwave diathermy, 219
    superficial, 217
    ultrasound, 219-221
    vs. cold therapy, 111
    whirlpools, 218
Heat-molded healing shoe, 347
Heel
    cushion, 355
    eversion, 64, 71-72
    flexibility, Sherman Coleman test,
        67
    inversion, 64
    pain, in basketball players, 272
Heel cord
    insertion, examination, 72
    passive stretching, 183
    tightness, 202
        testing, 62
Heel cord wedge, 211
Heel counter, of athletic shoe, 230
Heel flare, on footwear, 41
Heel spurs. *See* Plantar fasciitis
Heel-only extension, 355-356
Heel-toe footfall pattern (HT footfall
    pattern), 32
Heel-to-toe rocker sole, 353
Heiden board, 203

Hematomas, subungual. *See* Subun-
    gual hematomas
Herpes zoster, reflex sympathetic
    dystrophy and, 149
Heyman-Herndon procedure, 178
High voltage pulsed galvanic stimu-
    lation (HVPGS)
    blood flow and, 118
    edema reduction, 117-118
    vs. isometric exercise, 119
    wound healing and, 118-119
High-arched foot, overuse syn-
    dromes and, 300
Hilton's law, 97
Hindfoot
    angle, in running gait, 243-245
    bones, 26
    coordination of foot joint actions,
        30
    fixed varus deformity, examina-
        tion, 67
    joint, examination, 63-64
    ligaments and, 77
    pronation
        midsole density and, 41, 42
        stability devices, 41-42
    surgery, postoperative footwear
        for, 360-361
    valgus, 243
    valgus position, 73
    varus, 243
    varus position, 73
Hip
    range of motion assessment, of
        dancer, 312
    rotation, examination, 60
    symmetry, examination, 60
History, functional examination and,
    57-58
Home stretching program, for con-
    genital metatarsus adductus,
    178
Hosiery, 239
Hot packs, 217-218
    moist, 112, 113
HT footfall pattern (heel-toe footfall
    pattern), 32
HVPGS. *See* High voltage pulsed
    galvanic stimulation
    (HVPGS)
Hydration, soccer injuries and, 294
Hydrocollator packs, 217-218
Hydrotherapy, 112-113
    contrast baths, 114
Hypermobility, injury prevention
    measures for, 202
Hyperpronation
    pes cavus and, 253
    pes planus and, 253
    posture and, 252
    vs. structural abnormality, in
        chronic running injuries,
        242
Hypoglycemia, during exercise, in
    diabetes mellitus, 155, 164

Index

dorsiflexion, 84
neutral position, 26
plantarflexion, 84
range of motion, 26
Talocrural stress test, 323
Talonavicular joint, 7, 28
arthrodesis
with calcaneocuboid and subtalar arthrodeis, 381-382
isolated, 379
and calcaneocuboid arthrodesis,
380
Talonavicular ligament
dorsal, 85
Talus, 3, 26
anterior portion, 4
body of, 3-4
deformity, in talipes equinovarus,
174
distal ovoid articular surface, 4
head of, 4
inferior portion, 6
lateral articular surface, 4
medial articular surface, 4
neck of, 4
posterior plantar medial surface, 4
vertical. See Vertical talus
Taping, 337-338
of ankle sprain, 142
basketweave pattern, 331-332
dorsal checkreign, 332
high-tension, dynamic inversioin/
plantarflexion restraint, 331
with low-dye tape, 334
prophylactic ankle, for ankle
sprain treatment, 99-100
sideline, 332
spartan strip, 331-332
stirrups and horeshoes, 331
X-style longitudinal arch,
332-333
Tarsal coalition
clinical features, 180
extraarticular, 180
intraarticular, 180
pathophysiology, 180
treatment techniques, 180-181
Tarsal navicular, 5
Tarsal tunnel, 11
surgical treatment, postoperative
footwear for, 360-361
Tarsometatarsal joints, 8, 9, 85. See
also Lisfranc's joint
anatomy, 8, 9
arthrodesis, 377-379
axes, 28, 29
biomechanics, 28
examination, 64-66
ligaments, 87
TCI. See Total contact insert (TCI)
Teardrop-shaped metatarsal pad,
335
Tendinitis
high-arched foot and, 300
rehabilitation protocol, 209
in soccer players, 298-299

symptoms, 299
treatment, 299
Tendinosis, rehabilitation protocol,
209
Tendo calcaneus, 13
Tendon slips, 13
Tennis, foot and ankle in, 46-48
Tennis shoes. See Court shoes
TENS, 117, 209. See Transcutaneous electrical nerve stimulation (TENS)
Thera-Band
for ankle sprain rehabilitation, 206
for muscle strengthening, 212-
213, 214
Therapeutic exercise, 210-213
joint mobilization, 211-212
plyometric exercises, 213
proprioceptive retraining, 213
strengthening, 212-213
stretching, 211, 212
Therapeutic modalities, 122-123. See
also specific modalities
cryotherapy, 109-112
electrotherapy, 117-120
external compression, 120, 121
manual, 120-122
selection of, 109
thermal agents, 112-117
Thermal agents, 112-117
Thermography, of diabetic foot,
166
Thompson test, 72, 307-308
Threshold to detection measurements, 97
Throat, 340
of athletic shoe, 230
shoe fit and, 344
THT footfall pattern (toe-heel-toe
footfall pattern), 32
Tibia, 3
Tibial nerve, 19-20, 69
Tibial plafond, 3, 6
Tibialis anterior muscle
anatomy, 14, 78
physiology, 78, 79
Tibialis posterior muscle, 13, 31,
80-81
Tibiocalcaneal angle, in talipes equi-
novarus, 175
Tibiocalcanean ligament, 84
Tibiofibular syndesmosis, 3, 5-6
Tibionavicular ligament, 84
Tibiotalocalcaneal joint, arthrodesis,
384, 385
Tibulofibular syndesmosis, 6
TITF (transverse tibiofibular liga-
ment), 129
Toe(s)
crossover, 66
extension test, 59-60
function, in golf swing, 55
Morton's. See Morton's neuroma
"too many" sign, 59
Toe box, 340
of athletic shoe, 230

of court shoes, 235
shoe fit and, 344
Toe extensors, pressure-induced or
contact tendinitis, 263
Toe-heel-toe footfall pattern (THT
footfall pattern), 32
Toenail(s), 23
care of, in diabetes mellitus, 161
examination, 70
fungal infections, 161
hyperkeratotic, 161
surgery, postoperative footwear
for, 360
Toe-only rocker sole, 353
Toe-walking, idiopathic, 182-183
Tongue, of athletic shoe, 230
"Too many toes" sign, 59
Torque, 246
Total contact cast, for diabetic foot,
170-171
Total contact insert (TCI), 356-358
foot impression techniques for,
356-357
for free tissue transfer, 362
materials for, 357-358
objectives, 356
Traction apophysitis (Sever's disease),
300
Transcutaneous electrical nerve
stimulation (TENS), 117,
209
high-frequency, 222-224
low-frequency, 223, 224
for postoperative pain, 222
for reflex sympathetic dystrophy,
150-151
treatment duration, 223
units for, 222, 223
Transverse arch, 30-31
Transverse tarsal joint
axes, 28, 29
biomechanics, 28
examination, 64
Transverse tarsal joint (Chopart's
joint), 86
Transverse tibiofibular ligament,
129
Trauma, prescription footwear for,
361-362
Tread patterns
for court shoes, 235-236
of outersole, in athletic footwear,
231-232
Triceps surae, 80. See also Gastrocnemius muscle; Soleus
muscle
Triple arthrodesis, postoperative
footwear for, 361
Turf toe, 237, 259
morbid progression of, 259-260
in soccer, 296
treatment, 259-260, 309-310
orthotic device for, 260
padding, 336-337
in volleyball players, 309-310